BASIC Essentials

BASIC Essentials

A Comprehensive Review for the Anesthesiology BASIC Exam

Second edition

Edited by

Dharti Patel
Mount Sinai West and Morningside Hospitals, New York

Sang J. Kim
Hospital for Special Surgery, New York

Himani V. Bhatt
Mount Sinai West and Morningside Hospitals, New York

Alopi M. Patel
Rutgers Robert Wood Johnson Medical School, New Jersey

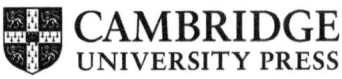
CAMBRIDGE
UNIVERSITY PRESS

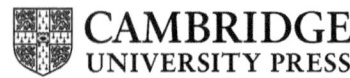

Shaftesbury Road, Cambridge CB2 8EA, United Kingdom

One Liberty Plaza, 20th Floor, New York, NY 10006, USA

477 Williamstown Road, Port Melbourne, VIC 3207, Australia

314–321, 3rd Floor, Plot 3, Splendor Forum, Jasola District Centre, New Delhi – 110025, India

103 Penang Road, #05–06/07, Visioncrest Commercial, Singapore 238467

Cambridge University Press is part of Cambridge University Press & Assessment, a department of the University of Cambridge.

We share the University's mission to contribute to society through the pursuit of education, learning and research at the highest international levels of excellence.

www.cambridge.org
Information on this title: www.cambridge.org/9781009334808

DOI: 10.1017/9781009334792

First published 2019
This Second Edition 2025

Printed in the United Kingdom by CPI Group Ltd, Croydon CR0 4YY

A catalogue record for this publication is available from the British Library.

A Cataloging-in-Publication data record for this book is available from the Library of Congress

ISBN 978-1-009-33480-8 Paperback

....

Contents

Contents

Contributors

Jordan Abrams, MD
Department of Anesthesiology, Perioperative & Pain
Medicine, Icahn School of Medicine at Mount Sinai
New York, NY

Vineet Aggarwal MD
Department of Anesthesiology Columbia University, NYPH
New York, NY

Diana Anca, MD
Weill Cornell Medicine
New York, NY

Ryan Barnette, MD
Cedars Sinai Medical Center
Los Angeles, CA

Jessica Brodt
Stanford University School of Medicine
Paolo Alto, CA

Ethan O. Bryson
Department of Anesthesiology, Perioperative and Pain
Medicine Department of Psychiatry Icahn School of Medicine
at Mount Sinai
New York, NY

Travis Burnett, DO
Department of Anesthesiology, Pain and Perioperative
Medicine Mount Sinai Morningside and West Hospitals
New York, NY

Maria Castillo, MD
Department of Anesthesiology, Perioperative & Pain
Medicine, Icahn School of Medicine at Mount Sinai
New York, NY

Kiang Lien Cheung, MD
Department of Anesthesiology Columbia University, NYPH
New York, NY

Jeffrey Ciccone, MD
Hospital for Special Surgery
Uniondale, NY

David Convissar, MD
Massachusetts General Hospital
Boston, MA

Christopher R. Cowart, MD
Department of Anesthesiology & Perioperative Medicine,
Penn State Milton S. Hershey Medical Center
Hershey, PA

Renee L. Davis, MD
Department of Anesthesiology, Perioperative & Pain
Medicine, Icahn School of Medicine at Mount Sinai
New York, NY

Johanna B. de Haan, MD
Division of Regional Anesthesiology, Acute Pain Medicine,
and Perioperative Ultrasound
UTHealth – McGovern Medical School
Houston, TX

Jeffrey Derham
Doylestown Health
Doylestown, PA

Jacqueline Donovan, MD
Department of Anesthesiology, Albany Medical Center
Albany, NY

Daphney Dorcius, MD
The Ohio State University Wesner Medical Center
Columbus, OH

Morgane Factor, MD
Department of Anesthesiology Stony Brook University
Hospital Stony Brook, NY

Shaji Faisal, MD
Lee Memorial Hospital
Fort Myers, FL

Devon Flaherty, MD
Department of Anesthesiology, Perioperative and Pain
Medicine
Brigham and Women's Hospital
Boston, MA

Kaitlin Flannery, MD
Stanford University School of Medicine
Palo Alto, CA

Jonathan Gal, MD
Department of Anesthesiology, Perioperative & Pain
Medicine, Icahn School of Medicine at Mount Sinai
New York, NY

Theresa A. Gelzinis, MD
Department of Anesthesiology and Perioperative Medicine,
University of Pittsburgh
Pittsburgh, PA

Andrew Glasgow Perez, MD
Sharp Chula Vista Medical Center
San Diego, CA

Regine Goh, MD
University of California San Diego
San Diego, CA

Nadia Hernández, MD
UTHealth - McGovern Medical School
Houston, TX

Bryan Hill, MD
The Ohio State Wexner Medical Center Columbus, OH

Jordan Holloway, MD
The Ohio State University Wexner Medical Center
Columbus, OH

Samuel Hunter, MD
Inova Fairfax Hospital
Fairfax, VA

Stefan A. Ianchulev, MD
Hunter Holmes McGuire Veterans Affairs Medical Center
Richmond, VA

Christina L. Jeng, MD
Icahn School of Medicine at Mount Sinai/The Mount Sinai
Medical Center
New York, NY

Kenneth John, MD
Department of Anesthesiology, Brown University/Rhode
Island Hospital
Providence, RI

Claire Joseph, MD
Montefiore Medical Center
Albert Einstein School of Medicine
Bronx, NY

Ishu Kant, MD
Mount Sinai Morningside and West
New York, NY

Daniel Katz, MD
Icahn School of Medicine at Mount Sinai
New York, NY

Yury Khelemsky, MD
Icahn School of Medicine at Mount Sinai
New York, NY

Hae-Young Kim
Boston Children's Hospital/Harvard Medical School
Boston, MA

Jung Kim, MD
Department of Anesthesiology, Perioperative & Pain
Management, Icahn School of Medicine at Mount Sinai
New York, NY

Nakiyah Knibbs, MD
Anesthesiology & Pain Management, Icahn School of
Medicine at Mount Sinai, New York, NY

Russell J. Krom, MD
Duke University Hospital
Durham, NC

Michael D. Lazar, MD
Department of Anesthesiology, Icahn School of Medicine
at Mount Sinai, Mount Sinai St. Luke's and West
Hospitals
New York, NY

Rebecca E. Lee, MD
Department of Anesthesiology, Perioperative & Pain
Medicine, Icahn School of Medicine at Mount Sinai
New York, NY

Matthew A. Levin, MD
Department of Anesthesiology, Perioperative and Pain
Medicine The Mount Sinai Health System
New York, NY

Hung-Mo Lin
School of Medicine
Yale Center for Analytical Science, School of Public Health
New Haven, CT

Sanford Littwin, MD
Butler Anesthesia Associates Butler Memorial Hospital
East Butler, PA

Katherine Loftus, MD
Mount Sinai Hospital Department of Anesthesiology and Pain
Medicine
New York, NY

Patrick Maffucci, MD
The Icahn School of Medicine at Mount Sinai
New York, NY

Daniel Mandell, MD
Department of Anesthesiology and Perioperative Medicine, University of Pittsburgh
Pittsburgh, PA

Aleksey Maryansky, MD
Mount Sinai Morningside and West
New York, NY

Jennifer Mardini, MD
Department of Anesthesiology & Perioperative Medicine, Penn State Milton S. Hershey Medical Center
Hershey, PA

Evida Mars-Holt, DO
Department of Anesthesiology & Perioperative Medicine, Penn State Milton S. Hershey Medical Center
Hershey, PA

Leena Mathew, MD
Department of Anesthesiology Columbia University, NYPH
New York, NY

Edward R. Mathney, MD
Department of Anesthesiology, Perioperative and Pain Medicine
Mount Sinai Health System
New York, NY

Megan Meyer, MD
University of California San Diego
San Diego, CA

Deborah C. Mokuolu, MD
Department of Anesthesiology, Perioperative & Pain Medicine, Icahn School of Medicine at Mount Sinai,
New York, NY

Christopher X. Muñoz, MD
Guthrie Corning Hospital
New York, NY

Victoria Nguyen
Medical City Healthcare
Dallas, TX

Lyle Nolasco, MD
The Icahn School of Medicine at Mount Sinai
New York, NY

Barbara Orlando, MD
Department of Anesthesiology McGovern Medical School at the University of Texas Health Science Center - Houston Memorial Hermann Hospital - Texas Medical Center
Houston, TX

Poonam Pai, MD
Mount Sinai West – Morningside Hospitals
New York, NY

Raj Parekh, MD
Icahn School of Medicine Mount Sinai St. Luke's and West Hospitals New York, NY

Joseph Park, MD
Maimonides Medical Center
New York, NY

Palak Patel, MD
Department of Anesthesiology and Pain Medicine, Mount Sinai Hospital
New York, NY

Charles P. Plant, MD
Hunter Holmes McGuire Veterans Affairs Medical Center
Richmond, VA

Kyle James Riley, MD
Massachusetts General Hospital
Boston, MA

Martha Schuessler, MD
Mount Sinai
New York, NY

Andrew J. Schwartz, MD
Mount Sinai
New York, NY

Giacomo Scorsese, MD
Stony Brook University Hospital
Stony Brook, NY

Ali Shariat, MD
Mount Sinai West – Morningside Hospitals
New York, NY

Evan Shawler, MD
University of California San Diego
San Diego, CA

Paul Shekane, MD
Mount Sinai Morningside and West Hospitals
New York, NY

Marc Sherwin, MD
The Icahn School of Medicine at Mount Sinai
New York, NY

Chris Sikorski, MD
Mount Sinai
New York, NY

Natalie Smith, MD
The Icahn School of Medicine at Mount Sinai
New York, NY

Daniel G. Springer, MD
Department of Anesthesiology and Perioperative Medicine, University of Pittsburgh
Pittsburgh, PA

Petrus Paulus Steyn, MD
Doylestown Health
Doylestown, PA

Kathirvel Subramaniam, MD
Department of Anesthesiology and Perioperative Medicine,
University of Pittsburgh
Pittsburgh, PA

Ben Toure, MD
Icahn School of Medicine at Mount Sinai
New York, NY

Sanjana Vig, MD
University of California San Diego
San Diego, CA

Joseph R. Williams, MD
Department of Anesthesiology and Perioperative Medicine,
University of Pittsburgh
Pittsburgh, PA

John Michael Williamson
McKing Consulting Corporation
Atlanta, GA

James Yeh, MD
Mount Sinai Hospital
New York, NY

John Yin, MD
Department of Anesthesiology and Perioperative Medicine,
University of Pittsburgh
Pittsburgh, PA

Connie Yue, MD
School of Medicine, Loma Linda University
Loma Linda, CA

Jeron Zerillo, MD
Memorial Sloan Kettering Cancer Center
New York, NY

Preface

The ABA Staged examinations consist of the BASIC, ADVANCED, and APPLIED Exams. The BASIC Exam was first introduced in 2014 in a series of exams that eventually allows resident anesthesiologists to become American Board of Anesthesiology (ABA) certified. Candidates can take the BASIC exam after completing their Clinical Anesthesia (CA) for one year. This exam focuses on the scientific basics of clinical anesthetic practice with a focus on pharmacology, physiology, anatomy, anesthesia equipment, and monitoring.

As with most examinations, the BASIC examination may induce a great deal of stress for resident anesthesiologists; however, with the appropriate resources, the candidates can pass the exam on their first attempt. Per the ABA, a diplomate of the Board must possess "knowledge, judgment, adaptability, clinical skills, technical facility, and personal characteristics sufficient to carry out an entire scope of anesthesiology practice without accommodation or with reasonable accommodation." The examination provides a means for the ABA to evaluate if a candidate has attained a certain level of proficiency to proceed with advanced training. The *BASIC Essentials* book is meant to provide a comprehensive review of the content for the ABA BASIC exam. Detailed information is also available on the ABA website (www.theaba.org) and the booklet of information published on the website.

Exam Structure

The BASIC examination is a computer-based test that is administered in numerous test centers across the country. The exam consists of 200 questions and examinees are given four hours to complete the examination. The questions consist of only A type. A-type questions are multiple choice questions with a single best answer out of four choices that require the application of knowledge as well as recall of factual information. The questions can be simply stated or include a brief clinical scenario. Some questions will require interpretation of an image.

Exam Content

The BASIC exam covers four content categories: basic sciences, clinical sciences, organ-based basic and clinical sciences, and special problems or issues in anesthesiology. The examination outline can be found on the ABA website. Per the ABA, the breakdown of the questions is as follows:

- Basic Sciences (24%): 44–52 questions
- Clinical Sciences (36%): 65–79 questions
- Organ-Based Basic and Clinical Sciences (37%): 66–82 questions
- Special Problems or Issues in Anesthesiology (3%): 4–8 questions

Test Preparation

This comprehensive review for the BASIC examination is based on the ABA content outline. Each chapter contains a thorough summary of each of the required content categories and subcategories. We recommend you use this book to annotate into as you learn more high-yield information from various resources. This book is meant to be an ultimate source of high-yield information as you take notes into it over three years of anesthesiology residency. The BASIC exam will focus on many facets of anesthetic management from basic pharmacology and physiology to the application of these details to clinical management. This book is a good foundation to obtain high-yield information; however, use of multiple resources including textbooks, articles, and question banks is recommended.

The key to being prepared for the BASIC exam is to start studying early. Start reading textbooks, doing questions, and annotating into this review book early on in residency, so when time comes to really start studying you will be well equipped with a great source of information – all in one place!

Test Day Tips

Just like most exams you've taken thus far, this exam can be anxiety provoking. The key is to stay calm and have faith in your preparation. As with any exam, start your day by eating a well-balanced and nutritious breakfast. Wear something comfortable. Go through the tutorial the day of the exam. It may seem like a waste of time but can help ease you into the exam by preparing you for how to use the tools on the screen rather than trying to find them later. Pace yourself during the exam even if it means leaving a question "marked" so you can return to it later. There will be questions to which you don't know the answers, and it is perfectly reasonable to return to those questions so you can move on to questions to which you may know the answers. There is no penalty for guessing, so do **NOT** leave an answer blank. There is a 25 percent chance that you pick the correct answer even if you cannot eliminate any answer choices. Read each question carefully and look for key words. When time comes for the break, use it. There is no reason to power through the entire exam without taking a break. Use this time to hydrate, eat a snack, or use the restroom even if you don't feel like you need to because that mental break will help you stay focused for the second half. If you have time left at the end of the exam, use it to review your marked questions or even the entire exam if you have time. Be hesitant to change your answers and second guess yourself.

Abbreviations

ACLS	Advanced Cardiac Life Support		IM	Intramuscular
AED	Automated External Defibrillator		IO	Intraosseous
AF	Atrial Fibrillation		ITD	Impedance Threshold Device
AV	Atrioventricular		IV	Intravenous
BLS	Basic Life Support		MAC	Minimum Alveolar Concentration
BP	Blood Pressure		MH	Malignant Hyperthermia
CBF	Cerebral Blood Flow		MV	Minute Ventilation
CMRO2	Cerebral Metabolic Rate		NMBD	Neuromuscular Blocking Drugs
CO	Cardiac Output		OHCA	Out-of-Hospital Cardiac Arrest
CPAP	Continuous Positive Airway Pressure		PEA	Pulseless Electrical Activity
CPR	Cardiopulmonary Resuscitation		PPV	Positive Pressure Ventilation
ECG	Electrocardiogram		RAP	Right Atrial Pressure
ECPR	Extracorporeal Cardiopulmonary Resuscitation		RBF	Renal Blood Flow
$EtCO_2$	End-Tidal Carbon Dioxide		RR	Respiratory Rate
Fa	Alveolar Concentration		TOF	Train of Four
FGF	Fresh Gas Flow		VF	Ventricular Fibrillation
Fi	Inspiratory Concentration		VT	Ventricular Tachycardia
ICP	Intracranial Pressure		Vt	Tidal Volume
IHCA	In-hospital Cardiac Arrest		WPW	Wolff–Parkinson–White Syndrome

Anatomy

Johanna B. de Haan and Nadia Hernández

Head and Neck

Vasculature

Internal Jugular Vein (IJV)

- Drains blood from the head, face, and brain.
- Lies deep to the sternocleidomastoid (SCM) muscle and lateral to the carotid artery, coursing inferiorly to join the subclavian vein to become the brachiocephalic (also known as innominate) vein.

External Jugular Vein (EJV)

- Carries blood from the face.
- Lies superficial to the SCM as it crosses obliquely from the angle of the mandible and dives posterior to the clavicle to join the subclavian vein.

Subclavian Vein (SCV)

- Posterior to the clavicle but anterior to the insertion of the anterior scalene muscle on the first rib (Figure 1.1).

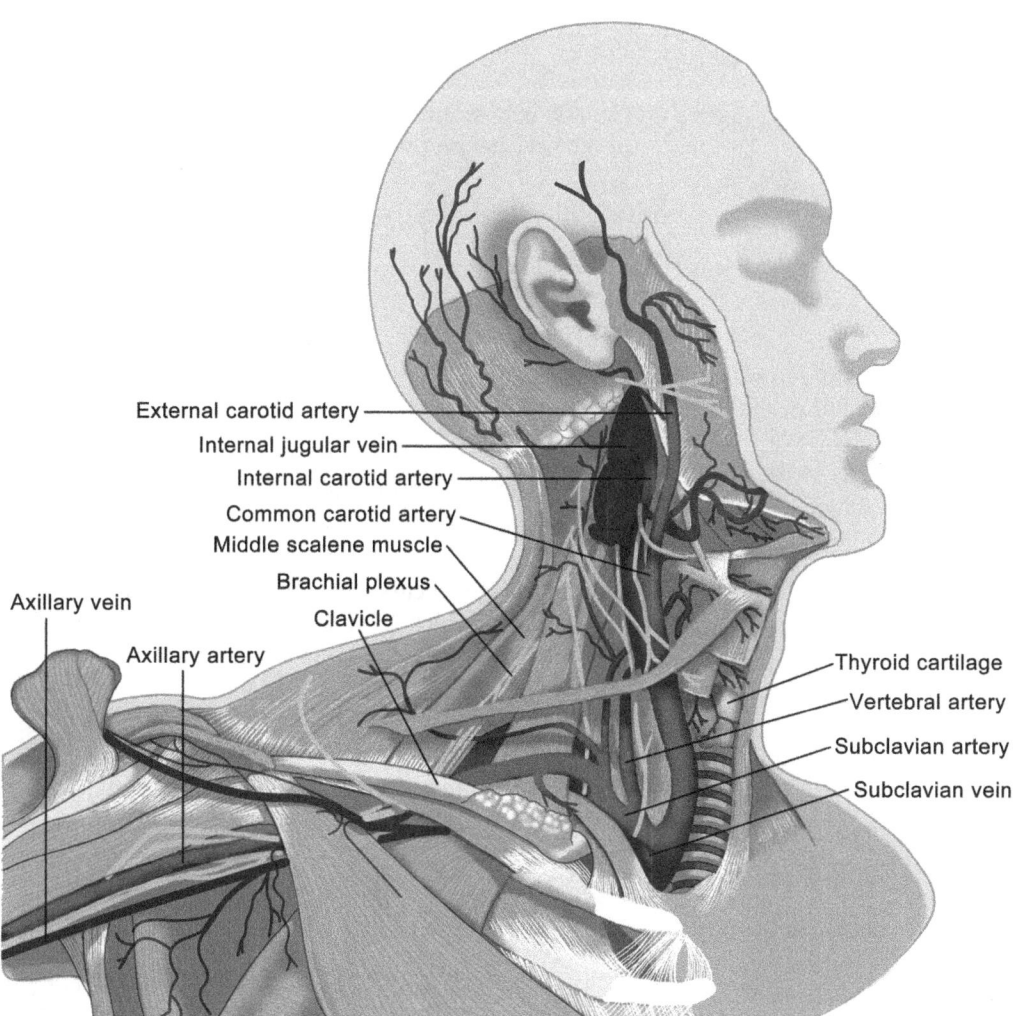

Figure 1.1 Normal anatomical relationships of the major vessels, nerves, bones, and muscles of the neck and axilla. A black and white version of this figure will appear in some formats. For the color version, please refer to the plate section.

External carotid artery
Internal jugular vein
Internal carotid artery
Common carotid artery
Middle scalene muscle
Brachial plexus
Axillary vein
Clavicle
Axillary artery
Thyroid cartilage
Vertebral artery
Subclavian artery
Subclavian vein

Vertebral Artery

- Branches from the subclavian artery, traveling cephalad to enter the spine deep to Chassaignac's tubercle.
- Travels through the transverse foramen of C1–C6 vertebrae before forming the basilar artery, supplying the posterior circle of Willis.
- Can inject into during interscalene block, causing seizures.

Carotid Artery

- Arises from brachiocephalic artery on the right, and aortic arch on the left.
- Bifurcates into internal and external carotid arteries at the level of C4 vertebra.
  - Carotid sinus:
    - Located at bifurcation of carotid artery.
    - Compression during carotid endarterectomy can cause a baroreceptor reflex resulting in bradycardia.

Thoracic Duct

- Lymphatic drainage of the body into the venous system.
- Formed at L2 level, ascends between aorta and azygos vein, crosses diaphragm posterior to esophagus.
- Crosses from right to left at T4–T5 and empties into the SCV just lateral to the IJV.
- Can be damaged during attempts for central access to the left SCV or IJV, leading to chylothorax.

Surface Landmarks

Thyroid Cartilage

- Motor and sensory innervation to the larynx is derived from CN X (vagus nerve) via the superior, inferior, and the recurrent laryngeal nerves bilaterally.
- Musculature of the larynx is innervated entirely by the recurrent laryngeal nerve except for the cricothyroid muscle, which is innervated by the external branch of the superior laryngeal nerve.

Cricothyroid Membrane

- Palpable as a soft, flat membrane in the anterior neck at the level of C6 between the rigid thyroid cartilage superiorly and cricoid cartilage inferiorly.
- Can be punctured with a needle, allowing for transtracheal injection of local anesthetic, insertion of a wire for retrograde intubation, or percutaneous cricothyroidotomy.

Chassaignac's Tubercle

- Name for the anterior tubercle of the transverse process of C6.
- Lies between the carotid artery anteriorly and the vertebral artery posteriorly.

- Used to identify the appropriate location to perform stellate ganglion blockade.

Vertebra Prominens

- Another name for spinous process of the C7.
- This spinous process is the most prominent in the majority of patients.

Stellate Ganglion

- Named for its "star-like" appearance.
- Is formed by the fusion of the inferior cervical and first thoracic sympathetic ganglia.
- Located lateral to the vertebral body of C7.
- Blockade of this structure is useful for the treatment of complex regional pain syndrome (CRPS) or Raynaud's phenomenon.
  - Side effect associated with stellate ganglion blockade is Horner's Syndrome (e.g., ptosis, anhidrosis, miosis), and may frequently occur following brachial plexus nerve blocks.

Brachial Plexus

- Provides sensory and motor innervation to the upper extremity.
- Courses between the anterior and middle scalene muscles in the neck before running down the arm.

Radiological Anatomy

See Figure 1.2.

Chest

Surface Landmarks

Trachea

- Begins at C6 and continues inferiorly until it bifurcates into the right and left main bronchi at the *carina*.
- This bifurcation occurs at the level of the *sternal angle*, or *angle of Louis*, which is the joint between the sternum and manubrium.

Lungs

- Are divided into their lobes by fissures.
- Three lobes on the right and two lobes on the left plus the lingual.
- Fissures
  - Bilaterally, the *oblique fissure* divides the *superior and inferior lobes* on the left and *superior and middle lobes* on the right.
  - The oblique fissures begin posteriorly at the level of T4, traveling caudally and laterally, and then around the

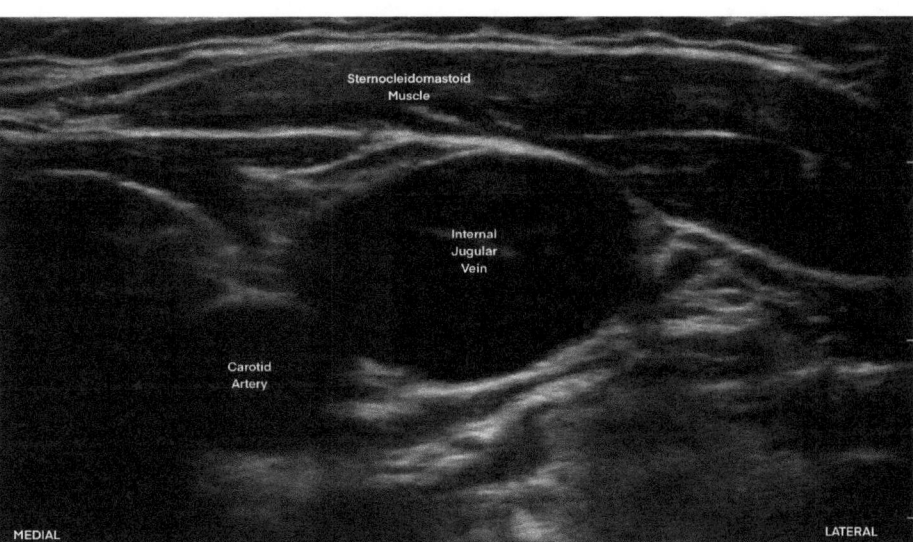

Figure 1.2 Ultrasound image of the lateral neck, displaying the internal jugular vein and the carotid artery.

torso to terminate anteriorly at approximately the level of the seventh rib on the midclavicular line.

- The right lung is divided a second time by the *horizontal fissure*, which begins anteriorly at approximately the fourth costal cartilage and traverses laterally to the anterior axillary line, where it intersects with the oblique fissure at the level of the fifth rib. This fissure demarcates the border between the inferior and middle lobes.

Heart

- **Point of maximal impulse (PMI)**
  - Landmark for the apex of the heart is the fifth intercostal space in the midclavicular line.

- **Coronary arteries**
  - Left and right main arise from the left and right aortic valve leaflets respectively.
  - Left main divides into the left anterior descending (LAD) and the circumflex (LCX).
  - LAD supplies the anterior wall of the left ventricle (LV) and the anterior two-thirds of the interventricular septum (IVS).
  - LCX supplies the lateral wall of the LV and part of the posterior wall.
  - Right coronary artery (RCA)
    - Supplies most of the right ventricle (RV) and usually both sinoatrial (SA) and atrioventricular (AV) nodes.
      - LAD supplies the apex of the RV.
      - Right atrium
      - Upper half of the interatrial septum
      - Posterior third of IVS
      - Inferior wall of LV
  - Posterior descending artery (PDA) arises from RCA in approximately 80% of patients. This is called "right-dominant" circulation.

Radiological Anatomy
See Figure 1.3.

Upper and Lower Extremities

Upper Extremity Vasculature

Basilic Vein

- Travels from the medial posterior forearm at the ulnar head proximally to the anterior elbow, where it lies *medial to the tendon of the biceps brachii muscle.*
- Becomes the axillary vein at the border of the *teres major muscle.*
- Becomes the subclavian vein at the outer border of the first rib.

Cephalic Vein

- Begins laterally at the wrist within the *anatomic snuffbox* – a triangle formed by the *radial head*, the *extensor pollicis longus tendon* and the *extensor pollicis brevis tendon.*
- At the elbow it is commonly found lateral to the biceps tendon. It then continues proximally in the arm lateral to the biceps brachii muscle before crossing anterior to the deltoid and diving deep to join with the axillary vein under the clavicle.

Axillary Artery

- Direct continuation of the subclavian artery, begins at the border of the 1st rib, coursing laterally until the border of the *teres muscle* where it becomes the brachial artery.

Brachial Artery

- The pulsation is typically felt just *medial to the biceps brachii tendon* at the cubital fossa.
- Subsequently bifurcates into the *radial and ulnar arteries* (Figure 1.4).

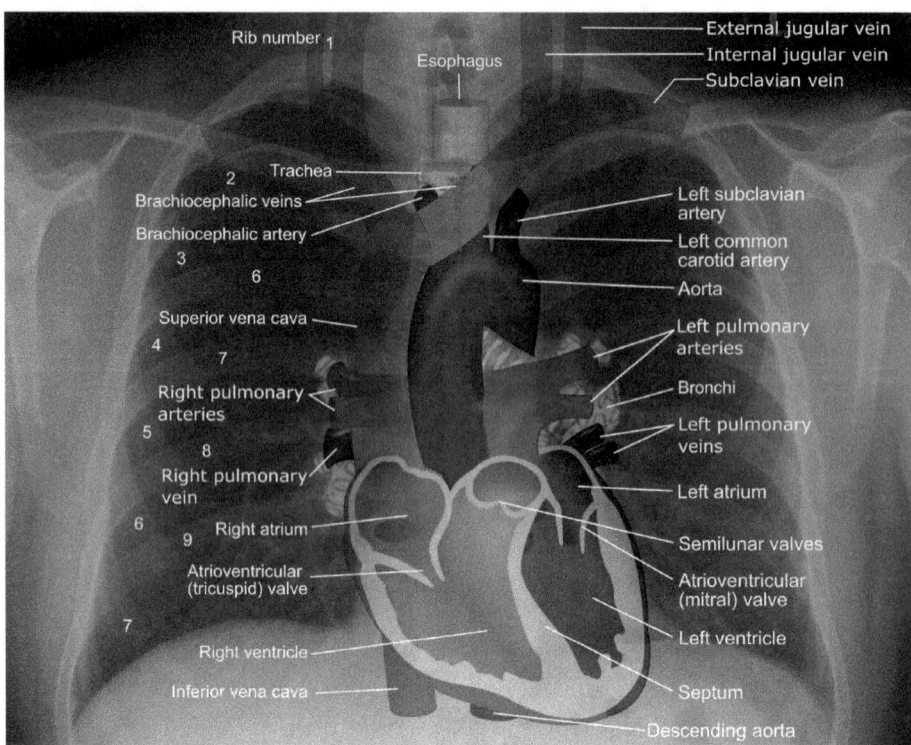

Figure 1.3 Normal radiograph of the chest. Superimposed on this image are outlines of some of the major topographical landmarks of the chest. A black and white version of this figure will appear in some formats. For the color version, please refer to the plate section.

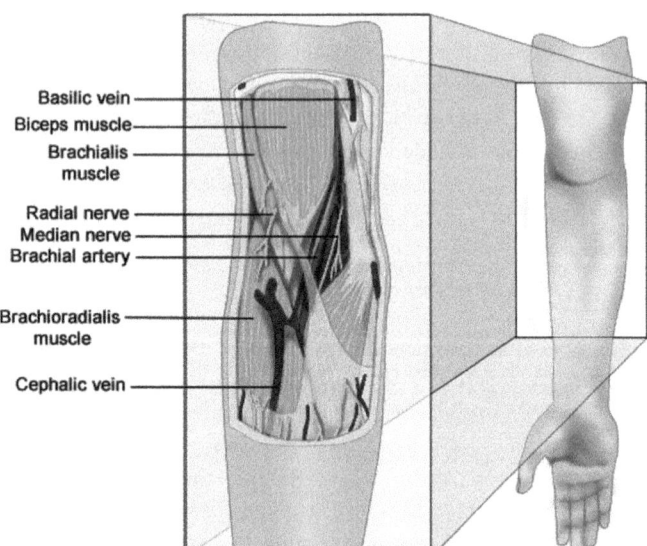

Figure 1.4 Normal anatomical relationships of the major vessels and nerves, bones, and muscles of the antecubital fossa. A black and white version of this figure will appear in some formats. For the color version, please refer to the plate section.

Upper Extremity Innervation

Brachial Plexus

- A complex network of nerves formed by ventral rami of *C5–T1*.
- Provides sensory and motor innervation of the upper extremities. Clinically, the anesthesiologist can provide surgical anesthesia to the upper extremity via blockade of the brachial plexus (see Table 1.1).
- ROOTS: exit the spinal column via the intervertebral foramen.
- TRUNKS: *roots (C5–T1)* combine to form the *trunks*, which lie between the anterior and middle scalene muscles.
  - *Superior trunk (C5–C6)* gives rise to the *suprascapular nerve*, which innervates 70% of the shoulder joint. Of the brachial plexus blocks, the interscalene block (ISB) is the only one that blocks this nerve. It is also the only block that can be used for shoulder surgery without supplementation.
  - *Middle trunk* is formed by the C7 nerve root.
  - *Inferior trunk* is formed by the C8 and T1 nerve roots.
  - *Roots/trunks* are blocked for the interscalene block.

Table 1.1 Upper extremity nerve block landmarks

Interscalene (i.e., brachial plexus: roots)	Between anterior and middle scalene muscles at level of C6
Supraclavicular (i.e., brachial plexus: trunks/divisions)	Lateral to the clavicular attachment of the sternocleidomastoid
Infraclavicular (i.e., brachial plexus: cords)	3 cm caudal to the midpoint of a line between the coracoid process and the medial clavicle
Axillary (i.e., brachial plexus: branches)	At the point of palpation of the axillary artery
Radial nerve	Between the brachioradialis and the biceps tendon
Ulnar nerve	Between the medial epicondyle and olecranon
Median nerve	Medial to the brachial artery at the antecubital fossa

- Due to proximity, *the phrenic nerve, stellate ganglion, superficial cervical plexus, recurrent laryngeal nerve and CN XI are frequently blocked with ISB.*
- DIVISIONS: *trunks* split into *anterior and posterior divisions.*
- CORDS: *divisions* recombine into the *lateral, medial and posterior cords*, which are named for their relationship to the *subclavian artery.*
- BRANCHES: *cords* split further to form the terminal *branches.*
  - There are five terminal branches of the brachial plexus, including:
    - axillary nerve (C5–C6)
    - musculocutaneous nerve (C5–C7)
    - radial nerve (C5–T1)
    - median nerve (C5–T1)
    - ulnar nerve (C8–T1)

Intercostobrachial Nerve

- Derived from the T2 intercostal nerve to innervate the skin of the axilla and medial upper arm.
- If not blocked, patient may experience tourniquet pain (Figure 1.5).

Lower Extremity Vasculature

Small Saphenous Vein

- Begins posterior to the lateral malleolus and extends proximally on the posterior lower leg until the popliteal fossa, where it drains into the popliteal vein.

Popliteal Vein

- Lies between the popliteal artery and the tibial nerve at the popliteal fossa (see Figure 1.5).
- The popliteal vein continues proximally through the adductor magnus muscle, where it becomes the femoral vein.

Great Saphenous Vein

- Longest vein the body. Typically found superficially anterior to the medial malleolus.
- Commonly cannulated in pediatrics for peripheral venous access.
- Courses proximally on the medial surface of the leg before entering the fossa ovalis to empty into the femoral vein on the anterior thigh near the inguinal crease.

Femoral Artery

- Arises as the direct continuation of the *external iliac artery.*
- Lies just lateral to the femoral vein at the inguinal ligament.
- Divides into superficial femoral artery and profunda femoris (also known as the deep artery of the thigh).
  - The profunda femoris provides vascular supply to the structures of the thigh.
  - The superficial femoral artery courses posteriorly and distally resurfacing at the popliteal fossa as the popliteal artery.

Popliteal Artery

- Divides into two branches: anterior and posterior tibial arteries.
- Anterior tibial artery:

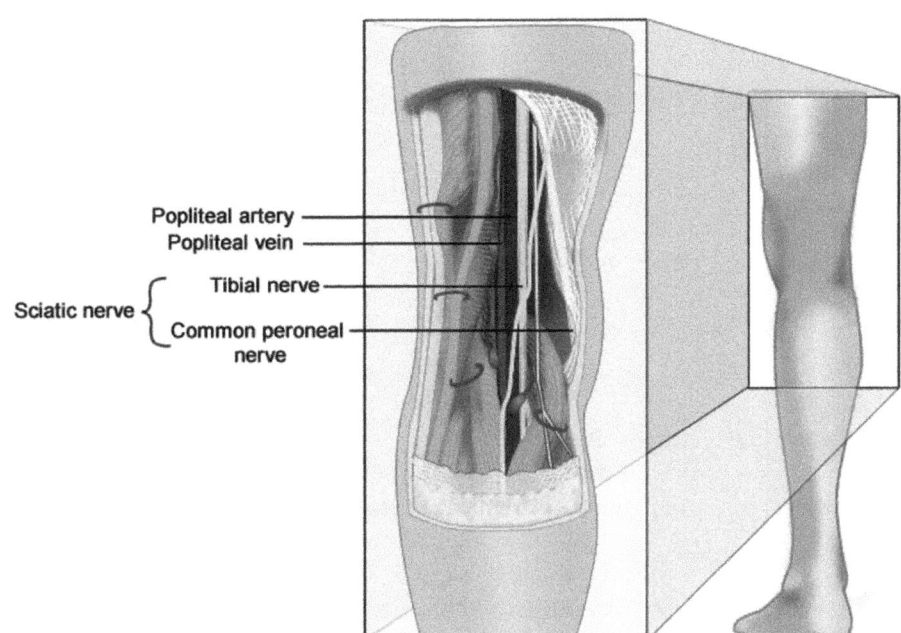

Figure 1.5 Normal anatomical relationships of the major vessels, nerves, bones, and muscles of the popliteal fossa (medial to lateral). A black and white version of this figure will appear in some formats. For the color version, please refer to the plate section.

Popliteal artery

Popliteal vein

Tibial nerve

Sciatic nerve

Common peroneal nerve

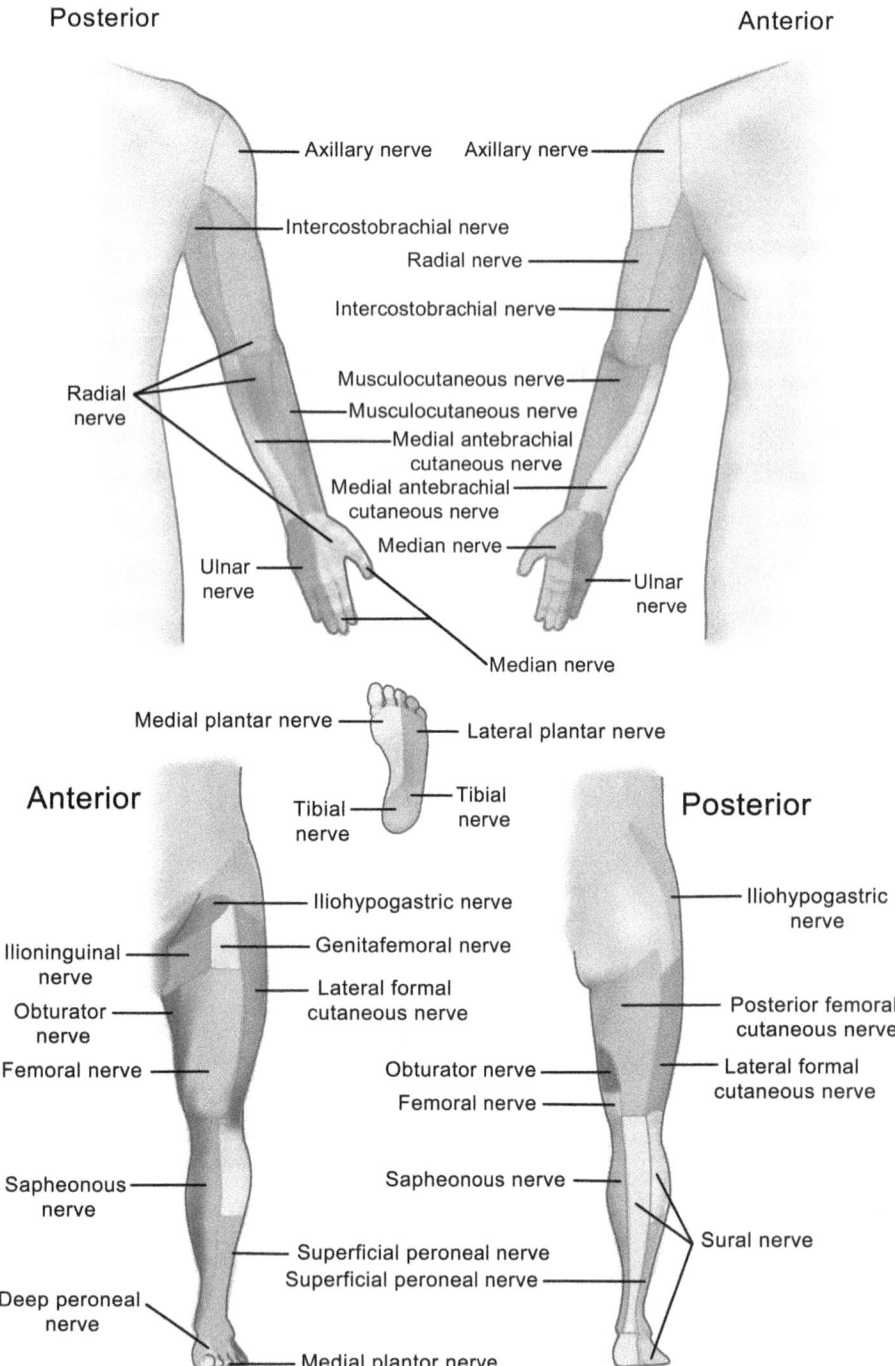

Posterior   Anterior

Axillary nerve   Axillary nerve

Intercostobrachial nerve

Radial nerve

Intercostobrachial nerve

Musculocutaneous nerve

Radial
nerve   Musculocutaneous nerve

Medial antebrachial
cutaneous nerve

Medial antebrachial
cutaneous nerve

Median nerve

Ulnar
nerve   Ulnar
                                              nerve

Median nerve

Medial plantar nerve   Lateral plantar nerve

Anterior   Tibial   Tibial   Posterior
              nerve   nerve

Iliohypogastric nerve   Iliohypogastric
                               nerve

Ilioinguinal   Genitafemoral nerve
nerve

Obturator   Lateral formal
nerve   cutaneous nerve   Posterior femoral
                                                 cutaneous nerve
Femoral nerve
                  Obturator nerve   Lateral formal
                  Femoral nerve   cutaneous nerve

Sapheonous   Sapheonous nerve
nerve

                                                 Sural nerve

                  Superficial peroneal nerve
                  Superficial peroneal nerve
Deep peroneal
nerve

              Medial plantor nerve

Figure 1.6 Distribution of the major cutaneous nerve branches of the upper and lower extremities. A black and white version of this figure will appear in some formats. For the color version, please refer to the plate section.

○ Terminates as the dorsalis pedis artery (DP).
○ Can be palpated on the dorsal surface of the foot between the extensor hallicus longus and extensor digitorum longus tendons.
○ DP pulse is a landmark for deep peroneal nerve blockade, which innervates the first dorsal webspace.
• Posterior tibial artery (PT):
○ Pulsation can be felt posterior to the medial malleolus (Figure 1.6).

Lower Extremity Innervation
Lumbar Plexus
• Formed by ventral rami of T12–L4.
• Gives rise to femoral, obturator, lateral femoral cutaneous, ilioinguinal, genitofemoral, and iliohypogastric nerves.
• **Femoral nerve** (L2–L4):
○ Found deep to the inguinal ligament lateral to the femoral artery.

- Provides motor innervation to the muscles for knee extension. Blockade of the femoral nerve results in 80% reduction in quadriceps strength.
  - Sensory innervation anterior and medial thigh via two anterior cutaneous branches.
- **Lateral femoral cutaneous nerve (LFCN)** (L2–L3):
  - Provides cutaneous innervation of the lateral thigh.
- **Obturator Nerve** (L2–L4):
  - Innervates the adductor muscles.
  - Sensory innervation varies:
    - One-third posterior knee, one-third medial thigh, one-third no innervation.

Sacral Plexus (L4–S4)

- **Sciatic nerve** (L4–S3)
  - Deep to piriformis muscle, travels distally toward the popliteal fossa.
  - Two branches:
    - **Tibial nerve**
      - Motor function of all muscles in the posterior compartment.

- **Common peroneal nerve**
  - Supplies the muscles of the anterior compartment.
    - Blockade or damage results in foot drop.

Cutaneous innervation of the ankle and foot is supplied by a combination of five nerves: four derived from the **sciatic nerve** and one derived from the **femoral nerve (Figure 1.7)**.

- Sciatic branches
  - **Tibial nerve**: provides sensory innervation to the heel and plantar surface of the foot.
    - Blocked by injection next to PT pulsation posterior to medial malleolus.
  - **Superficial peroneal nerve**: sensory to the dorsum of the foot.
    - Blocked by superficial infiltration of local anesthetic between medial and lateral malleoli.
  - **Deep peroneal nerve**: sensory to the web space between first and second toes.
    - Blocked at the dorsum of the foot by injecting next to DP pulsation.
  - **Sural nerve**: derived from both the tibial and common peroneal nerves. Provides sensory innervation to the posterior lower leg and lateral ankle.

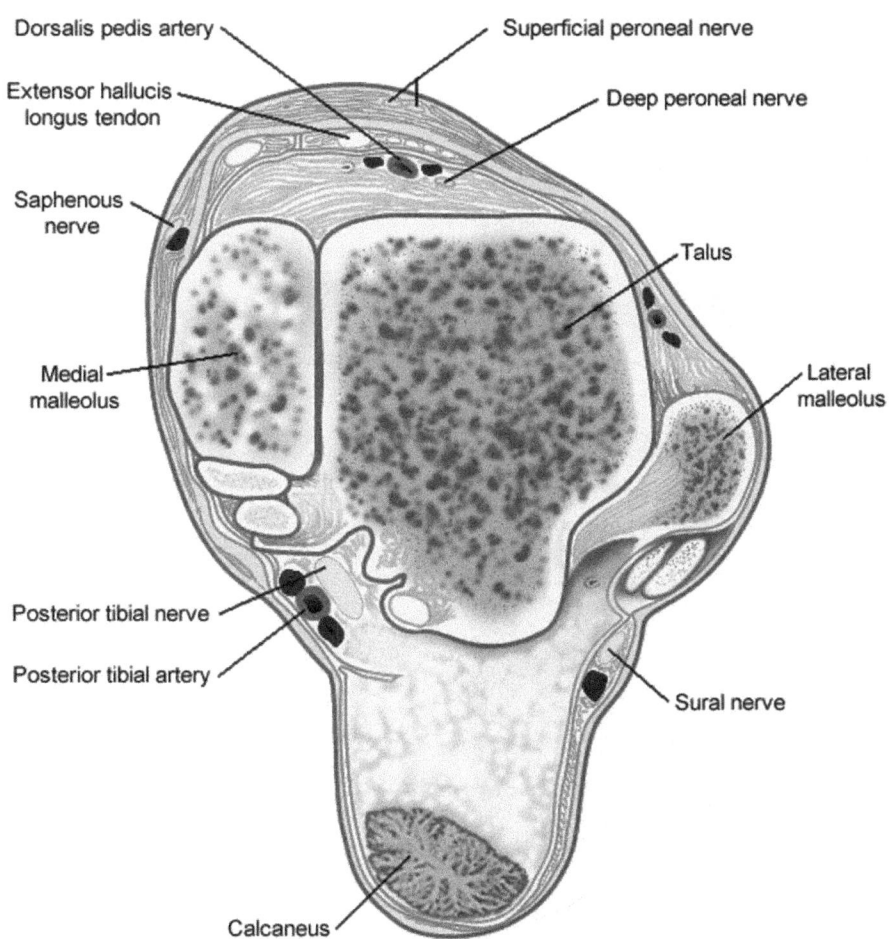

Figure 1.7 Normal anatomical relationship of the major vessels, nerves, bones, and the ankle. A black and white version of this figure will appear in some formats. For the color version, please refer to the plate section.

Table 1.2 Lower extremity nerve block landmarks

Femoral nerve	Lateral to the pulsation of femoral artery at the inguinal ligament
Lateral femoral cutaneous nerve	Medial to anterior superior iliac spine
Sciatic nerve	4 cm distal to the midpoint of a line between the greater trochanter and posterior superior iliac spine
Saphenous nerve	Anterior to the medial malleolus near the saphenous vein
Superficial peroneal nerve	Anterior to the lateral malleolus
Deep peroneal nerve	Near the pulsation of the dorsalis pedis artery at the ankle
Posterior tibial nerve	Posterior to the pulsation of the posterior tibial artery
Sural nerve	Posterior to the lateral malleolus

- Blocked by injection of local anesthetic between lateral malleolus and Achilles tendon.
- Femoral branch
  - **Saphenous nerve** provides sensory innervation at the medial lower extremity.
    - Blocked by injection anterior to medial malleolus next to saphenous vein.

Table 1.2 lists some of the normal anatomical relationships and topographic landmarks associated with nerve blocks of the lower extremities.

Radiological Anatomy

See Figures 1.8–1.12.

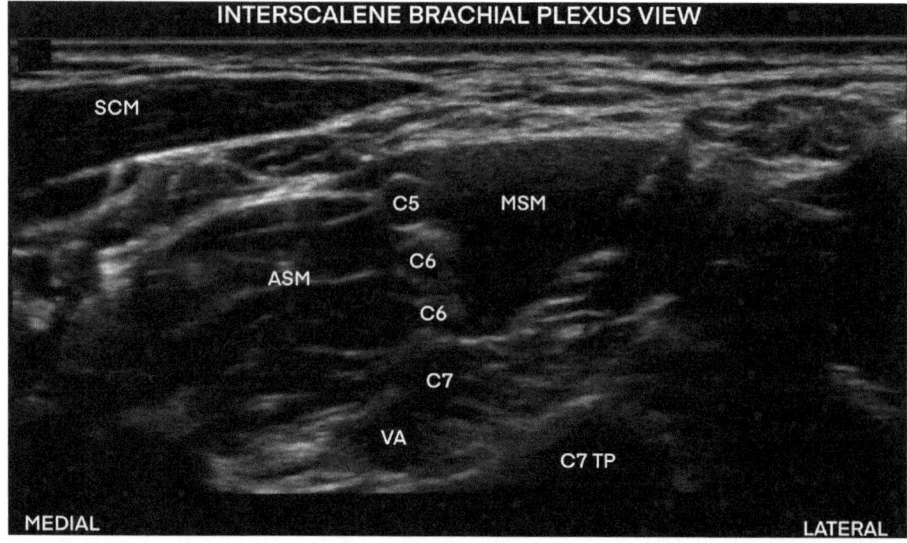

INTERSCALENE BRACHIAL PLEXUS VIEW

Figure 1.8 Ultrasound image of the brachial plexus at the location for the interscalene block. At this level, the roots of C5, C6, and C7 appear as hypoechoic circles between the anterior (ASM) and middle (MSM) scalene muscles, deep to the sternocleidomastoid muscle (SCM). Also seen is the vertebral artery (VA) and C7 transverse process (TP).

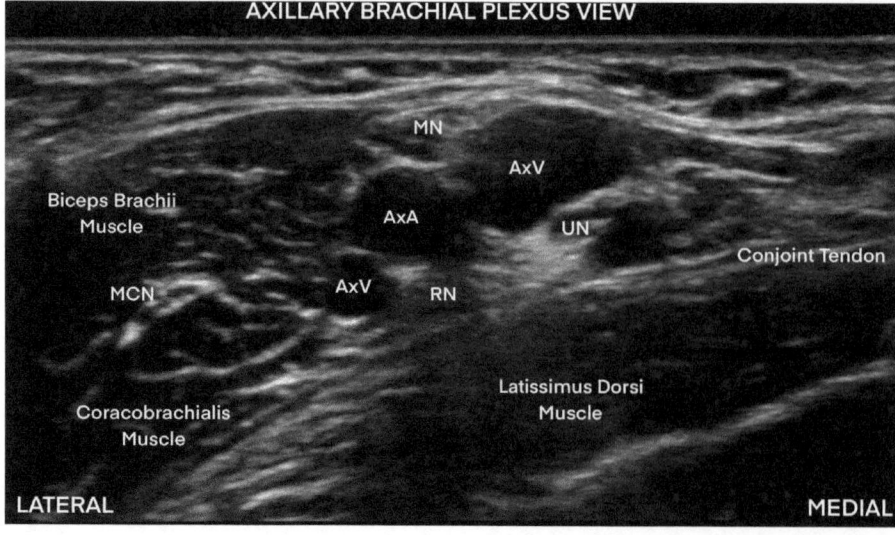

AXILLARY BRACHIAL PLEXUS VIEW

Figure 1.9 Ultrasound image of the brachial plexus at the location for the axillary block. The axillary artery (AxA) is surrounded by the ulnar (UN), median (MN), and radial (RN) nerves. The musculocutaneous nerve (MCN) is seen laterally within the coracobrachialis muscle. Also seen is the axillary vein (AxV).

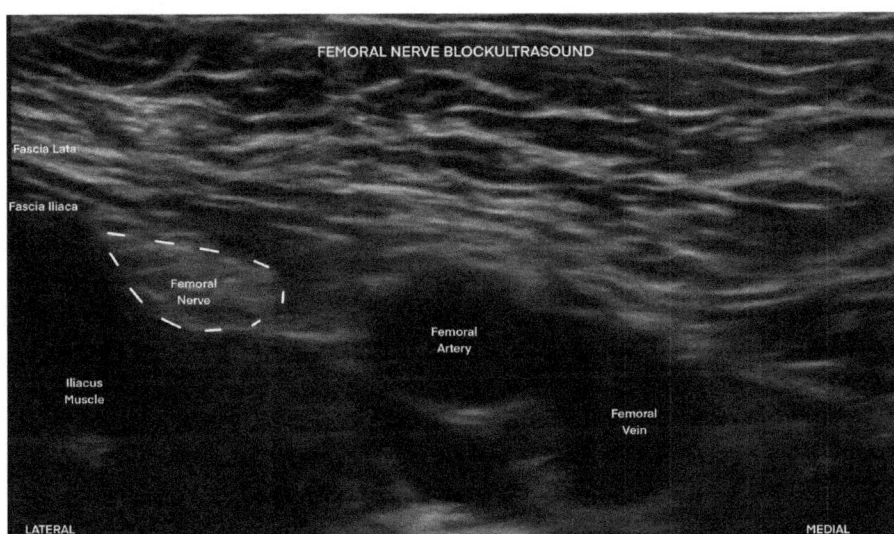

Figure 1.10 Ultrasound image of the inguinal area, depicting the normal relationship between the femoral vein, femoral artery, and femoral nerve. The mnemonic "VAN" can be used to remember the orientation of these structures in the medial to lateral direction.

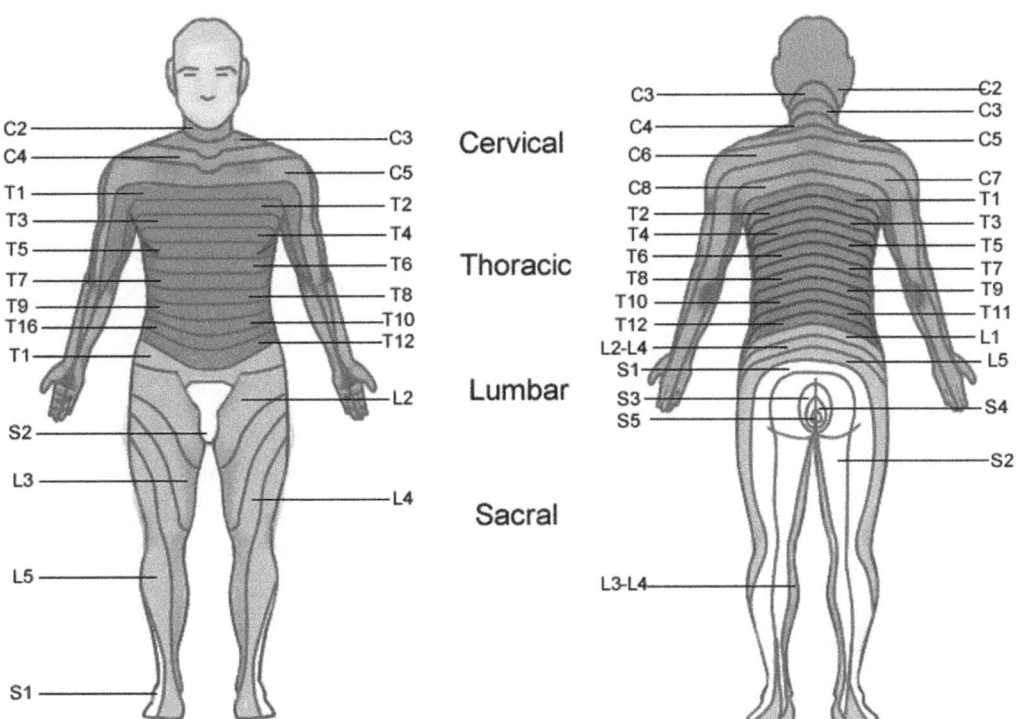

Figure 1.11 Dermatome map. A black and white version of this figure will appear in some formats. For the color version, please refer to the plate section.

Spinal Anatomy, Landmarks, and Dermatomes

Surface Landmarks

Table 1.3 describes some of the clinically relevant surface landmarks, and important key sensory and motor areas of innervation.

Spinal Anatomy

Vascular Supply

- Anterior two-thirds of the spinal cord receives its blood supply from a single *anterior spinal artery*, which arises from the vertebral arteries.

- ○ Receives branches from six to eight radicular arteries, most important of which is the *artery of Adamkiewicz*, arising most commonly at T9–T12.
- ○ Damage to artery of Adamkiewicz causes *anterior spinal cord syndrome.*
  - ▪ Flaccid paralysis of the lower extremities.
  - ▪ Bowel and bladder dysfunction.
  - ▪ Proprioception and sensation spared.
    - • Occurs most commonly in emergent repair of dissecting or ruptured thoracic aortic aneurysm (40%).

Table 1.3 Clinically relevant topographic landmarks

Mastoid process	Cervical 1
Thyroid cartilage	Cervical 5
Vertebral prominens	Cervical 7
Suprasternal notch	Thoracic 2–3
Sternal angle	Thoracic 4–5
Inferior angle of the scapula	Thoracic 7
Xyphoid process	Thoracic 9–10
Inferior costal margin	Lumbar 2–3
Iliac crest	Lumbar 4–5
Anterior superior iliac spine	Sacral 1–2
Greater trochanter	Distal coccyx
Symphysis pubic	2.5 cm inferior to distal coccyx

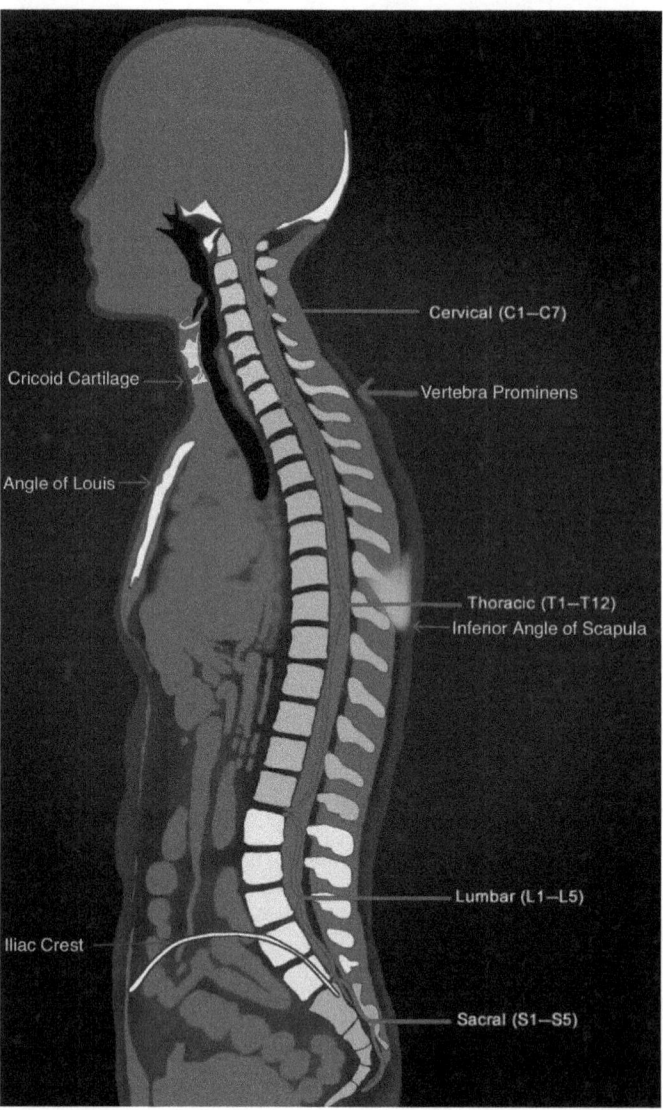

Figure 1.12 Spinal anatomy and relevant surface anatomy. A black and white version of this figure will appear in some formats. For the color version, please refer to the plate section.

- Posterior third of the spinal cord receives its blood supply from two *posterior spinal arteries*.
  - Conversely, *posterior spinal cord syndrome* (very rare) is characterized by loss of sensation and proprioception and spares motor innervation.

Cauda Equina

- Nerve roots of the lumbosacral plexus that arise following the termination of the spinal cord at the *conus medullaris*.
- Conus medullaris terminates at L1–L2 in adults and L3–L4 in infants.
- Damage to this structure can result in *cauda equina syndrome*, characterized by pain, paralysis of the lower extremities, and loss of bowel and bladder function.

Caudal Space

- Lowest part of the epidural space.
- Dural sac ends at S2 (S3–S4 at birth) where it fuses to filum terminale.
- Sacral hiatus is a defect in the lower part of the posterior wall of the sacrum due to failure of S4–S5 laminae to fuse at midline.
- Roofed by the *sacrococcygeal ligament*, an extension of ligamentum flavum.

Further Reading

Gray H. *Anatomy of the Human Body*, 20th ed. 1918. Online edition from Bartleby.com. Published May 2000. Available at: www.bartleby.com/br/107/ (accessed March 2017).

Miller RD, Pardo M, Stoelting RK. *Basics of Anesthesia*. Elsevier/Saunders, 2011.

NYSORA – The New York School of Regional Anesthesia. Available at: www.nysora.com/ (accessed March 2017).

Anesthesia Delivery Systems

Giacomo Scorsese, Bryan Hill, Jeron Zerillo, and Morgane Factor

Components of the Anesthesia Machine

a. **Pressure regulating component** – regulators that serve to safely decrease gas pressures
b. **Gas supply system** – divided into three sections for each gas (oxygen, air, and nitrous oxide).
  i. High pressure – only gas cylinders are "high" pressure (i.e., oxygen and nitrous oxide)
  ii. Intermediate pressure – begins at either the hospital pipeline or the stepped-down input from the size E cylinders and extends to the flowmeter control valves
  iii. Low pressure – begins at the flowmeter control valves, includes the flowmeters and anesthetic vaporizer, and ends at the fresh gas outlet
c. **Compressed gases** – oxygen, air, and nitrous oxide
  i. Gases are most often delivered to the anesthesia machine from a central supply source located in the hospital (i.e., pipeline).
  ii. Gas delivery from central source requires adequate pressurization (ranges from 40 to 50 psi).
  iii. Diameter index safety system (DISS) – quick coupler system connecting pipeline hose to wall and/or anesthesia machine
    1. Noninterchangeable gas-specific diameter fittings
    2. Prevents pipeline misconnection
    3. Gases can also be delivered via auxiliary compressed gas cylinders located on back of workstation (i.e., E cylinders – most common tank you will encounter).
      a. Cylinders of compressed gas on machine in case of central supply failure
  iv. **Pin index safety system (PISS)** – designed to prevent incorrect gas cylinder connections in the anesthesia workstation
    1. Two metal pins in cylinder valve casing that connect via hanger yoke

  v. Calculation of E cylinder contents
    1. Pressure and volume directly proportional in oxygen and air cylinder
    2. $P_1V_1 = P_2V_2$
    3. Pressure and volume NOT proportional in nitrous oxide cylinder
      a. Pressure begins to decrease after all liquid nitrous oxide is vaporized.
      b. ~ 75% of nitrous oxide cylinder content must been used
      c. Must weigh cylinder and subtract from tare weight to calculate contents (Table 2.1)
d. **Oxygen flush valve**
  i. Allows manual delivery of 100% oxygen at a high flow rate (35–75 L/min) directly to the breathing circuit
  ii. Supplied directly from intermediate pressure segment and bypasses vaporizers
  iii. May cause barotrauma if utilized during inspiratory cycle of mechanical ventilation
e. **Pneumatic safety system**
  i. Oxygen supply failure alarm sensor – audible and visual alarm that sounds when oxygen pressure drops below acceptable standard
  ii. Oxygen supply failure protection device (aka "fail safe valves") – either shuts off (binary valve) or reduces (proportional valve) the flow of other gases such as nitrous oxide or air when oxygen pressure drop < 30psi
f. **Proportioning system (GE/Datex-Ohmeda Link-25)** – provides mechanical integration of the nitrous oxide and oxygen flow control valves to ensure a minimum nitrous oxide–oxygen flow ratio of 3:1
g. **Flow control assembly (aka flowmeters)** – allows the operator to select a *total fresh gas flow* that enters the low-pressure section of the anesthesia workstation

Table 2.1 E cylinder contents

Gas	Color	State in cylinder	Volume (L)	Pressure (psi)	Weight empty (kg)	Weight full (kg)
Oxygen	Green	Gas	625	2,000	5.9	6.8
Nitrous oxide	Blue	Liquid/gas	1,590	750	5.9	8.8
Carbon dioxide	Grey	Liquid/gas	1,590	838	5.9	8.9
Air	Yellow	Gas	625	1,800	5.9	–

i. These valves separate the intermediate-pressure section from the low-pressure section.

ii. Flow tubes (rotameter) – a tapered, transparent flow tube known as a *variable orifice flowmeter* or *Thorpe tube* that measures the volumetric flow of fluid (gas) in a closed circuit

   1. Narrowest at the bottom and widens at the top

   2. The rotameter (aka bobbin) floats at equilibrium between gravitational forces and gas flow. Must be rotating if functioning properly. Will not function if the tube is broken or not vertical.

   3. Proportional flow and pressure affected by:

     a. Resistance (tube shape)

     b. Gas density

     c. Gas viscosity

   4. The flowmeter → manifold (mixing chamber) → vaporizer → breathing circuit

     a. Oxygen should be the last gas in the manifold (i.e., closest to patient). This will decrease chances that proximal leak will decrease concentration of delivered oxygen.

Vaporizers

- Vaporization: conversion of liquid to vapor
- Vaporizer: closed container where vaporization occurs
- Volatile anesthetics: liquid at atmospheric pressure (760 mmHg) and room temperature (22°C)
- **Physics of vaporization**
  - Asymmetrical arrangement of intermolecular forces at liquid-oxygen interface for volatile anesthetic in vaporizer
    - Net attractive force keeps molecules in liquid phase (cohesion).
    - Heat energy can be applied so that the molecules can overcome the force to enter the gaseous phase (latent heat of vaporization).
    - Heat energy requirement increases as liquid temperature decreases.
  - Vaporization stops when there is a liquid–gas equilibrium.
  - Molecules in vapor phase collide and create vapor pressure.
    - Vapor pressure and temperature are directly proportional.
- **Vaporizer classification and design**
  - In-circuit vs. out-of-circuit vaporizers
    - Virtually all modern vaporizers are "out-of-circuit," meaning their controlled output is introduced into the breathing circuit through a fresh gas line.
  - Type of vaporizers
    - *Variable-bypass* – total fresh gas flow is split into two portions

- One portion enters vaporizer and becomes saturated with volatile anesthetic vapor → referred to as *flow-over*.
- Second portion travels via bypass chamber of vaporizer and meets at patient outlet of anesthesia machine.
- Delivered anesthetic concentration is determined by control dial.

- *Dual-circuit vaporizer* – Tec 6 vaporizer (aka desflurane vaporizer)
  - Desflurane's vapor pressure (669 mmHg) at sea level approximates barometric pressure (760 mmHg). Thus, small changes in ambient temperature could potentially alter the saturated vapor pressure.
  - Vaporizer is electrically heated to 39°C, which produces a consistent vapor pressure of 1,300 mmHg.
  - Allows for more predicted volatility

- **Vaporizer safety mechanisms**
  - Agent specific – only one volatile anesthetic can be placed in a vaporizer. Key filler adapter is specific to each agent and each vaporizer.
  - Temperature-compensated = Constant vaporizer output over a range of temperatures
  - Controlled by temperature-sensitive bimetallic strip = If liquid anesthetic temperature decreases → vapor pressure decreases → increased gas inflow will occur to help raise the pressure.
  - Vaporizer interlock system – Prevents fresh gas flow through more than one vaporizer at a time.

Anesthesia Breathing Systems

Serves as a conduit to deliver anesthetic and other gases to a patient. Classified based on the presence or absence of a gas reservoir bag in the circuit, rebreathing of exhaled gases, unidirectional valves, a means to chemically neutralize exhaled carbon dioxide, and fresh gas flow rates.

a. Open system – has no reservoir bag, no functional rebreathing of exhaled gases, no unidirectional valves, and no means of neutralizing exhaled CO_2. *These systems include insufflation and open-drop anesthesia.*

b. Semi-open circle system – has a reservoir bag, no functional rebreathing of exhaled gases, may or may not have unidirectional valves, no CO_2 absorber and has high fresh gas flows. *These include Mapleson breathing systems.*

c. Semi-closed circle system – has a reservoir bag, partial rebreathing of exhaled gases, unidirectional valves, neutralizing carbon dioxide, and moderate fresh gas flows. *These include circle systems with an adjustable pressure-limiting (APL) valve that is at least partially open.*

d. Closed circle system – has a reservoir bag, total rebreathing of exhaled gases, unidirectional valves, and neutralize carbon dioxide. *These include circle systems with the APL valve closed. See Table 2.2.*

Table 2.2 Breathing flow

Type of circuit	Reservoir bag	Rebreathing	Unidirectional valves	CO$_2$ absorber	Fresh gas flow rate
Open	–	–	–	–	Unknown
Semi-open (Mapleson)	+	–	+/–	–	High
Semi-closed (APL partially open)	+	Partial	+	+	Moderate
Closed (APL closed)	+	Total	+	+	Low

Table 2.3 Absorbents

Absorbent	KOH %	NaOH %	Ca(OH)$_2$ %	Ba(OH)$_2$ %	H$_2$O %
Baralyme	4.6	–	70		14
Soda lime	2.6	1.3	80	–	15
Dragersorb 800 Plus	0.003	2.0	82	–	16
Medisorb	0.003	2.6	81	–	16
Sodasorb	0.0005	3.8	90	–	16
Amsorb Plus	–	–	83.2	–	14.4

Carbon Dioxide (CO$_2$) Absorbents

CO$_2$ absorbents minimize waste by reducing fresh gas flow to allow exhaled anesthetic agents to be rebreathed.

a. Absorbent formulations typically consisted of calcium hydroxide Ca(OH)$_2$ combined with strong bases like sodium and potassium hydroxide.
   i. $CO_2 + Ca(OH)_2 \rightarrow CaCO_3 + H_2O + heat$
   ii. CO$_2$ does not react quickly with Ca(OH)$_2$; therefore, water and small amounts of strong base catalysts are required to speed up the reaction.

b. All halogenated anesthetic agents can undergo chemical degradation in the setting of carbon dioxide absorbents.
   i. For example, soda lime can degrade sevoflurane into compound A, which at high doses is a nephrotoxin in rats.

c. Carbon dioxide absorbents that contain great quantities of "strong bases," such as KOH or NaOH, will tend to produce greater amounts of carbon monoxide, compared with "weak bases," such as Ba(OH)$_2$ or Ca(OH)$_2$.
   i. $KOH > NaOH \gg Ba(OH)_2 > Ca(OH)_2$
   ii. Typically, this is greatest with Desflurane, dry absorber and low flows.

d. Baralyme and soda lime have the highest proportion of KOH and therefore the highest potential.
   i. Baralyme was withdrawn from the market in 2004.
   ii. Soda lime is still in use today and has the greatest risk of carbon monoxide production.
   iii. Amsorb has the least risk of carbon monoxide production.

See Table 2.3.

Mapleson Breathing Systems

a. Classifies five different semi-open breathing systems (Mapleson A, B, C, D, and E)
b. Absence of valves to separate inspired and expired gases
   i. Rebreathing when inspiratory flow > fresh gas flow (FGF)
c. Absence of chemical neutralization of carbon dioxide
   ○ **Mapleson F** = Jackson-Rees modification of Mapleson D
     ▪ Uses a reservoir bag and APL valve distal to the reservoir bag
     ▪ Must adjust mode of ventilation and APL valve to prevent rebreathing
     ▪ Can be used when transporting intubated patients
     ▪ Disadvantages include lack of humidity, need for high FGF to prevent rebreathing, possible barotrauma if APL valve is occluded (Figure 2.1)
   ○ **Bain system**
     ▪ Modification of Mapleson D circuit
     ▪ Fresh gas supply tube runs concentrically within expiratory tubing
     ▪ Exhaled gas vented out the overflow valve near reservoir bag
     ▪ Fresh gas inflow is warmed by the surrounding exhaled gases
     ▪ Easy to scavenge waste via overflow valve
     ▪ Often difficult to recognize problems with inner fresh gas tube such as disconnection
   ○ **Circle system**
     ▪ Most widely used in the United States
     ▪ Components arranged in circular fashion: fresh gas inlet, unidirectional inspiratory and expiratory valves, inspiratory and expiratory tubing, Y piece

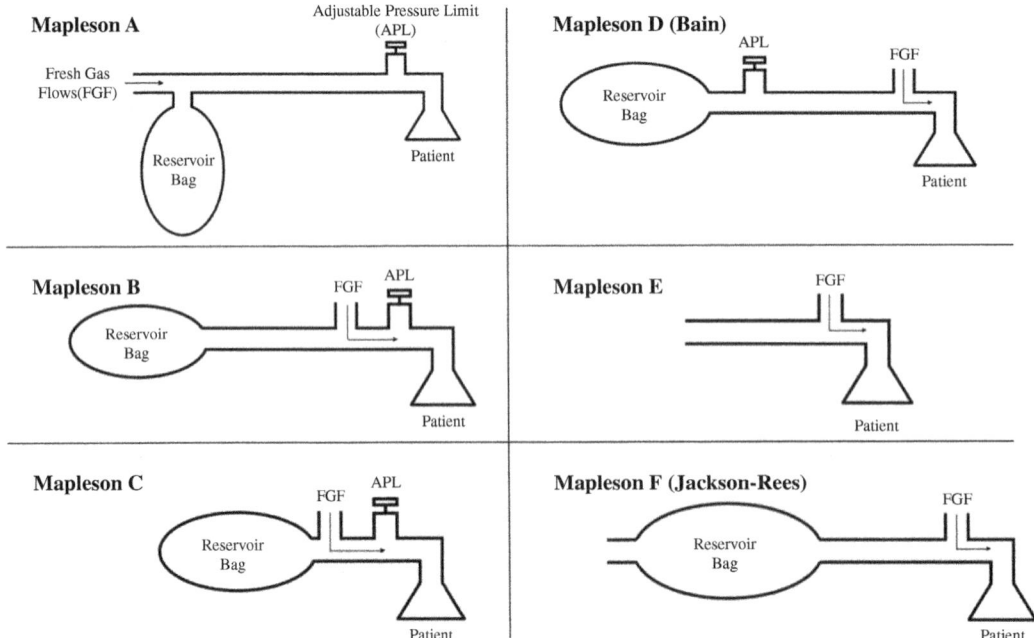

Figure 2.1 Mapleson breathing systems.

connector, APL valve, reservoir bag, carbon dioxide absorbent canister, bag/vent switch, mechanical ventilator

- Allows for chemical neutralization of carbon dioxide to prevent rebreathing
- Can be closed, semi-closed, or semi-open depending on fresh gas inflow
- Semi-closed is most popular, can rebreathe exhaled gases
- Allows for conservation of body heat and moisture in circuit
- Increased circuit resistance from unidirectional valves and carbon dioxide absorbent

○ **Closed anesthetic breathing system**
- Total rebreathing of exhaled gases after carbon dioxide is absorbed
- Maximizes humidification, economizes use of volatile anesthetics
- Unable to rapidly change delivered amounts of anesthetic and oxygen
- Risk of delivering unpredictable concentration of oxygen and unknown amounts of volatile anesthetic

Anesthesia Machine Checkout

a. The most important part of the checkout procedure is to verify the presence of a self-inflating resuscitation bag and that an alternative oxygen source (E-cylinder) is available and functioning.

b. American Society of Anesthesiologists' *2008 Recommendations for Pre-Anesthesia Checkout Procedures*
   i. Perform daily: 15-item checklist that serves as a template for the creation of machine-specific checkout procedures

Physiological Monitoring

a. Qualified anesthesia personnel are present in the room throughout all general anesthetics, regional anesthetics, and monitored anesthesia care.

b. The patient's oxygenation, ventilation, circulation, and temperature are continually evaluated.
   i. Oxygenation – ensure inhaled concentrations of oxygen, carbon dioxide, inhaled anesthetics as well as blood concentrations
      1. Plethysmography (i.e., pulse oximetry)
   ii. Ventilation – exhaled concentrations of oxygen, carbon dioxide, inhaled anesthetics
      1. Capnography
   iii. Circulation –
      1. Electrocardiogram
      2. Arterial blood pressure measurement, either noninvasive and/or invasive
   iv. Body temperature

Anesthesia Equations:
   I. Vapor output. This equation will give you the volume of vapor leaving the circuit (in mL).

$$VO = (CG \times SVP)/(Pb - SVP)$$

VO = Vapor output

SVP = Saturated vapor pressure (mmHg at room temp)

CG = Carrier gas

Pb = barometric pressure (mmHg)

II. Percentage concentration of volatile anesthetic. Once the total volume of vapor leaving the circuit is known you can solve for % concentration delivered

$$\%Va = [Va/(FGF + Va)] \times 100$$

Va = Volatile anesthetic

FGF = fresh gas flow

III. (Anesthesia circuit) time constant

$$(\tau) = V_{circ}/(FGF)$$

τ = Time constant

V_{circ} = Volume of circuit

FGF = Fresh gas flow

Further Reading

American Society of Anesthesiologists. *Check-Out: A Guide for Preoperative Inspection of an Anesthetic Machine.* American Society of Anesthesiologists, 1987; pp 1–14.

American Society of Anesthesiologists. Standards for basic anesthetic monitoring. (Last affirmed October 20, 2020; original approval October 21, 1986.) Available at: www.asahq.org/standards-and-guidelines/standards-for-basic-anesthetic-monitoring.

ASA Committee on Equipment and Facilities. *2008 Recommendations for Pre-Anesthesia Checkout Procedures.* American Society of Anesthesiologiest, 2008. Available at: https://psnet.ahrq.gov/issue/2008-recommendations-pre-anesthesia-checkout-procedures

Brockwell RC, Andrews JJ. Delivery systems for inhaled anesthetics. In Barash PG, Cullen BF, Stoetling RK, editors. *Clinical Anesthesia*, 5th ed. Lippincott Williams & Wilkins, 2006; pp 557–594.

Bokoch MP, Weston SD. Inhaled anesthetics: delivery systems. In Gropper MA, editor. *Miller's Anesthesia*, 9th ed. Elsevier, 2020; chapter 22, pp 572–637.

Conway CM. Anaesthetic breathing systems. *Br J Anaesth* 1985 Jul;**57**(7):649–657. doi: 10.1093/bja/57.7.649. PMID: 3925973.

Kharasch ED, Fink EJ Jr, Artru A, et al. Long-duration low-flow sevoflurane and isoflurane effects on postoperative renal and hepatic function. *Anesth Analg* 2001;**93**(6):1511–1520, table of contents.

Miller, RD, Roth P. Anesthesia delivery systems. In Pardo MC, editor. *Basics of Anesthesia*, 7th ed. Elsevier, 2018; chapter 15, pp 220–238.

Chapter 3

Monitoring Methods

Aleksey Maryansky

General Monitors

Blood Pressure Monitoring

Arterial Line[1]

An invasive continuous blood pressure monitoring method.

Indications: Repetitive blood sampling, severe cardiovascular disease with expected hemodynamic instability, titration of vasopressors or antihypertensives, respiratory disturbance requiring persistent arterial blood gas monitoring, inability to obtain blood pressure with a noninvasive cuff.[1]

- Arterial cannula transmits mechanical pressure wave through fluid-filled noncompliant tubing to transducer, which converts mechanical energy into kinetic energy and is displayed as a waveform on the monitor.[1]
- The arterial waveform is composed of a series of sine waves, which are analyzed by Fournier analysis. The arterial pressure system must be able to transmit high-frequency waves in order to obtain a precise arterial blood pressure reading. The natural frequency (or the frequency at which the system oscillates freely) must be set higher (at least 25 Hz but usually 100–200 Hz) than the frequency of any possible sine wave in order to prevent resonance and thus signal deformation.[2]
- Natural frequency can be changed by: changing diameter, density, compliance or length. *Increasing the length* of the tubing will *decrease natural frequency*.[2]
- The arterial line is "zeroed" to ensure negligible effect by atmospheric pressure on the pressure reading by opening the transducer to air. The arterial line transducer is normally placed at the level of the heart to measure arterial pressure. It can also be placed at the level of the circle of Willis if measuring cerebral perfusion pressure.[1]
- A 10-cm change in the height of the level of the transducer will change the reading by 7.5 mmHg opposite of the direction of change. A change in the level of the arterial cannula is negligible as long as the transducer remains at the same level of measurement.[1]
- An arterial pressure system can be overdampened or underdampened, which is due to interference resulting in change in the amplitude of the wave and thus incorrect blood pressure readings. Dampening can occur due to bubbles, kinks, the addition of stopcocks and tubing. In an overdampened system, the systolic blood pressure will be underestimated and the diastolic blood pressure will be overestimated. The reverse will occur in an underdampened system. The mean arterial pressure will remain accurate.[1]

Noninvasive Blood Pressure (NIBP)

- By ASA guidelines, blood pressure must be measured at least every 5 minutes during any case where an anesthetic is provided.[3]
- Oscillometric: Internal pressure transducer senses oscillations after cuff is inflated; if no oscillations are sensed than the cuff deflates and senses again at the next level. Once oscillations are sensed, a microprocessor within the system compares oscillation amplitudes. The *systolic blood pressure* is obtained at the point *where oscillation amplitude first increases*. The *mean arterial pressure* (MAP) is obtained at *the maximum amplitude of oscillations*. The *diastolic blood pressure* is obtained at the point where the *oscillation amplitude drops off.*[4]
- This method is reliable for obtaining MAP and diastolic blood pressure but can underestimate systolic blood pressure.[4]

Pulse Oximetry

Used to continuously monitor a patient's saturation but appreciable pulse must be present to achieve accuracy. The pulse oximeter can thus also measure and display heart rate. In low blood-flow conditions, pulse oximetry may not be reliable. Pulse oximetry correlates predictably with PaO_2.[4]

- The probe detects two wavelengths of light: *red (660 nm) and infrared (940 nm)*. Oxyhemoglobin absorbs more infrared light and deoxyhemoglobin absorbs more red light. The ratio of infrared to red light determines the SpO_2.[4]
- The pulse oximeter does not differentiate between oxyhemoglobin and other types of hemoglobin such as carboxyhemoglobin, and methemoglobin. Therefore, in the presence of one of these conditions, the SpO_2 may not correlate to the PaO_2. In methemoglobinemia, the SpO_2 will be displayed as 85%, whereas in carboxyhemoglobinemia it may be falsely elevated. In

order to clinically differentiate between these hemoglobins, a co-oximeter should be employed instead.[4]

- The pulse oximeter is not a good measure of assessing ventilation, especially if a patient is breathing 100% oxygen as this can significantly prolong apnea time.
- Other entities that can affect pulse oximeter readings are *methylene blue, hypothermia, indigo carmine, and nail polish.*[4]

Temperature

As per ASA guidelines, temperature should be continuously monitored during any anesthesia case where clinically significant changes in body temperature are intended, suspected, or anticipated.[4]

- Temperature can be monitored in a variety of locations. Skin temperature can differ depending on where the temperature probe is placed and is not a good reflection of core temperature.[4]
- Esophageal or nasopharyngeal temperatures are most reflective of core temperature but can often only be used under general anesthesia.[4]
- Bladder temperature, as commonly attached to a Foley catheter, is also reflective of core temperature but is dependent on urine flow.[4]

Neuromuscular Function

A nerve stimulator monitor used intraoperatively after muscular blockade.[4]

- The nerve stimulator is commonly placed at the *adductor pollicis (ulnar nerve)* or the *orbicularis oculi (facial nerve).* Monitoring at the orbicularis oculi during induction allows for faster intubation as laryngeal blockade occurs at the same time.[4]
- Nerve stimulators can be qualitative and quantitative:
  - Qualitative: rely subjectively on tactile or visual analysis of stimulation. Reliable for assessing twitch count and "depth" of paralysis but poor for estimating train-of-four (TOF) ratio. Twitches correspond to the percentage of receptor blockade: four twitches (0–75% blocked), three twitches (75% blocked), two twitches (80% blocked), one twitch (90% blocked), zero twitches (100% blocked).[4] Most nerve stimulators provide the ability to assess for sustained tetanus. Five seconds of sustained tetanus at 50 Hz correlates to a TOF ratio > 0.7.[5] However, this still does not meet the threshold of TOF ratio > 0.9 for extubation. No qualitative method can reliably assess readiness for extubation.
  - Quantitative: directly measures and divides the amplitude of the first twitch by the amplitude of the fourth twitch and thus provides the ability to objectively calculate TOF ratio. A TOF ratio > 0.7 classically corresponds with full return of neuromuscular function. A TOF ratio > 0.9 is ideal criteria for extubation and reduces postoperative complications.[4]

Bispectral Index (BIS)

A monitor usually placed on the forehead, which detects raw electroencephalographic (EEG) data and converts them into a BIS number. It is presumed to be useful in the titration of anesthesia to an appropriate level to try to ensure that the patient is not awake.[4]

- A BIS # of 91–100 correlates with the patient being awake. A BIS # of 61–90 correlates with light anesthesia. A BIS # of 41–60 correlates with acceptable general anesthesia. A BIS # of 1–40 correlates with deep anesthesia and a BIS # of 0 correlates with electrical silence.[4]
- The raw EEG waveform and thus the BIS # are susceptible to artifact from any electrical (i.e., cautery, defibrillator) devices that are close to the BIS monitoring site.[4]
- The BIS # can also become inaccurate due to muscle activity thus the BIS sensor allows you to monitor EMG activity as well. A greater level of EMG is inversely proportional to the accuracy of the BIS #.[4]
- Some anesthetic agents such as ketamine or etomidate may falsely elevate the BIS reading. The former due to an increase in high-frequency EEG activity and the latter due to an increase in high-frequency EMG activity.[4]

Electrocardiogram (ECG)

Critical monitor in the perioperative setting for both diagnosing and monitoring cardiovascular function, including the preoperative setting for risk stratification and guiding the need for more invasive tests.[4]

- Electrical activity emanates from the heart and can be recorded from multiple sites. Leads placed on the skin measure electrical potentials. Bipolar leads utilize two electrodes at two different sites to measure a potential difference. Unipolar leads measure the absolute potential difference at one site relative to a control reference site.[4]
- Standard 12-lead ECG: three bipolar leads (I, II, III), six unipolar leads (V1–V6), and three modified unipolar limb leads (aVR, aVL, aVF).[4]
- P wave: Represents atrial depolarization. Normally proceeds from right to left, so wave is biphasic in V1 and V2 and upright in lateral leads.[4]
- PR interval: Represents conduction through the AV node, bundle branches, bundle of His and intraventricular conduction systems. Relative delay due to slow conduction through AV node. Normally 120–200 ms.[4]
- QRS complex: Represents left and right ventricular depolarization. Begins in the septum and spreads toward free walls of the ventricles. The main QRS vector in the frontal plane determines the axis, which is normally –30 to +90. Normal QRS complex lasts 120 ms.[4]
- ST/T wave: Represents ventricular repolarization. Usually begins at epicardial surface and spreads toward endocardium. Normally, QRS and T waves both deflect in the same direction. QT interval starts at Q wave and ends at conclusion of T wave and is highly rate-dependent, hence the use of the QTc,

which is corrected for heart rate. Prolonged QTc intervals predispose to malignant ventricular arrhythmias. The ST segment is the most sensitive marker of ischemia on the EKG. ST elevations classically represent transmural ischemia and ST depressions represent subendocardial ischemia, but there is considerable overlap.[4]

- Q waves: when pathological, can represent areas of myocardial scarring, usually from prior ischemic events. They more commonly represent a prior transmural infarct and often correlate on the ECG to the specific area involved. V1–V3 usually localize to anteroseptal and apical segments of the left ventricle, V4–V6 to the apical and lateral segments and II, III, and aVF to the inferior segments.[4]

- Monitoring: Three-lead systems utilize RA, LA, LL, and RL (reference) electrodes and represent the simplest form of measuring real-time ECG. This system allows for three bipolar leads (I, II, III) and ideally measures heart rate and R waves, and detects ventricular fibrillation. It is inadequate in the diagnosis and monitoring of more complex arrhythmias and detecting myocardial ischemia. Five-lead systems utilize LA, RA, LL, RL electrodes and one precordial lead (V1 through V6). This allows for leads I, II, III, aVR, aVL, and aVF and is better at detecting left ventricular ischemia in the operating room when leads V3–V5 are chosen (ideal position for detecting the bulk of left ventricular tissue).[4]

Ventilation Monitors

Respirometer – A part of the anesthesia machine that allows for the measurement of tidal volumes and minute volumes. Classically, in the case of the original Wright respirometer, expired gas into a chamber would cause the rotation of a rotor attached to a needle on an indicator dial displaying tidal volume.[4]

Inspiratory force – Negative inspiratory force (NIF) is often measured in anticipation of extubation. Generally, a negative inspiratory force of more than –25 cm H_2O is required before extubation. NIF corresponds to the negative inspiratory pressure generated by inspiratory musculature during a maximal inhalation. This can be performed actively by asking the vented patient to perform a maximal inhalation and measuring pressure. It can also be performed passively by steadily increasing the ventilator trigger setting to –25 cm H_2O and seeing if the patient is able to trigger a breath.[4]

Spirometry – With most modern anesthesia machines, spirometry measures airway flow, volume, compliance and pressure with each breath. Flow/volume and pressure/volume loops are dynamically displayed. These measurements allow for a more intricate detection of potential problems during the anesthetic as characteristic patterns will be seen. For example, in the case of a leak the expiratory loop will remain open at the end of exhalation. In obstruction, pressure will be high and volume will be low.[4]

Gas Concentrations

O_2 – Oxygen analyzers are critical to anesthesia practice and are usually located in the inspiratory limb or at the common gas outlet. They exist to ensure that the inspired gas mixture contains an adequate amount of oxygen to prevent hypoxia.[4]

○ Exhaled patient oxygen is monitored as well and is useful for assessing whether a patient is adequately pre-oxygenated. These analyzers consist of two chambers, one that samples gas and one that is used as a reference. An electromagnetic field agitates oxygen molecules in the sampling chamber and this is converted into a pressure that is then transduced and essentially displayed as a concentration on the monitor.[4]

CO_2 – Exhaled carbon dioxide monitors allow a practitioner to be able to measure adequate ventilation and avoid hypercapnia. They are also useful in detection of rebreathing and can be utilized as a monitor or cardiac output.[4]

○ Changes in end-tidal (ET) CO_2 can alert a practitioner to acute problems. $ETCO_2$ can be pathologically increased in a variety of scenarios; that is, hypoventilation, hypermetabolic state, obstructive respiratory disease, insufflation during laparoscopy or exhausted CO_2 absorbent. In other scenarios, it can be pathologically decreased, that is, hyperventilation, circuit disconnection or obstruction, pulmonary embolism and shock/cardiac arrest.[4]

○ CO_2 analyzers employ infrared absorption. The more CO_2 present in a sample, the more infrared light can be absorbed. The CO_2 concentration displayed is thus proportional to the amount of infrared light detected by the analyzer to be absorbed. The machine then displays this as both a number and a waveform called a capnogram.[4]

As pictured in Figure 3.1, a capnogram is divided into four phases:

- The inspiratory baseline (the point at which exhalation begins and is zero in normal patients due to the expired gas at this point coming from respiratory dead space; it is greater than zero in cases of rebreathing and inadequate fresh gas flow)[6]

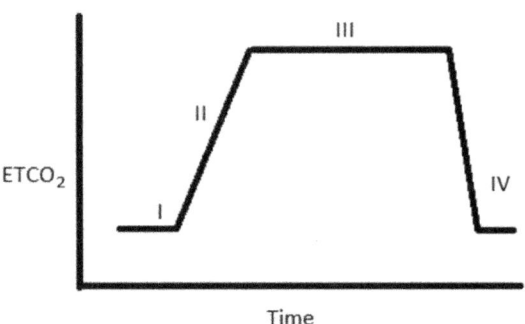

Figure 3.1 Capnogram.

- Expiratory upstroke (at this point, dead space gas ends and CO_2-containing gas from the alveoli begins to be exhaled). In obstructive lung disease (such as COPD) or an incompetent expiratory valve, this phase is prolonged.[6]
- Plateau phase (only CO_2-containing gas from the alveoli is exhaled at this point), if a patient is spontaneously breathing during mechanical ventilation, a notch called the "curare cleft" can be seen in the middle of the plateau.[6]
- Inhalation (gas is no longer exhaled at this point so in a normal situation the $ETCO_2$ falls back to zero; During rebreathing (such as in the case of an exhausted CO_2 absorbent), the $ETCO_2$ does not return back to zero at this point.[6]

Nitrogen – Many modern anesthesia machines monitor ET nitrogen. This can be useful in assessing adequate denitrogenation (pre-oxygenation). An abrupt increase in end-tidal nitrogen has been studied as an early sign of venous air embolism.[7]

Volatile anesthetics – Monitoring the concentration of volatile anesthetic delivered to the patient is important to ensure that the patient is at an adequate depth of anesthesia. Vapor concentrations are commonly measured either by Raman scattering or mass spectrometry (the most accurate method). In Raman scattering, a laser beam is directed toward a sample of gas in a chamber. When the light from the laser beam comes in contact with a molecule of a gas, the light scatters. The light is then passed through a variety of filters (each individual gas has its' own special filter) and into a detector/processing unit. The concentration of the gas is proportional to the number of photons passing through that gas' specific filter. In mass spectrometry, a gas sample passes into a low-pressure chamber and then into a high-pressure chamber which results in the ionization of the molecules of gas. Electromagnets separate the ions by mass and charge. The ions are then filtered and processed and a concentration of gas is displayed. Most modern anesthesia machines will convert the concentration into a minimum alveolar concentration (MAC) reading (for each respective gas and sometimes incorporating patient age).[4]

References

1. Weiner R, Ryan E, Yohannes-Tomicich J. Arterial line monitoring and placement. In Oropello JM, Kvetan V, Pastores SM, editors. *LANGE Critical Care.* McGraw-Hill/Medical, 2016; chapter 89.

2. Stoker MR. Principle of pressure transducers, resonance, damping and frequency response. *Anaesth Intensive Care Med* 2004;5(11):371–375.

3. American Society of Anesthesiologists Committee of Origin. *Standards and Practice Parameters. Standards for Basic Anesthetic Monitoring.* (Last amended October 20, 2010.)

4. Barash PG, Cullen BF, Stoelting RK, et al., editors. *Clinical Anesthesia*, 7th ed. Lippincott Williams & Wilkins, 2011.

5. Ali HH, Savarese JJ, Lebowitz PW, Ramsey FM. Twitch, tetanus and train-of-four as indices of recovery from nondepolarizing neuromuscular blockade. *Anesthesiology* 1981 Apr;**54**(4):294–297. doi:10.1097/00000542-198104000-00007. PMID: 6452074.

6. Ortega R, Connor C, Kim S, Djang R, Patel K. Monitoring ventilation with capnography. *N Engl J Med* 2012;367(19):e27.

7. Sprung J, Whalley D, Schoenwald PK, O'Hara PJ, O'Hara J. End-tidal nitrogen provides an early warning of slow, ongoing, venous air embolism. *Anesthesiology* 1996;85(5):1203–1206.

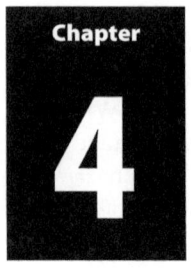

Ventilators, Alarms, and Safety Features

Michael D. Lazar

Ventilators

Phase variables:[1] Three main ventilator phase variables that make up a ventilator mode

What is the trigger of breath initiation (i.e., what will cause *start of inhalation*)?

- Time: Initiation of breath after a fixed interval of time, after which ventilator delivers a breath such as in controlled mechanical ventilation (MV)
- Flow: Patient inhalation efforts as sensed by flow in the circuit during assisted mechanical ventilation
- Pressure: Patient inhalation efforts as sensed by negative pressure during assisted mechanical ventilation

What is the limit of breath phase (i.e., what is the *quality of inhalation*)?

- Flow limited: There is a set rate of flow, and the ventilator will not allow any flow greater than this during inspiration.
- Volume limited: There is a set volume, and the ventilator will not allow any increase in volume than this during inspiration.
- Pressure limited: There is a set pressure, and the ventilator will not allow any further increase in pressure during inspiration.
- Of note, these variables are fixed if controlled MV and variable if assisted MV.

How long is the cycle of breath transition (i.e., *end of inhalation, beginning of exhalation*)?

- Time cycled: Inspiration and expiration according to the time set by ventilator such as in controlled mechanical ventilation
- Flow cycled: Once the flow decreases, the ventilator allows exhalation such as in pressure support.
- Volume cycled: Once target volume reached, the ventilator allows exhalation.
- Pressure cycled: Once peak inspiratory pressure reached, the ventilator allows exhalation.

Modes

Noninvasive ventilation:[2] Noninvasive alternatives to intubation

Continuous Positive Airway Pressure (CPAP)

- Mechanism: Continuous positive pressure administered throughout inhalation and exhalation via facemask (although nasal administration is also possible).

- Purpose: CPAP is administered to recruit and stent open alveoli and increase available surface area for gas exchange. It also encourages patency of the upper airway. Commonly used for obstructive sleep apnea (OSA) and respiratory distress syndrome of infancy.

Biphasic Positive Airway Pressure (BiPAP)

- Mechanism: The clinician sets an *inspiratory peak airway pressure* (serving as a form of pressure support) and an *expiratory peak airway pressure*. The difference between the two is equal to positive end-expiratory pressure (PEEP).
- Purpose: Administered for recruitment and maintenance of airway patency, augmenting tidal volume and eliminating carbon dioxide. May be implemented in an attempt to avoid invasive ventilation for patients with exacerbations of reactive airway disease, pneumonia, or acute heart failure.

Total controlled mechanical ventilation:[3] No patient-initiated breaths. Time triggered, volume or pressured limited and time cycled.

Volume Control (VC)

- Mechanism: Delivers constant flow to provide set tidal volume, regardless of characteristics of patient airway.
- Limitations: Opening airway pressure is dependent on patient characteristics, which could result in creation of excessive peak airway pressures (Figure 4.1).

Pressure Control (PC)

- Mechanism: Delivers set pressure to airway opening. Inhalational flow decreases progressively (see also Figure 4.1), which allows lower peak airway pressures.
- Limitations: In cases of decreased lung compliance, there is a risk of under-ventilation with variable tidal volumes.

Assisted Mechanical Ventilation

Volume Modes

Assist Control (AC)

- Mechanism: The patient may trigger the ventilator at a set negative pressure or flow threshold, otherwise the ventilator will deliver a breath according to a backup frequency (i.e., time trigger). Each breath is assisted or controlled by the

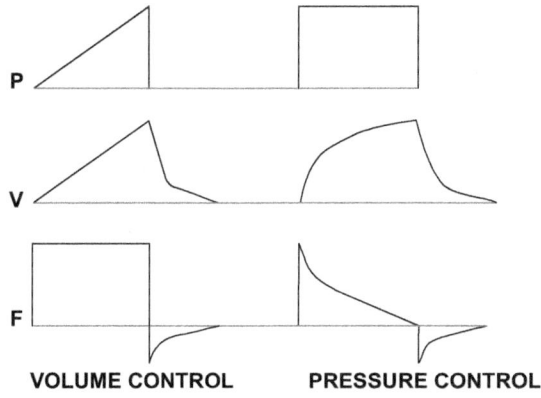

Figure 4.1 Pressure, volume, and flow curves for the two modes of controlled mechanical ventilation: volume control (left) and pressure control (right). P = pressure, V = volume, F = flow.

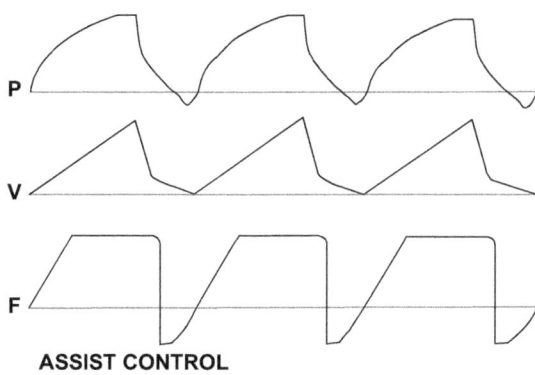

Figure 4.2 Sample pressure, volume, and flow curves representative of assist control ventilation.

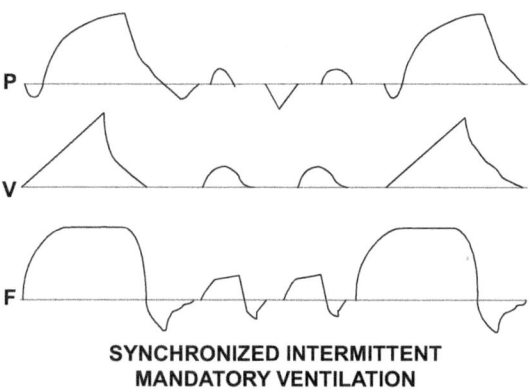

Figure 4.3 Examples of pressure, volume, and flow curves for synchronized intermittent mandatory ventilation. Note that patient-initiated breaths above the set respiratory rate are not supported by additional positive pressure.

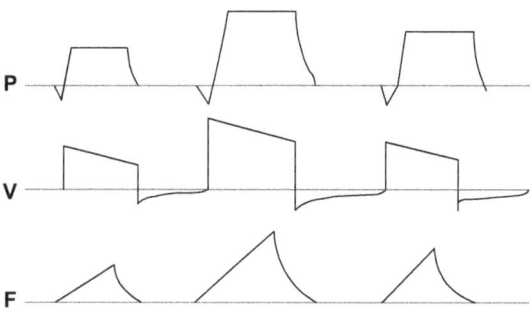

Figure 4.4 Pressure, volume, and flow curves illustrating pressure support ventilation.

ventilator, and all delivered tidal volumes are *equal*. Pressure, volume, and flow curves are shown in Figure 4.2.

- Limitations: With inadequate expiratory time or excessive respiratory rates, *hyperinflation* may occur. AC is the assisted mode with the most *asynchrony*, as peak inspiratory flows rarely match patient requirements, resulting in *increased work*. Risk of *air trapping* and *respiratory alkalosis*, especially with hyperinflation disease processes (i.e., COPD and asthma) or tachypneic disease processes (i.e., sepsis and hypermetabolic states).[1,3]

Synchronized Intermittent Mandatory Ventilation (SIMV)

- Mechanism: The mandatory ventilation in SIMV refers to a *guaranteed number of breaths*, which can be machine- or patient-initiated and which will achieve a *set tidal volume*. This is similar to AC; however, mandatory breaths are synchronized with *spontaneous* efforts. May be volume- or pressure-cycled. During attempts to wean patients from the ventilator, the number of mandatory breaths can be decreased to facilitate an increasing proportion of spontaneous breaths.

- Limitations: Additional patient inspiratory efforts beyond the set rate are not supported, as shown in Figure 4.3 (unless a combination SIMV–Pressure Support mode is selected). There is evidence that SIMV may reduce cardiac output in certain patient populations and prolong time to extubation during intensive care unit (ICU) weaning attempts.[4,5]

Pressure Modes

Pressure Support (PS)

- Mechanism: Triggered by the patient's negative pressure breath, limited by inspiratory pressure, and cycled by inhalational flow rate. PEEP may be added. Useful intraoperatively to supplement spontaneous breathing or during ventilator weaning trials in the ICU to compensate for circuit and endotracheal tube resistance. Decreases work of breathing. Example pressure, volume, and flow curves are demonstrated in Figure 4.4.

- Limitations: Clinician must change ventilator settings to achieve desired tidal volumes if there is a change in the mechanical properties of the lungs.

Pressure-Regulated Volume Control (PRVC)

- Mechanism: Clinician sets a baseline minute ventilation, and the patient may provide a negative pressure or flow trigger in order to initiate a breath. Uses a closed-loop algorithm to automatically measure the static compliance of the respiratory system and adapt the airway opening pressure to match a target tidal volume on a breath-by-breath basis. Intent is to use minimal pressure to achieve tidal volume and thereby reduce incidence of barotrauma, as illustrated by the progressively increasing pressures in Figure 4.5.[3]
- Limitations: Risk of auto-PEEP.

Interactive Modes

Proportional-Assisted Ventilation (PAV)

- Mechanism: Uses internal sensors measuring pressure and flow in order to adjust to patient effort. A benefit of PAV, as compared to PSV, is that tidal volumes (as opposed to respiratory rate) can adapt over time to stimuli such as hypercapnia.
- Limitations: Errors in evaluating elastance and resistance may result in inadequate ventilation.[4,6]

Neurally Adjusted Ventilatory Assist (NAVA)

- Mechanism: Designed to improve neuroventilatory coupling. Electrodes are placed through a nasal or oral gastric tube into the lower esophagus in order to use sensory information to correlate diaphragmatic movement with ventilator-assisted breaths.[4]
- Limitations: Limited clinical applicability to patients.

Ventilator Manipulation Techniques

Positive End-Expiratory Pressure (PEEP)

- Mechanism: Applied at *end-exhalation*, in contrast to CPAP, which is applied throughout inhalation and exhalation. PEEP is intended to expand collapsed alveoli to participate in gas exchange, reduce shunt, and increase

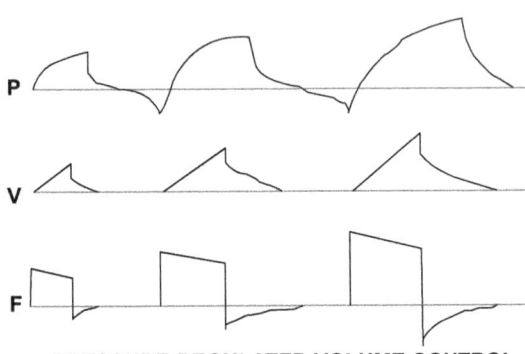

PRESSURE-REGULATED VOLUME CONTROL

Figure 4.5 Pressure-regulated volume control mode pressure, volume, and flow curves. Note, in particular, the gradual adjustment in pressure is required to achieve the desired tidal volume.

functional residual capacity. Up to 10 cm H_2O of PEEP, there is a linear increase in alveolar diameter. PEEP may be increased up to 20 cm H_2O for severe hypoxia secondary to acute respiratory distress syndrome (ARDS).

- Limitations: In the absence of collapsed alveoli available for recruitment, PEEP may result in *hyperinflation* and *increased dead space*. Increased intrathoracic pressure from PEEP may *decrease venous return*, although the clinical significance of this is dependent on patient characteristics (i.e., volume status) and comorbidities.[5]

Inverse Ratio Ventilation (IRV)

- Mechanism: A form of pressure control ventilation with an increased inspiratory:expiratory ratio, intended to improve oxygenation through reduced peak airway pressures. May be used in refractory cases of ARDS.[4,6]
- Limitations: Mean airway pressures may actually be elevated with resultant *reduction in venous return*. Associated with *risk of auto-PEEP*.

Airway Pressure Release Ventilation (APRV)

- Mechanism: A form of IRV with a very high inspiratory:expiratory ratio and very short expiratory time. Used in ARDS for refractory hypoxia. The prolonged inspiratory phase at high pressure followed by a short expiratory time, during which this pressure is released, creates a gradient that improves exhalation quality. Allows for superimposed spontaneous ventilation.[7]
- Limitations: Concern for hemodynamic compromise due to high inspiration pressures. Requires increased sedation.

Periodic Sigh

- Mechanism: Also described as *periodic hyperinflation*, this consists of an increased tidal volume (approximately 1.5–2 × set tidal volume) delivered approximately once every 6 to 10 minutes. Goal of technique is intermittent alveolar recruitment, but PEEP administration has been demonstrated as superior for this purpose.
- Limitations: Avoid with baseline tidal volumes greater than 7 mL/kg or with peak airway pressures greater than 30 cm H_2O.[1,3]

Alternative Ventilation

High-Frequency Ventilation

- Mechanism: Unlike the mechanical ventilation modes described above, high-frequency ventilation uses tidal volumes (1 to 2 mL/kg) that are less than dead space volume. These low volumes are delivered at frequencies of approximately 5 to 15 Hz at high flows and pressures with an oscillatory piston. Mean airway pressures are typically high.
- Limitations: Enough time must occur between breaths to allow passive expiration of carbon dioxide.

Monitoring Parameters[4]

- *Peak pressure*: Peak airway pressure is the highest pressure throughout the respiratory cycle and reflects a combination of all the *resistance* in both physiologic (patient) and mechanical (endotracheal tube, circuit, etc.) airways.
- *Plateau pressure*: Plateau pressure is obtained during an inspiratory pause on the ventilator (which eliminates airway resistance) and represents the pressure in the *small airways and alveoli*. Plateau pressure is typically indicative of *lung compliance*, whereas peak pressure is generally proportional to airway resistance. Figure 4.6 depicts peak and plateau pressures on a ventilator pressure curve. With decreased compliance or increased tidal volumes, both plateau and peak pressures should rise.
- *Increased peak and plateau pressure*: Increased tidal volume or decreased compliance (i.e., pneumothorax, abdominal insufflation, Trendelenburg position, pulmonary edema, pleural effusion, ascites).
- *Increased peak, unchanged plateau pressure*: Increased gas flow rate or airway resistance (i.e., bronchospasm, kinked or herniated endotracheal tube, secretions, mucous plugs, foreign body aspiration).
- *Static compliance*: Static compliance (normal 50–100 mL/cm H_2O) = Tidal volume/(plateau pressure – PEEP)
- *Dynamic compliance*: Dynamic compliance (always lower than or equal to static compliance) = Tidal volume/(peak pressure – PEEP).
- *Assisted ventilation monitoring*: Vigilant observation of patient–ventilator interaction is necessary during assisted ventilation.
  - *Asynchrony*: May occur secondary to inhalation time discrepancy (i.e., the ventilator is still delivering an inhalational pressure, but the patient has started to exhale), ineffective inspiratory triggering (i.e., ventilator is unable to sense the patient's breath despite adequate effort)
  - *Work of breathing* (WOB): Breath-by-breath analysis of patient work is ideal, but a more practical evaluation may be made by computing the work (pressure × volume) of breathing per minute and per liter of minute ventilation. Normal WOB at rest is approximately 0.3–0.6 joules/L. Use of any invasive ventilation requires additional work to be exerted by patient in order to trigger the ventilator and overcome the resistance of the circuit and endotracheal tube.

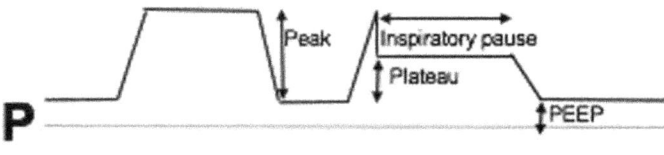

PRESSURES FOR COMPLIANCE ASSESSMENT

Figure 4.6 Extrapolation of peak and plateau pressure from ventilator pressure curves, which can be used to calculate dynamic and static compliance, respectively. Note that inspiration must be held in order to determine plateau pressure.

Alarms and Safety Features

General Alarm Concepts

- *Design*: Although there is no single organization that regulates alarms pertinent to monitoring for anesthesiology, at the International Standards Organization meeting in 2003, alarm severity was classified into high, medium, and low priorities.[8,9] See Table 4.1.
- *Alarm fatigue*:[8,10] Alarm fatigue is a product of the sheer number of alarms encountered, and in particular by excessive false positives, leading to the tendency to ignore meaningful information when it is provided. A significant reduction in false positives can occur by individualizing alarm limits for each patient, although caution must be taken, as limits that are excessively wide can result in false negative data. Innovations in technology have begun to reduce the incidence of false positive alarms (i.e., an EKG monitor automatically switching leads if an electrode is removed or pulse oximeters with algorithms designed to compensate for motion artifact). However, it is the clinician's responsibility to remain vigilant and prevent alarm fatigue from causing inattention to monitor alerts.

Operating Room Safety

- *Alarm sources*: There are a multitude of alarms and alerts within the operating room that can generate background noise. It is the anesthesiologist's responsibility to distinguish these from alarms that are specific to the anesthesia machine and its integrated monitor. Some examples include convection warming devices, electrocautery equipment, laser devices, and personal communications equipment such as pagers and phones.
- *Line isolation monitor*: Most grounded electrical systems outside of the operating room only require one fault to deliver a potential shock. With the addition of an isolation monitor

Table 4.1 Organization of medical monitoring alarm priorities

	High priority	**Medium priority**	**Low priority**
Intended response	**Immediate action**	**Prompt action**	**Awareness**
Visual alert	Red, Flashing at high frequency	Yellow, flashing at low frequency	Yellow/blue, no flash
Auditory alert	Loud, complex	Loud, monotone	Relatively muted
Examples	Severe hypoxia, malignant dysrhythmia (ventricular tachycardia/fibrillation, asystole)	Hypo/hypercarbia, Hypo/hypertension	Temperature probe disconnect

Data obtained from General Requirements, Tests and Guidelines for Alarm Systems in Medical Electrical Equipment and in Medical Electrical Systems (ISO-IEC 60601-1-8).[9]

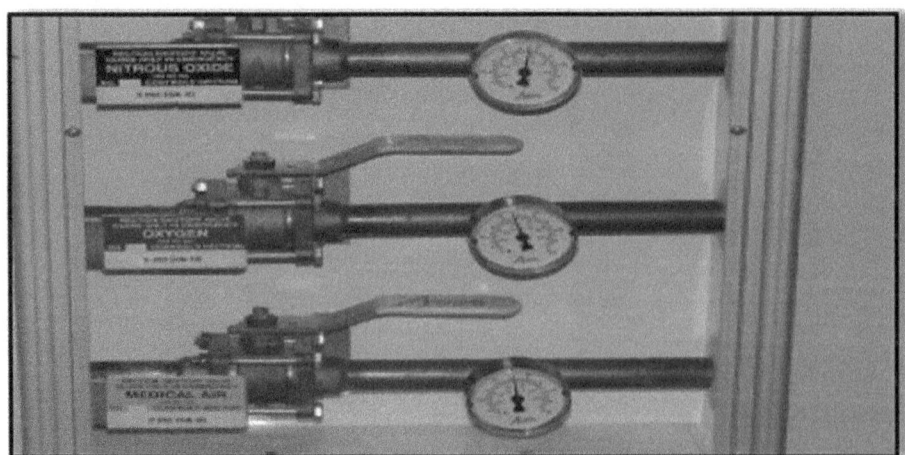

Figure 4.7 Gas-specific shutoff valves, required to be located outside of each operating room to enable control of pipeline supply in the event of emergencies such as fires. A black and white version of this figure will appear in some formats. For the color version, please refer to the plate section.

and transformer, electrical surgery equipment has an added protective layer, as it requires two faults to shock a patient. An alarm will sound if a hazardous amount of current could be transmitted to the patient in the event of a second fault, or the system becoming grounded. The last device or instrument added to the system before the alarm was initiated is typically the culprit and should be removed and analyzed.[3]

- *Air contamination*: The air in operating rooms is changed approximately 12 times per hour. National Institute for Occupational Safety and Health requirements: Volatile anesthetic concentrations must be <= 2 ppm; nitrous oxide must be <= 25 ppm (or <= 50 ppm in dentistry offices or where used without volatile gases).[11] Concentrations are measured with infrared analyzers, which can detect volatiles in ranges from 0 to 30 ppm and nitrous oxide in ranges from 0 to 100 ppm.

- *Gas control*: The gas-specific supply pressures must be displayed in close proximity to operating room clusters. This information is used to convey alarms to gas suppliers automatically so that stores can be replaced before supply pressures fall excessively. In the event of fires or suspected gas delivery errors, there are master shutoff valves for oxygen, air, and nitrous oxide outside each operating room (Figure 4.7).

Anesthesia Machine Safety

- Gas pressures:[8] First-stage regulators decrease pressures from approximately 85 PSIG inside bulk storage containers to 50 PSIG throughout all pipelines delivering gas into operating rooms and anesthesia machines. Second-stage regulators, located just upstream of flowmeters, further reduce gas pressures to 12–16 PSIG in order to reduce the risk of patient barotrauma.

- *Hypoxic mixture avoidance*:[10] Several mechanisms exist in order to prevent delivery of a hypoxic gas mixture to the patient, the most important of which is the *end-tidal oxygen level determined from the circuit's gas-sampling line*. Another feature designed to achieve the same goal is the *oxygen analyzer*, a fuel cell located in the inspiratory circuit limb. It is calibrated to room air but beware, if calibrated at sea level but used at altitude, the reading will be less than 21% because the ambient partial pressure of oxygen is less than 159 mmHg. Fail-safe systems are well known to be poorly named, because they are pressure-sensitive (not gas-sensitive) and would not prevent a hypoxic gas mixture in the event of a pipeline switch outside of the operating room. It is worth mentioning that GE-Ohmeda Pressure Sensor Shutoff Valves completely stop the flow of nitrous oxide if oxygen pressure falls below 26 PSIG in the high-pressure system. Conversely, Draeger Oxygen Failure Protection Devices reduce nitrous oxide flows in a stepwise manner in proportion to decreasing oxygen supply pressures. Finally, there is a high-priority Low Oxygen Supply Pressure alarm that is activated if oxygen pressures fall below 30 PSIG in the high-pressure system.

References

1. Cairo JM. *Pilbeam's Mechanical Ventilation*. 5th ed. Mosby, 2012.

2. Boldrini R, Fasano L, Nava S. Noninvasive mechanical ventilation. *Curr Opin Crit Care* 2012;**18**:48–53.

3. Hess DR, Kacmarek RM. Ventilator mode classification. In Moyer A, Thomas C, editors. *Essentials of Mechanical Ventilation*, 3rd ed. McGraw-Hill Education, 2014; chapter 5.

4. Miller RD, Cohen NH, Eriksson LI, et al. *Miller's Anesthesia.*, 8th ed. Saunders, 2015.

5. Goligher EC, Ferguson ND, Brochard LJ. Clinical challenges in mechanical ventilation. *Lancet* 2016;**387**:1856–1866.

6. Marini JJ. Mechanical ventilation: past lessons and the near future. *Crit Care* 2013;17:S1.

7. Daoud EG. Airway pressure release ventilation. *Ann Thorac Med* 2007;2:176–179.

8. Dorsch J, Dorsch S. *A Practical Approach to Anesthesia Equipment*. Wolters Kluwer/ Lippincott Williams & Wilkins Health, 2011.

9. General Requirements, and Tests Guidelines for Alarm Systems in Medical Electrical Equipment and in Medical Electrical Systems (ISO-IEC 60601-1-8). International Standards Organization, 2003.

10. Ehrenworth J, Eisenkraft J, Berry J. *Anesthesia Equipment: Principles and Applications*. Saunders, 2013.

11. OSHA Directorate of Technical Support and Emergency Management. Anesthetic Gases: Guidelines for Workplace Exposures. Available at: www.osha.gov/dts/osta/ anestheticgases/.

Chapter

5

Defibrillators

Matthew A. Levin

Definition and Types

A defibrillator is a device designed to treat ventricular arrhythmias by delivery of an electrical shock that terminates the arrhythmia and restores a normal cardiac rhythm. Defibrillators can be external or internal/implanted.

External

External devices consist of electrocardiogram (ECG) leads to sense the rhythm, a battery and capacitor to generate the charge, and paddles/adhesive pads to deliver therapy. There may or may not be a monitor. The paddles/pads can also be used for sensing. External devices can be classified as follows:

- Manual External Defibrillator
  Displays an ECG on a monitor, which the user is required to interpret. The user is also required to choose the amount of energy used and the timing of when to deliver the shock.
- Automated External Defibrillator (AED):
  Detects and analyzes the heart's rhythm automatically.[1] If a shockable rhythm is found, the user is prompted to press a button to deliver a shock. There is usually no monitor. Some AEDs are fully automated and will deliver a shock without requiring user intervention. AEDs are now commonly found in airports and other public spaces and are designed to be used by lay persons.
- Wearable Cardioverter Defibrillator
  A defibrillator worn by the patient that looks like a vest. An example is the LifeVest, manufactured by Zoll.[2] The vest continuously monitors the heart's rhythm, and if a shock is needed, sounds an alarm. If the patient fails to respond, a shock is automatically delivered. Usually used as a bridge to permanent therapy, or to recovery of heart function.[3-7]

Internal/Implantable (Figure 5.1)

An implantable cardioverter defibrillator (ICD) is a type of cardiovascular implantable electronic device (CIED). An ICD consists of *generator* (sometimes called a *can* because of the metal enclosure) containing a battery, capacitor, central processing unit (CPU), and one or more *leads* (wires) that are used to sense arrhythmias. The leads are also used to deliver therapy in the form of an electrical shock that terminates the arrhythmia and restores a normal rhythm. All modern ICDs are also pacemakers. Lead placement can vary as follows:

- Transvenous
  The leads are placed transvenously via the subclavian vein and superior vena cava directly into the right heart. There are usually two leads, one in the right atrium for pacing and one in the right ventricle for defibrillation. The ventricular lead has two defibrillation coils (Figure 5.1) that are used to deliver a shock. The generator is located subcutaneously, usually on the left upper chest wall.
- Bi-ventricular Leads for Cardiac Resynchronization Therapy (CRT)
  A third lead is placed in the coronary sinus to enable bi-ventricular pacing.
- Epicardial
  The leads are placed directly on the surface of the heart. Generator location is usually the same as above.
- Subcutaneous
  A subcutaneous ICD is a completely extrathoracic device.[8] There is no direct vascular access. The subcutaneous ICD has been shown to be non-inferior to a transvenous ICD.[9]
  - A single lead with two sensing electrodes and a coil is tunneled underneath the skin, usually along the right parasternal border. The generator is located subcutaneously, usually on the left mid-axillary line.
  - Benefits are reduced risk of endocarditis, lead fracture or lead malfunction requiring lead extraction.

Manufacturers and Identification

- External
  There are many manufacturers. Zoll is a commonly seen brand.
- Internal/Subcutaneous
  The major current manufacturers of ICDs are Boston Scientific, Biotronik, Medtronic, and St. Jude Medical. Devices can often be identified by their silhouette on chest X-ray (Figure 5.1).[10] There is a validated application (Pacemaker) for iOS and Android that can be used to easily and rapidly identify most devices.[11-13]
  - Historically, an ICD could be distinguished from a pacemaker by the thicker coils on the ventricular lead. Newer devices may not have a thicker lead.

Indications

Indications for ICD Placement

Indications can be divided into primary and secondary prevention.[14-17]

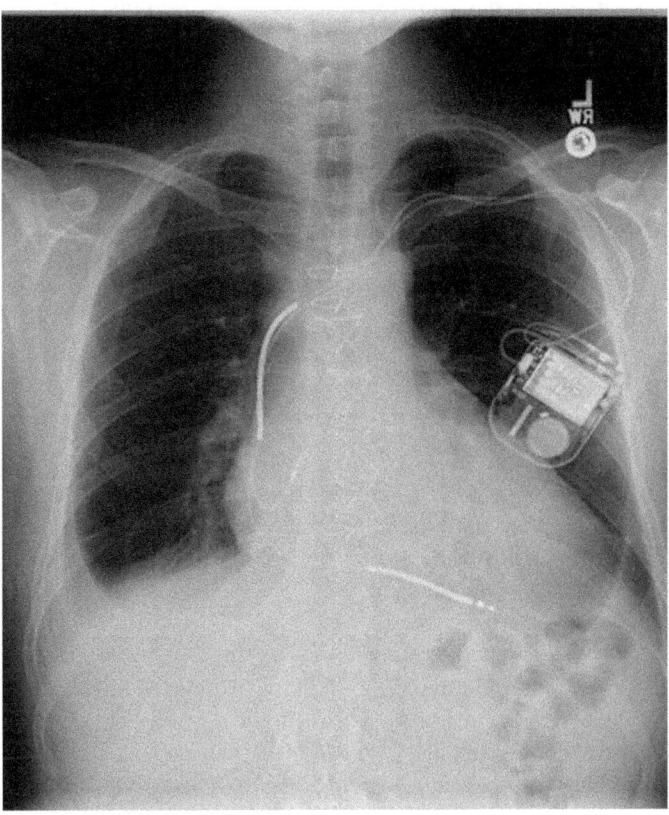

Figure 5.1 Chest X-ray of a patient with an ICD. Note the thick defibrillation coils, one in the superior vena cava and one in the right ventricle. Also note the thinner pacing lead in the right atrium. Used with permission from Stone ME, Salter B, Fischer A. Perioperative management of patients with cardiac implantable electronic devices. *Br J Anaesth* 2011;107 Suppl 1:i16–26. doi:10.1093/bja/aer354.

- Primary Prevention
  For patients who are at risk for but have not yet had an episode of sustained ventricular tachycardia (VT), ventricular fibrillation (VF), or resuscitated cardiac arrest.
- Class I indications include:
  ○ Left ventricular ejection fraction (LVEF) ≤ 35% due to prior MI ≥ 40 days post-MI and NYHA Class II or III (symptomatic)
  ○ LVEF ≤ 30% due to prior MI, > 40 days post-MI (asymptomatic)
  ○ LVEF ≤ 40% due to prior MI, with inducible VT/VF on Electrophysiologic (EP) study
  ○ LVEF ≤ 35% and NYHA Class II or III
  ○ Structural heart disease causing sustained VT
  ○ Syncope of undetermined origin with inducible VT/VF on EP study
- Secondary Prevention
  For patients who are survivors of cardiac arrest attributable to ventricular fibrillation or unstable ventricular tachycardia.

Indications for External Defibrillation

- Pulseless ventricular tachycardia (pVT)

- VF
- Cardiac arrest (excluding asystole or pulseless electrical activity)

Indications for External Cardioversion

- VT with a pulse
- Atrial fibrillation
- Atrial flutter

Modes/Therapies

Electrode Size and Position

Electrodes can be either self-adhesive pads or handheld paddles.

- Size
  Recommended pad size is 8–12 cm.[18] A larger size is associated with higher success rate because the pad impedance is lower and more current is delivered. Adult-sized pads can be used on pediatric patients (less than 8 years old or < 25 kg) but may misinterpret the rhythm, deliver too much current, or the current delivered may bypass the heart because the pad is larger than the heart.[19] Pediatric-sized pads and AEDs have been developed. Typical size of a pediatric pad is 4–5 cm.[20,21]
- Position
  Pads should be placed so that the path of electrical current from one pad to the other passes through the heart. There are two generally accepted positions:[18,22]
- Antero-apical
  ○ One pad is place on the right upper chest wall just to the right of the sternum and just below the clavicle over the 2nd or 3rd intercostal space.
  ○ The other pad is placed laterally on the left anterior or mid-axillary line at the 5th or 6th interspace, over the cardiac apex.
- Antero-posterior
  ○ One pad is placed on the back in the left or right infrascapular region.
  ○ The other pad is placed over the cardiac apex as above, or on the left mid-clavicular line over the precordium.
  ○ Antero-posterior placement is preferable in patients with an ICD/CIED, to avoid damaging the device.[23–25]

Defibrillation versus Cardioversion

- Cardioversion
  Used when there is an intrinsic cardiac rhythm sensed. Delivery of the shock is timed (synchronized) to coincide with the sensed R wave.
  Use of an unsynchronized shock when there is an intrinsic rhythm can result in an "R on T" phenomenon and trigger Torsades de pointes (polymorphic VF).
- Defibrillation
  Used when no intrinsic cardiac rhythm is sensed (wide complex VT, VF). Delivery of the shock is unsynchronized and may fall on any part of the cardiac cycle.

Energy and Waveforms for External Defibrillators

The electrical waveform used can be *monophasic* or *biphasic*. The amount of energy delivered depends on the mode.

- Biphasic
  Current flows in both directions. Current delivery is more consistent. *All modern devices use a biphasic waveform.*
- Monophasic
  Current flows in only one direction. Only much older devices use a monophasic waveform.
- Energy Requirements
  Depend on the underlying rhythm and the presence or absence of a pulse. The 2020 Adult Basic and Advanced Life Support guidelines published by the American Heart Association provide the following recommendations.[22] Dosing for pediatric patients is weight based, 2–4 J/kg, not to exceed 10 J/kg or the adult maximum dose.[18]
- VT with Pulse (Unstable)
  - Biphasic – Manufacturer recommendation, typically 50–200 J, *synchronized*. Start with the lowest energy and then double if unsuccessful.
  - Monophasic – 200 J
- VF/Pulseless VT
  - Biphasic – Manufacturer recommendation, typically 120–200 J. If unknown use maximum dose available.
  - Monophasic – 360 J

Atrial dysrhythmias are treated in the same way as VT with a pulse, with synchronized cardioversion.[8] Increase the energy in a stepwise fashion if the initial shock is unsuccessful.

- Atrial Fibrillation
  - Biphasic – 120–200 J
  - Monophasic – 200 J
- Atrial Flutter
  - Biphasic – 50–100 J
  - Monophasic – 100 J
- Energy Levels Delivered by an ICD
  The amount of energy delivered by an ICD is much lower, typically less than 30 J, increasing to up to 45 J.
- Energy Levels Delivered by a Subcutaneous ICD The amount of energy delivered by a subcutaneous ICD is 80 J.[26]

Perioperative Management

The Heart Rhythm Society (HRS) and American Society of Anesthesiologists (ASA) Expert Consensus Statement on the perioperative management of patients with CIEDs was published in 2011 and reaffirmed in 2021.[27,28]

Major Risks

Perioperative management of the patient with a ICD/CIED can be challenging.[29–31] The major risk during the perioperative period is that Electromagnetic Interference (EMI) will disrupt normal device operation. *The most common source of EMI in the operating room is monopolar electrocautery.* Use of monopolar electrocautery below the umbilicus is unlikely to cause interference. Bipolar electrocautery will not cause EMI unless it is applied directly to the device. Radio frequency (RF) energy such as that used in surgical sponge counting systems is another source of EMI that may cause ICD/CIED malfunction.[32] Some possible effects of EMI are:

- Inhibition of pacemaker function due to oversensing
- Pacemaker mediated tachycardia
- Delivery of inappropriate therapy (i.e., shock)
- Direct damage to the ICD/CIED

Management Strategy

The primary recommendation of the HRS/ASA Expert Consensus document is to consult with the patient's CIED care team pre-operatively, to obtain a prescription for the most appropriate management for the specific device and procedure. However, there is a simple algorithm that can be used to guide intraoperative management.[29]

(a) Determine Whether There Will Be a Source of EMI during the Procedure
  If yes, deactivate the ICD by disabling anti-tachycardia therapy using a magnet or by reprogramming the device. Reprogramming should only be done by a credentialed practitioner.

(b) Determine Whether the Patient Is Pacemaker Dependent
  If yes, determine whether the source of EMI will be ≤ 15 cm from ICD. **The distance should be measured to the closest part of the ICD, including the leads.** Ventricular leads will be closer to the diaphragm than the ICD generator.
  If EMI is within 15 cm, reprogram the ICD to an asynchronous pacing mode. This should only be done by a credentialed practitioner.

Magnet Application

Application of a magnet directly over the ICD will temporarily suspend anti-tachycardia (VT/VF) detection/therapy and prevent inadvertent shock delivery. Detection/therapy will resume when the magnet is removed. A magnet will not affect the pacemaker function of an ICD, that is, it will not place an ICD in an asynchronous pacing mode.

Pros

- Easy to use. A sterile magnet can be placed in the operative field.

Cons

- Some devices may not respond as expected because they can be programmed to ignore the magnet.[27]
- Deeply implanted subcutaneous ICDs may not respond to a magnet.[33]
- *A magnet cannot be used to change the pacemaker mode of an ICD.*

Reprogramming

The device can be reprogrammed using a programmer. Programmers are manufacturer specific.

Pros

- The device can be reprogrammed to any mode. An ICD can be placed in an asynchronous pacing mode using a programmer.
- The device can be interrogated and a detailed report on the device mode, function and therapy history can be printed for reference.

Cons

- Requires a programmer and specialized knowledge/expertise, neither of which may be readily available in the perioperative setting.
- In most institutions, only a credentialed practitioner, typically a cardiologist, will be allowed to interrogate and reprogram a device.

Non-Operating Room Locations

The guidelines for management of an ICD in a non-operating room anesthetizing location are generally the same.

Colonoscopy/Endoscopy

There is no evidence that either procedure interferes with ICD operation. If electrocautery is used the standard guidelines should be followed.

MRI

The historical recommendation was that MRI be avoided in patients with an ICD/CIED, because of concerns for magnetically induced heating of the leads that could result in myocardial injury, and/or changes in the lead properties.[34] The exception was devices that have been tested by their manufacturer to be MRI safe and labeled "MRI-conditional".

However, a recent prospective, registry-based study of non-certified devices ("non-MRI conditional") found no device or lead failures among 500 patients who had a non-thoracic MRI and had their device reprogrammed appropriately prior-to and after the MRI.[34]

The 2022 Joint British Society consensus statement on best practice management of patients with CIEDs requiring MRI recommends the following:[35]

- A full device interrogation immediately prior to the MRI scan, followed by reprogramming to an MRI mode as per manufacturer/device guidelines.
- This will include disabling anti-tachycardia shock therapies.
- After the scan is completed, the device should be interrogated again and set back to its original mode of operation.
- Device interrogation and reprogramming should only be done by an appropriately trained and credentialed practitioner.

References

1. Center for Devices, Radiological Health. Automated External Defibrillators (AEDs). U.S. Food & Drug Administration, 2022. Available from: https://www.fda.gov/medical-devices/cardiovascular-devices/automated-external-defibrillators-aeds

2. ZOLL LifeVest Wearable Defibrillator. Available from: https://lifevest.zoll.com

3. Klein HU, Goldenberg I, Moss AJ. Risk stratification for implantable cardioverter defibrillator therapy: the role of the wearable cardioverter-defibrillator. *Eur Heart J* 2013 Aug;**34**(29):2230–2242.

4. Kutyifa V, Moss AJ, Klein H, et al. Use of the wearable cardioverter defibrillator in high-risk cardiac patients: data from the Perspective Registry of Patients Using the Wearable Cardioverter Defibrillator (WEARIT-II Registry). *Circulation* 2015 Oct;**132**(17):1613–1619.

5. Olgin JE, Pletcher MJ, Vittinghoff E, et al. Wearable cardioverter-defibrillator after myocardial infarction. *N Engl J Med* 2018 Sep 27;**379**(13):1205–1215.

6. Masri A, Altibi AM, Erqou S, et al. Wearable cardioverter-defibrillator therapy for the prevention of sudden cardiac death: a systematic review and meta-analysis. *JACC Clin Electrophysiol* 2019 Feb;**5**(2):152–161.

7. Olgin JE, Lee BK, Vittinghoff E, et al. Impact of wearable cardioverter-defibrillator compliance on outcomes in the VEST trial: as-treated and per-protocol analyses. *J Cardiovasc Electrophysiol* 2020 May;**31**(5):1009–1018.

8. Kamp NJ, Al-Khatib SM. The subcutaneous implantable cardioverter-defibrillator in review. *Am Heart J* 2019 Nov;**217**:131–139.

9. Knops RE, Olde Nordkamp LRA, Delnoy P-PHM, et al. Subcutaneous or transvenous defibrillator therapy. *N Engl J Med* 2020 Aug 6;**383**(6):526–536.

10. Jacob S, Shahzad MA, Maheshwari R, Panaich SS, Aravindhakshan R. Cardiac rhythm device identification algorithm using X-rays: CaRDIA-X. *Heart Rhythm* 2011 Jun;**8**(6):915–922.

11. Weinreich M, Weinreich B, Chudow J, et al. Computer-aided detection and identification of implanted cardiac devices on chest radiography utilizing deep convolutional neural networks, a form of machine learning. *J Am Coll Cardiol* 2019 Mar 12;**73**(9_Supplement_1):307.

12. Weinreich B. Pacemaker-ID. Available from: https://www.pacemakerid.com/

13. Weinreich M, Chudow JJ, Weinreich B, et al. Development of an artificially intelligent mobile phone application to identify cardiac devices on chest radiography. *JACC Clin Electrophysiol* 2019 Sep;**5**(9):1094–1095.

14. Epstein AE, DiMarco JP, Ellenbogen KA, et al. ACC/AHA/HRS 2008 Guidelines for device-based therapy of cardiac rhythm

abnormalities: a report of the American College of Cardiology/ American Heart Association Task Force on Practice Guidelines (Writing Committee to Revise the ACC/AHA/ NASPE 2002 Guideline Update for Implantation of Cardiac Pacemakers and Antiarrhythmia Devices) developed in collaboration with the American Association for Thoracic Surgery and Society of Thoracic Surgeons. *J Am Col Cardiol* 2008;**51** (21):e1–62.

15. Epstein AE, DiMarco JP, Ellenbogen KA, et al. 2012 ACCF/ AHA/HRS focused update incorporated into the ACCF/AHA/ HRS 2008 guidelines for device-based therapy of cardiac rhythm abnormalities: a report of the American College of Cardiology Foundation/American Heart Association Task Force on Practice Guidelines and the Heart Rhythm Society. *J Am Coll Cardiol* 2013;**61**(3): e6–75.

16. Russo AM, Stainback RF, Bailey SR, et al. ACCF/HRS/AHA/ASE/HFSA/ SCAI/SCCT/SCMR 2013 appropriate use criteria for implantable cardioverter-defibrillators and cardiac resynchronization therapy: a report of the American College of Cardiology Foundation appropriate use criteria task force, Heart Rhythm Society, American Heart Association, American Society of Echocardiography, Heart Failure Society of America, Society for Cardiovascular Angiography and Interventions, Society of Cardiovascular Computed Tomography, and Society for Cardiovascular Magnetic resonance. *Heart Rhythm* 2013 Apr;**10**(4):e11–58.

17. Kusumoto FM, Calkins H, Boehmer J, et al. HRS/ACC/AHA expert consensus statement on the use of implantable cardioverter-defibrillator therapy in patients who are not included or not well represented in clinical trials. *Circulation* 2014 Jul 1;**130**(1):94–125.

18. Link MS, Atkins DL, Passman RS, et al. Part 6: electrical therapies: automated external defibrillators, defibrillation, cardioversion, and pacing: 2010 American Heart Association Guidelines for Cardiopulmonary

Resuscitation and Emergency Cardiovascular Care. *Circulation* 2010 Oct;**122**(18_suppl_3):S706–S719.

19. Samson RA, Berg RA, Bingham R, et al. Use of automated external defibrillators for children: an update: an advisory statement from the pediatric advanced life support task force, International Liaison Committee on Resuscitation. *Circulation* 2003;**107**(25):3250–3255.

20. Atkins DL, Jorgenson DB. Attenuated pediatric electrode pads for automated external defibrillator use in children. *Resuscitation* 2005 Jul;**66**(1):31–37.

21. Atkins DL, Scott WA, Blaufox AD, et al. Sensitivity and specificity of an automated external defibrillator algorithm designed for pediatric patients. *Resuscitation* 2008 Feb;**76** (2):168–174.

22. Panchal AR, Bartos JA, Cabañas JG, et al. Part 3: adult basic and advanced life support: 2020 American Heart Association Guidelines for Cardiopulmonary Resuscitation and Emergency Cardiovascular Care. *Circulation* 2020 Oct 20;**142** (16_suppl_2):S366–S468.

23. Botto GL, Politi A, Bonini W, Broffoni T, Bonatti R. External cardioversion of atrial fibrillation: role of paddle position on technical efficacy and energy requirements. *Heart* 1999 Dec;**82**(6):726–730.

24. Ambler JJS, Sado DM, Zideman DA, Deakin CD. The incidence and severity of cutaneous burns following external DC cardioversion. *Resuscitation* 2004 Jun;**61**(3):281–288.

25. Lüker J, Sultan A, Plenge T, et al. Electrical cardioversion of patients with implanted pacemaker or cardioverter-defibrillator: results of a survey of German centers and systematic review of the literature. *Clin Res Cardiol* 2018 Mar;**107**(3):249–258.

26. Emblem MRI S-ICD System. Available from: https://www.bostonscientific.co m/en-US/products/defibrillators/emble m-s-icd-system.html

27. Heart Rhythm Society. 2011 HRS/ASA Expert Consensus Statement on the Perioperative Management of Patients with Implantable Defibrillators, Pacemakers, and Arrhythmia Monitors: Facilities and Patient Management.

2011. Available from: https://www.hrsonline.org/guidance/cli nical-resources/2011-expert-consensus-statement-perioperative-management-patients-implantable-defibrillators

28. Crossley GH, Poole JE, Rozner MA, et al. The Heart Rhythm Society (HRS)/ American Society of Anesthesiologists (ASA) Expert Consensus Statement on the Perioperative Management of Patients with Implantable Defibrillators, Pacemakers and Arrhythmia Monitors: Facilities and Patient Management. *Heart Rhythm* 2011 Jul;**8**(7):1114–1154.

29. Stone ME, Salter B, Fischer A. Perioperative management of patients with cardiac implantable electronic devices. *Br J Anaesth* 2011 Dec;**107** (Suppl):i16–26.

30. Izrailtyan I, Schiller RJ, Katz RI, Almasry IO. Perioperative pacemaker-mediated tachycardia in the patient with a dual chamber implantable cardioverter-defibrillator. *Anesth Analg* 2013 Feb;**116**(2):307.

31. Thompson A, Neelankavil JP, Mahajan A. perioperative management of cardiovascular implantable electronic devices (CIEDs). *Curr Anesthesiol Rep* 2013 Sep 1;**3**(3):139–143.

32. Williams MR, Atkinson DB, Bezzerides VJ, et al. Pausing with the gauze: inhibition of temporary pacemakers by radiofrequency scan during cardiac surgery. *Anesth Analg* 2016 Nov;**123** (5):1143–1148.

33. Richman T, Stanton T, Fryer M, Dayananda N, Tung M. Evaluating the magnet response in deep subcutaneous implanted cardioverter defibrillator implants. *Pacing Clin Electrophysiol* 2023 Oct 21;**46** (2):93–99.

34. Russo RJ, Costa HS, Silva PD, et al. Assessing the risks associated with MRI in patients with a pacemaker or defibrillator. *N Engl J Med* 2017 Feb;**376**(8):755–764.

35. Bhuva A, Charles-Edwards G, Ashmore J, et al. Joint British Society consensus recommendations for magnetic resonance imaging for patients with cardiac implantable electronic devices. *Heart* 2024;**110**(4): e3.

Electrical, Fire, and Explosion Hazards: Basic Electronics

Andrew J. Schwartz

Electrical Considerations

Static Electricity

- Electricity or discharge generated by the movement of electrons across an interface
- Occurs when two distinctly charged items are brought into contact
- Leads to organization of oppositely charged particles on adjacent surfaces
- Magnitude of charge is dependent on material type, contact surface area and temperature.
- Separation of oppositely charged particles leads to a potential difference.
- If field strength exceeds a critical level, there is atmospheric ionization.
- Discharge to a less charged object can create a spark that is responsible for most operating room (OR) fires/explosions.

Static Electricity as an Ignition Source

- Requires the presence of four elements:
  - Accumulation of static electricity
  - The accumulated static must be insulated from any grounding body
  - The discharged spark must be of adequate ignition energy
  - The spark must occur in an atmosphere containing a fuel source within range[1]

Bonding

- Connection of one conductor to another
- Prevents the accumulation of static charge
- Allows the equalization of charge over the entire conducting system
- Allows an exit of the accumulated charge, eliminating it as an ignition source

Grounding

- Specific type of bonding
- Links conductive material to the ground
- The ground has an unlimited ability to accept electrons
- Any conductive system connected to the ground is devoid of charge
- Prevents the passing of charge within the system to a transient conductor[1]

- Transient conductors include patients and other operating room personnel
- Faulty equipment may provide errant currents to patients

Line Isolation Monitor (LIM)

- OR safety device that will alarm if a faulty ground connection occurs
- Typically alarms with current generation of > 2 mA that may be conducted to a patient[1]

Isolation Transformers:

- All electrical power sources in the OR are isolated from the ground
- Prevents passage of dangerous current through the patient[1]

***

Macro and Micro Current Hazards

Macro Shock

- Externally applied current across a surface with high resistance and large spatial distribution (i.e., skin)
- Leads to the disturbance of neural or muscular function.
- Current is spread throughout the body/less concentrated impulse
- Requires high energy to be harmful (10–100 mA)
- Degree of injury is affected by resistance of the skin
- Wet/broken skin has 1% the resistance of dry intact skin
- 5–10 mA: sustained muscle contraction and inability to "let go"
- 50–100 mA: mechanical injury
- 100–500 mA: ventricular fibrillation
- > 6,000 mA: sustained myocardial contraction and respiratory paralysis[1]

Micro Shock

- Directly applied current concentrated at one point (small spatial distribution)
- Typically applied to the heart
- Acceptable safety limit of 10 microA
- Maximum level of current allowable through catheters or electrodes in contact with heart. Generally caused by leakage current in line-operated equipment.

- Since LIM warning occurs at 2 mA, it will not protect against micro shock.

***

Operating Room Fire Considerations

Background

- Unknown incidence (no centralized reporting), but estimated at 500–700 OR fires/year[2]
- ASA Closed Claim Database reports 103 claims for OR fires since 1985.
- Eighty-five percent of OR fires occur during the delivery of MAC anesthesia for head, neck and upper chest surgery
- Fifteen percent of claims were for airway fire mainly occurring during tracheostomy and tonsillectomy
- Electrocautery was the ignition source in 90% of claims

The Fire Triad

- Fire requires a fuel source, an oxidizing agent, and an ignition source.
- Fire can be prevented or extinguished by the removal of any of these three critical components.[3]

Fuel

- Substance that produces heat from chemical combustion
- Surgical preparation solution (particularly alcohol based)
- PVC endotracheal tubes; also laryngeal mask airways (LMA) and O_2 masks
- Hair, tissue, patient gowns, linens
- Surgical drapes, sponges/gauze (when dry), packing materials, dressings

Oxidizer

- Oxygen enrichment is the most significant factor contributing to surgical fires.
- Facilitates the chemical reaction of combustion
- Nitrous oxide functions equally as well as oxygen at facilitating combustion.
- Many items that will not burn in air will readily ignite in the presence of enriched O_2.

Ignitions Sources

- Current, heat, friction
- Electrocautery is the ignition source in > 90% of claims for OR fires.[4]
- Other sources: Lasers, drills, argon beam, light cables, defibrillator paddles

Risk Factors for Intraoperative Fire

- Procedures involving an ignition source in proximity to oxidizer-rich environment
- Head and neck procedures
- Ophthalmic procedures
- MAC with supplemental O_2 that involves surgical draping leading to oxygen pooling

***

OR Fire Prevention

Communication and Education

- Communication between surgeon, anesthesiologist, and OR staff is critical.
- Recognition of high-risk procedures
- Preemptive discussion of strategy to mitigate risk for OR fires should be held prior to each case.
- ASA practice advisory: fire safety education is necessary for all OR personnel.[5]

Prep Solution

- Alcohol-based prep solution burns easily in room air.
- Allow sufficient time for prep solution to completely dry.
- ChloraPrep is 70% alcohol and is highly flammable.
- ChloraPrep: 3 minutes to dry on skin and up to 1 hour on hair
- Betadine solution is generally preferred for high-risk procedures.
- The large 30 mL ChloraPrep is contraindicated for head and neck surgery (high fire risk) because of pooling of the solution.

MAC for High-Risk Procedures (Head/Neck/Upper Chest)

- Recommend avoidance of open delivery of oxygen (i.e., nasal cannula)
- Always ask, "Is supplemental oxygen really necessary?"
- If supplemental O_2 is required, then use laryngeal mask airway or endotracheal tube.
- Securing the airway prevents accumulation of oxygen in surgical field.

Special Cases (Supplemental O_2 Required via Open Delivery)

- Surgery that requires the patient be able to communicate
- Carotid artery surgery, neurosurgery, some pacemaker implantations
- Minor surgery when risk of securing airway is > risk of open delivery
- Use blended O_2 supply in order to keep supplemental O_2 to a minimum.
- Use minimum necessary FiO_2 to maintain acceptable oxyhemoglobin concentration.
- Consider the delivery of 5–10 L/min of air under drapes for washout effect.
- Alternate surgical tool: scalpel, bipolar, harmonic scalpel
- Open draping techniques

OR Fire Management

- Immediately remove any source of oxygen.
- Remove all burning drapes from the patient.
- Douse fire and patient with saline.
- Use a fire extinguisher to eliminate any remaining fire on drapes once removed.

***

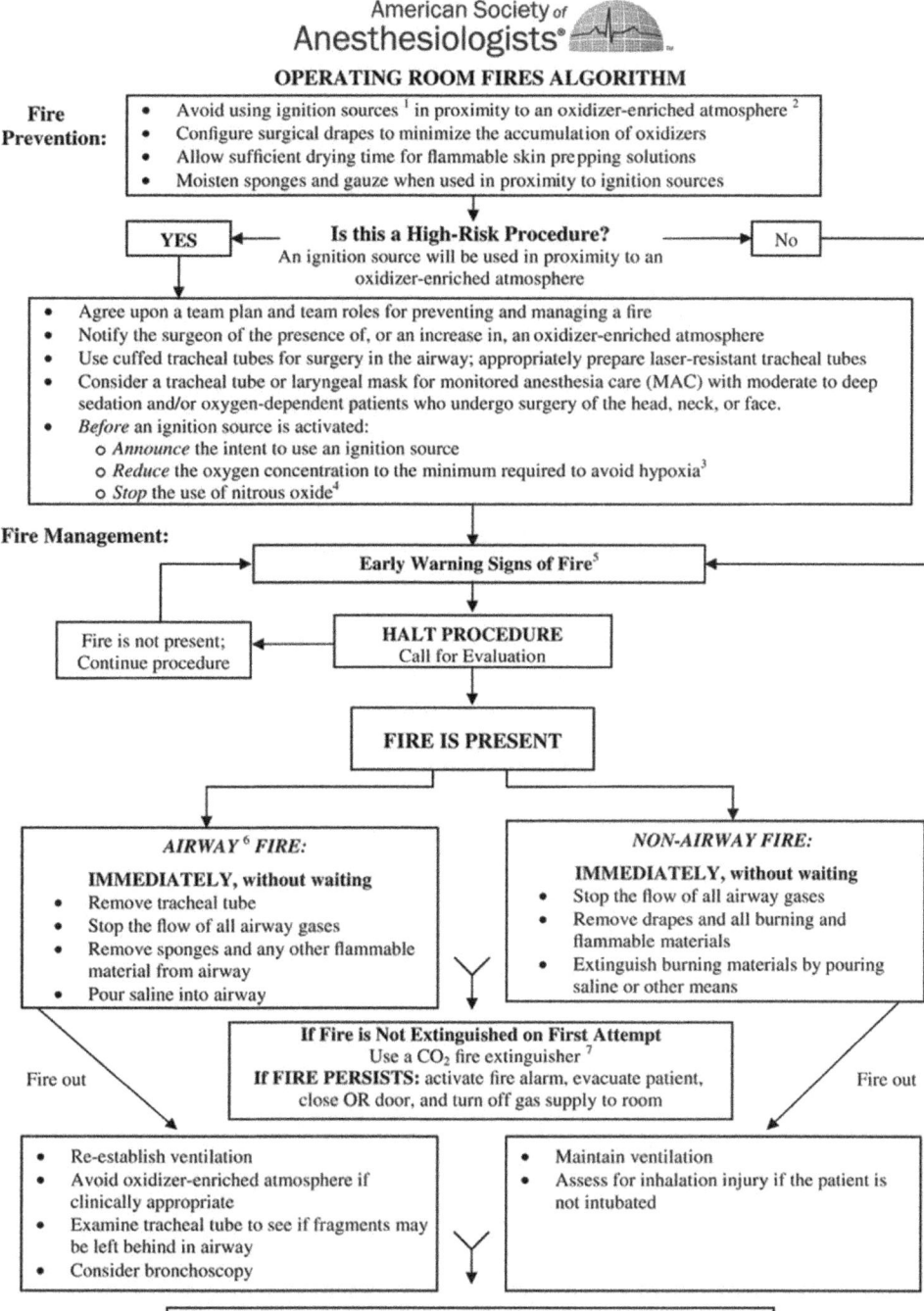

American Society of Anesthesiologists®

OPERATING ROOM FIRES ALGORITHM

Fire Prevention:
- Avoid using ignition sources [1] in proximity to an oxidizer-enriched atmosphere [2]
- Configure surgical drapes to minimize the accumulation of oxidizers
- Allow sufficient drying time for flammable skin prepping solutions
- Moisten sponges and gauze when used in proximity to ignition sources

Is this a High-Risk Procedure?
An ignition source will be used in proximity to an oxidizer-enriched atmosphere

YES / No

- Agree upon a team plan and team roles for preventing and managing a fire
- Notify the surgeon of the presence of, or an increase in, an oxidizer-enriched atmosphere
- Use cuffed tracheal tubes for surgery in the airway; appropriately prepare laser-resistant tracheal tubes
- Consider a tracheal tube or laryngeal mask for monitored anesthesia care (MAC) with moderate to deep sedation and/or oxygen-dependent patients who undergo surgery of the head, neck, or face.
- *Before* an ignition source is activated:
  o *Announce* the intent to use an ignition source
  o *Reduce* the oxygen concentration to the minimum required to avoid hypoxia[3]
  o *Stop* the use of nitrous oxide[4]

Fire Management:

Early Warning Signs of Fire[5]

Fire is not present; Continue procedure

HALT PROCEDURE
Call for Evaluation

FIRE IS PRESENT

AIRWAY[6] FIRE:

IMMEDIATELY, without waiting
- Remove tracheal tube
- Stop the flow of all airway gases
- Remove sponges and any other flammable material from airway
- Pour saline into airway

NON-AIRWAY FIRE:

IMMEDIATELY, without waiting
- Stop the flow of all airway gases
- Remove drapes and all burning and flammable materials
- Extinguish burning materials by pouring saline or other means

If Fire is Not Extinguished on First Attempt
Use a CO_2 fire extinguisher [7]
If FIRE PERSISTS: activate fire alarm, evacuate patient, close OR door, and turn off gas supply to room

Fire out / Fire out

- Re-establish ventilation
- Avoid oxidizer-enriched atmosphere if clinically appropriate
- Examine tracheal tube to see if fragments may be left behind in airway
- Consider bronchoscopy

- Maintain ventilation
- Assess for inhalation injury if the patient is not intubated

Assess patient status and devise plan for management

[1] Ignition sources include but are not limited to electrosurgery or electrocautery units and lasers.

[2] An oxidizer-enriched atmosphere occurs when there is any increase in oxygen concentration above room air level, and/or the presence of any concentration of nitrous oxide.

[3] After minimizing delivered oxygen, wait a period of time (e.g., 1–3 min) before using an ignition source. For oxygen-dependent patients, *reduce* supplemental oxygen delivery to the minimum required to avoid hypoxia. Monitor oxygenation with pulse oximetry, and if feasible, inspired, exhaled, and/or delivered oxygen concentration.

[4] After stopping the delivery of nitrous oxide, wait a period of time (e.g., 1–3 min) before using an ignition source.

[5] Unexpected flash, flame, smoke or heat, unusual sounds (e.g., a "pop," snap, or "foomp") or odors, unexpected movement of drapes, discoloration of drapes or breathing circuit, unexpected patient movement or complaint.

[6] In this algorithm, airway fire refers to a fire in the airway or breathing circuit.

[7] A CO_2 fire extinguisher may be used on the patient if necessary.

Figure 6.1 Operating room fires algorithm. Courtesy of Practice Advisory for the Prevention and Management of Operating Room Fires.[3]

Airway Fire Safety

High-Risk Procedures

- Tonsillectomy
- Tracheostomy
- Laser laryngeal surgery (see below)

Prevention

- Reduction of oxidizer-rich environment as possible
- Eliminate ignition sources as possible (use scalpel or coblation)
- Manage fuel sources
- Use cuffed endotracheal tubes

Reduction of FiO$_2$

- Reduce FiO$_2$ < 30% during high-risk cases.[5]
- Recognize the significance of expired gas concentration.
- It will take several minutes of air flow to reduce ETO$_2$ < 30% after pre-oxygenation.[6]
- Questionable evidence on efficacy of suction to reduce oxidizer concentration[5]

Laser Procedure Safety

- Utilize laser resistant endotracheal tubes.
- Utilize a double cuff system in order to prevent O$_2$ leak in case of single cuff rupture.
- Fill endotracheal tube (ETT) cuffs with saline or methylene blue: extinguishes and alerts surgeon.
- Open communication: no use of laser until exhaled O$_2$ < 30%

- Laser airway surgery risk has been lowered considerably secondary to awareness, vigilance and communication by OR personnel.

Airway Fire Management

- Eliminate oxygen source by disconnecting circuit and turning off oxygen flow.
- Remove ETT while attached to oxygen source may result in further fire/injury
- ETT should be removed following disconnection.
- Remove ignition source (electrocautery).
- Flood field and oropharynx with saline and suction debris/chemical irritants.
- Re-secure airway as rapidly as possible.
- Endotracheal intubation may prove difficult given the thermal injury; follow ASA difficult airway algorithm.
- Consider emergent tracheostomy early on when intubation proves difficult.[7]
- The goal is to extinguish fire, maintain oxygenation/ventilation, and manage hemodynamics (Figure 6.1).

Smoke Inhalation Injury Management

- High morbidity and mortality
- Airway edema, mucosal necrosis, inflammation[8]
- Investigate degree of injury with laryngoscopy, bronchoscopy, and endoscopy.
- Lavage and debris removal may be warranted.
- Inhaled bronchodilation to relieve bronchospasm
- Humidified air may relieve excessive airway drying from thermal injury.
- Prophylactic antibiotics and steroids have not been shown to improve outcomes.[9]

References

1. Miller RD, editor. *Miller's Anesthesia*, 8th ed. Churchill Livingstone/Elsevier, 2016.

2. White PF, Eng MA. Intravenous anesthetics. In Barash PG, Cullen BF, Stoelting RK, et al., editors. *Clinical Anesthesia*, 6th ed. Lippincott Williams & Wilkins, 2009; chapter 18, pp 185–190.

3. Barnes AM, Frantz RA. Do oxygen-enriched atmospheres exist beneath surgical drapes and contribute to fire hazard potential in the operating room? *AANA J* 2000;68:153–161.

4. Mehta SP, Bhananker SM, Posner KL. Domino KB. Operating room fires: a closed claims analysis. *Anesthesiology* 2013;118:1133–1139.

5. Apfelbaum JL, Caplan RA, Barker SJ, et al. Practice advisory for the prevention and management of operating room fires: an updated report by the American Society for Anesthesiologists Task Force on Operating Room Fires. *Anesthesiology* 2013;118:271–290.

6. Eichhorn JH, Eisenkraft JB. Expired oxygen as the unappreciated issue in preventing airway fires: getting to "never." *Anesth Analg* 2013; 117:1042–1044.

7. Demaria S, Schwartz AD, Narine V, Yang S, Levine AI. Management of intraoperative airway fire. *Simul Healthc* 2011;6:360–363.

8. Rogers ML, Nickalls RW, Brackenbury ET, et al. Airway fire during tracheostomy: prevention strategies for surgeons and anaesthetists. *Ann R Coll Surg Engl* 2001;83: 376–380.

9. Cha SI, Kim CH, Lee JH, et al. Isolated smoke inhalation inj uries: acute respiratory dysfunction, clinical outcomes, and short-term evolution of pulmonary functions with the effects of steroids. *Burns* 2007;33:200–208.

Basic Mathematics and Statistics

Hung-Mo Lin, Hae-Young Kim, and John Michael Williamson

Logarithm

Logarithm is the inverse operation to exponentiation. It is the power to which the base must be raised to produce a given number. For example, as $81 = 3^4$, then $\log_3(81) = 4$. The *logarithm* to base 10 is called the *common* logarithm and the logarithm to base e (≈ 2.72) is called the *natural* logarithm (ln).

Graph of Simple Equation

The simplest equation for a biological model is of the linear form $y = a + bx$, where the y and x can be described by a linear relationship with slope b and intercept a. The slope represents the amount of change in y for every unit increase in x and is typically the primary interest of analysis (Figure 7.1).

Analysis of Biological Curves

Biological curves are often nonlinear. In medical research, three types of biological curves are often encountered.

Analysis of Dose Response Curve: A method used to depict the relationship between the dose of a drug administered and its pharmacological response. The abbreviation for the median effective dose is *ED50*, the dose required to produce efficacy in half of the population (Figure 7.2).

Analysis of Pharmacokinetic Modeling: A mathematical modeling technique for predicting the absorption, distribution, metabolism and excretion of synthetic or natural chemical substances in humans and other animal species.

Analysis of Growth Curves: The modern use of the term *growth curve model* typically refers to statistical methods that allow for the estimation of inter-individual variability in intra-individual patterns of change over time.[1] Often the within-person patterns of change are referred to as *growth curves*, or *trajectories*.

Analysis of Survival Curves: A survival curve is a plot of probability that an individual survives longer than time t, or has not experienced the event of interest. In survival analysis, not all individuals continue in the study until the event of interest occurs (they are called *censored*). The Kaplan–Meier survival curve is the most familiar method in medical discipline for depicting the survival probability when some individuals are subject to being censored (Figure 7.3).[2]

Sample and Population

Population: A complete set of elements (persons or objects) that possess some common characteristic defined by the sampling criteria established by the researcher.

Sample: The selected elements (people or objects) chosen for participation in a study and are referred to as subjects or participants.

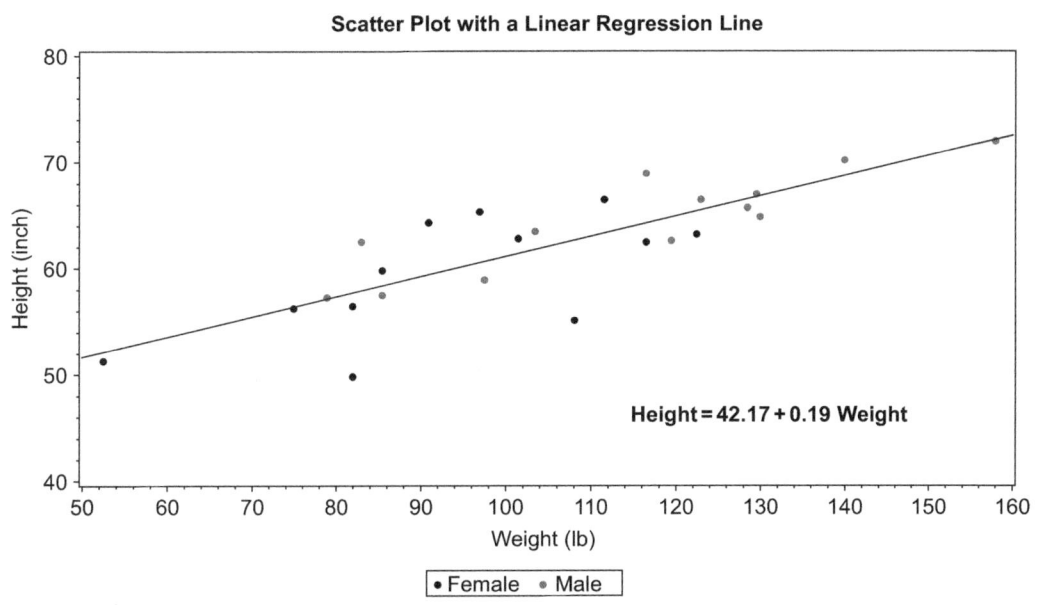

Scatter Plot with a Linear Regression Line

Height = 42.17 + 0.19 Weight

Height (inch) vs. Weight (lb)

• Female • Male

Figure 7.1 Example of a linear equation used to model the relationship between height (in.) and weight (lb) in children aged 11–17. A black and white version of this figure will appear in some formats. For the color version, please refer to the plate section.

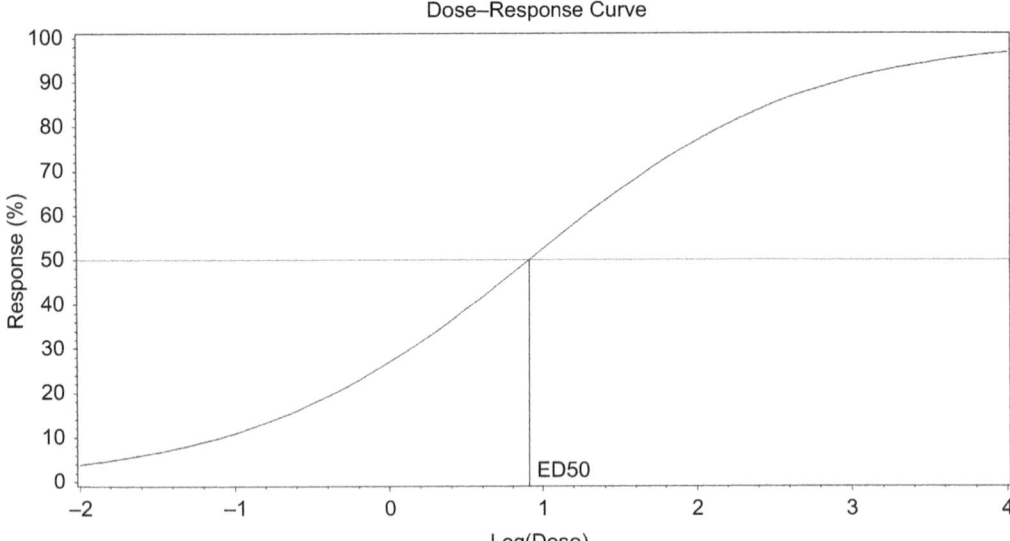

Figure 7.2 Example of a dose response curve. The *y*-axis is the percentage of response and the *x*-axis the amount of dose in logarithmic scale. ED50 is the medium effective dose.

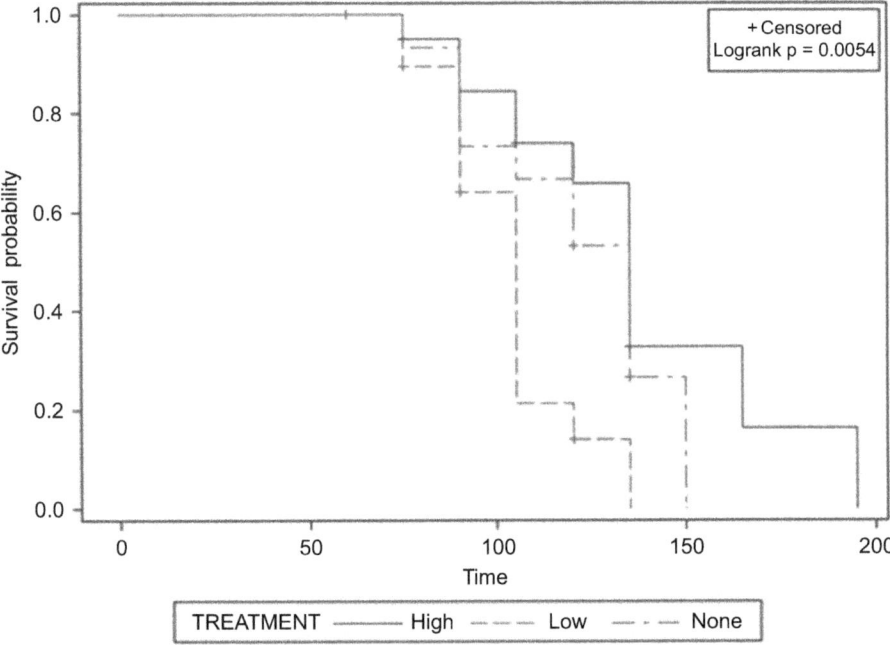

Figure 7.3 Example for a Kaplan–Meier survival curve for three treatment arms with none, low, and high dose. Censoring is indicated by the + symbol.

Probability

The proportion of times an event is expected to occur in the long run. Probabilities are numbers between 0 and 1 with 0 corresponding to "never" and 1 corresponding to "always." With probabilistic events, individual occurrences are uncertain, but occurrences over the long term are predictable.

Mean, Median, and Mode

Mean: The arithmetic average. This is the most common measure of central location. To calculate the mean, add up all the values in the data set and divide by the number of

Observations: $\overline{x} = \frac{x_1 + x_2 + \cdots + x_n}{n} = \frac{\sum\limits_{i=1}^{n} x_i}{n}$

- *n* represents the sample size.
- x_i denotes the value of the *i*th observation in the data set.

Median: The middle value of a distribution and the central value in the order array of the data. To find the median, arrange all the numbers from smallest to greatest.

- If there are an odd number of observations, the middle one is picked. For example, consider the set of numbers: 1, 2, 3, 6, 8, 9, and 10. The median is the fourth number, which is 6.
- If there is an even number of observations, then the median is usually defined to be the mean of the two

middle values. For example, in the data set: 1, 2, 3, 4, 5, 6, 8, and 9. The median is the mean of the middle two numbers: this is $(4 + 5) \div 2$, which is 4.5.

Mode: It is the most frequently occurring value in the data set. For example, the following data set[3] has a mode of 7: 4, 7, 7, 7, 8, 8, 9.

Standard Deviation and Error

Standard Deviation (SD): It is the most common measure of spread. This statistic is based on the average squared distance of values around the data sets mean. It is calculated as follows:

- Determine the deviation of each data point. A deviation is the data point minus its mean: $x_i - \overline{x}$.
- Sum the squared deviations. This is the sum of squares (SS): $SS = (x_1 - \overline{x})^2 + (x_2 - \overline{x})^2 + \cdots + (x_n - \overline{x})^2$
- Divide the sum of squares by n minus 1. This is the variance:

$$s^2 = \frac{SS}{n-1}$$

- Take the square root of the variance. This is the standard deviation:

$$s = \sqrt{s^2} = \sqrt{\frac{SS}{n-1}}$$

- The percentage of data in one standard deviation above and below the mean is 68% in a bell curve. It is 95% for two standard deviations above and below, and 99% for three standard deviations above and below (Figure 7.4).

Standard Error (SE): The standard deviation of the sampling distribution of the sample mean, $\overline{x}$, is often referred to as the standard error of the mean (SEM). SEM is the standard deviation of the sample mean's estimate of a population mean. SEM is usually estimated by the sample estimate of the population standard deviation (sample standard deviation) divided by the square root of the sample size (assuming statistical independence of the values in the sample):

$$SE_{\overline{x}} = \frac{s}{\sqrt{n}}$$

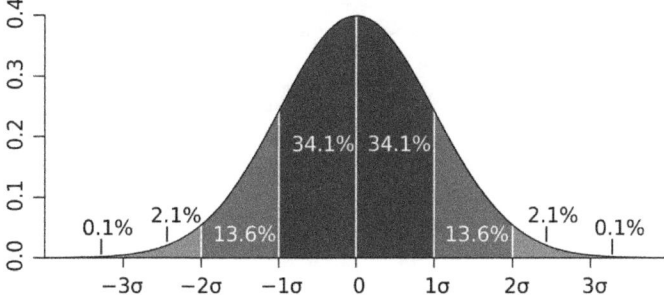

Figure 7.4 Bell curve.

- s is the sample standard deviation
- n is the size (number of observations) of the sample

Types of Data

- Categorical: Values that can be sorted into groups or categories, cannot be measured
- Nominal: Values that can be *sorted but cannot be placed in an order* (i.e. gender, eye color)
- Ordinal: Values that can be *counted and placed in order* (i.e. residency training year, house number)
- Binary: One of two values (i.e., yes or no)
- Numerical: Values that can be *measured* and placed in *order*
- Discrete: Values that are a finite whole number (i.e., number of calls a month)
- Continuous: Values that are a number on a spectrum or continuum (i.e. temperature)

t-test

A *t*-test is a statistical examination of one or two population means. The *t*-test is commonly used when the variances of normally distributed variables are unknown. This test is used with *numerical data*.

- A one-sample *t*-test examines whether one population mean is equal to a specified value. For one sample *t*-test:
    - The null hypothesis is H_0: $\mu = \mu_0$, where μ_0 represent the mean under the null hypothesis.
    - The alternative hypothesis is either $H_A : \mu > \mu_0$ (one sided to the right), $H_A : \mu < \mu_0$ (one sided to the left), or $H_A : \mu \neq \mu_0$ (two sided).
    - The one-sample *t*-test statistic is $T = \frac{(\overline{x} - \mu_0)}{s/\sqrt{n}}$, where s is the standard deviation.
- With a paired sample, each data value in one sample is matched to a unique one in the second sample (e.g., observations made on the left and right eyes of the same person).
- A two-sample *t*-test examines whether two population means are different.

Chi-Square

The chi-square test is used to test the association between the row (R) and column (C) variables that comprise an R by C contingency table. This test is use with *categorical data*.

- The null hypothesis is H_0: no association between the row and column variables in the source population.
- The alternative hypothesis is H_A: association.

Regression Analysis/Correlation

Regression analysis and correlations are methods used to assess the relationship between explanatory variables (X) and the continuous response variable (Y).[3]

Regression Analysis: Linear regression finds the best fitting line for the data using a least squares method. The relationship is described by the linear regression equation $\hat{y} = a + bx$.

Correlation: The Pearson correlation coefficient (r) is used to assess the linear dependence between two variables X and Y (Figure 7.5).

Odds Ratio

The odds ratio (OR) is a parameter that measures the relationship between a categorical explanatory variable and a binary response variable. The OR takes on non-negative values. See Table 7.1 for the example of a 2 by 2 table. Group 1 can be persons exposed to a certain agent and group 2 can be the nonexposed persons.

- The odds of an event is the proportion of disease divided by the proportion of no disease.
- The point estimator for the odds ratio ($\widehat{OR}$.) is
  $\frac{Odds\ in\ Group\ 1}{Odds\ in\ Group\ 2} = \frac{a_1/b_1}{a_2/b_2} = \frac{a_1 b_2}{b_1 a_2}$.
- $OR = 1$ indicates that the exposure is not related to disease. $OR > 1$ indicates that the exposure is positively related to disease $OR < 1$ indicates that the exposure is negatively related to disease.

Risk Ratio

A risk ratio (RR) is a parameter that measures the relationship between a categorical explanatory variable and a binary response variable. The RR takes on nonnegative values. See Table 7.1 for an example of a 2 by 2 table.[3]

- The point estimator for the risk ratio ($\widehat{RR}$) is $\frac{\hat{p}_1}{\hat{p}_2}$, where $\hat{p}_1$(a risk of Group 1) $= \frac{a_1}{n_1}$ and $\hat{p}_2$(a risk of Group 2) $= \frac{a_2}{n_2}$ are the point estimators of population proportions, p_1 and p_2.
- $RR = 1$ indicates that the risk in exposed is equal to the risk in non-exposed. $RR > 1$ indicates that the risk in exposed is greater than the risk in non-exposed. $RR < 1$ indicates that the risk in exposed is less than the risk in non-exposed.

Analysis of Variance

Analysis of variance (ANOVA) tests the *equality of group means*, not variances. ANOVA can be used for multiple variables with *numerical data*.

Table 7.1 Example of a 2 by 2 table for odds ratio and risk ratio

	Disease	No disease	Total
Group 1 (Exposed)	a_1	b_1	n_1
Group 2 (Nonexposed)	a_2	b_2	n_2

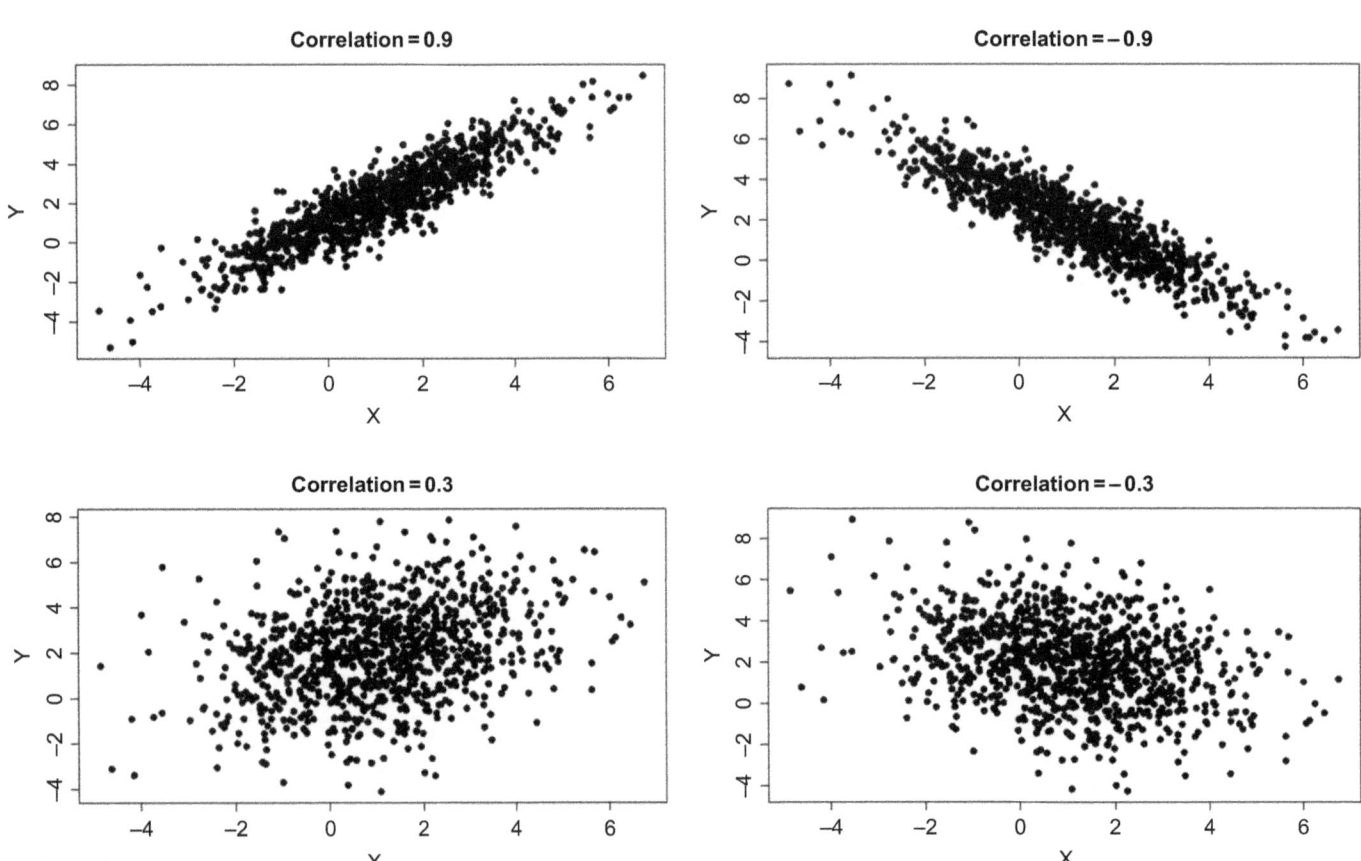

Figure 7.5 Example of the different correlations to assess the relationship between X and Y.

Power Analysis

The power of a statistical test is its ability to detect an effect if it actually exists. More formally, it is the probability that the test correctly rejects the null hypothesis (H_0) when the alternative hypothesis (H_1) is true. Power calculations are conducted to determine the minimum sample size required so that one can be reasonably confident of detecting an effect of a given size. Power analysis can also be used to calculate the minimum effect size that is likely to be detected in a study using a specified sample size. Power analysis is usually conducted before the research study and is used for calculating the sample size required to achieve sufficient power (usually 80% or 90%).

> Power = 1 – beta, where beta is the type II error (i.e., false negative). Increasing the beta value will decrease the power of the study.

Ways to increase power: Increase the alpha value (i.e., false positive or type I error) to lower the chance of false negatives, decrease population variability, increase sample size (most feasible)

Meta-Analysis

Meta-analysis attempts to estimate a common parameter across conceptually similar studies by deriving a pooled estimate that takes into account the error within each study. There are different methods for deriving the weighted average of parameter estimates from the results of the individual studies, although almost always the sample sizes of the smaller studies are taken into account. Meta-analysis has greater statistical power and a more robust point estimate of the parameter than is possible from a single study due to the larger sample size. However, meta-analysis does not inherently correct for bias or flawed study design in the original smaller studies.

Confidence Intervals

A confidence interval (CI) is a range of values that seeks to capture the parameter of interest. For example if we are estimating the population mean μ with the sample average $\bar{x}$, then a CI for μ will be $\bar{x} \pm$ a margin of error. For the usual 95% confidence interval, the margin of error is 1.96 times the standard error of the mean. A 95% confidence level means that 95% of the intervals obtained from such samples will contain the true parameter, although any particular interval will either contain the true parameter or not. A larger sample size will typically lead to a smaller confidence interval, and thus a better estimate of the population parameter.

Bland–Altman Plot

A Bland–Altman plot is a method of data plotting used in analyzing the agreement between two different *continuous variables*, often different assays or instruments or measurement techniques. The plot lets the viewer note any systematic difference between the paired values (i.e., fixed bias) or possible outliers. The differences between the paired measurements are plotted against the averages of the paired measurements. A horizontal line is drawn at the mean difference allowing the viewer to ascertain any systematic difference between the measurements. Horizontal lines are also drawn at the limits of agreement, the mean difference plus and minus 1.96 times the standard deviation of the differences, allowing the viewer to detect potential outliers.

Types of Error

Type I Error (Alpha Error): Incorrectly rejecting the null hypothesis – false positive
- Alpha value historically has been used as .05, meaning that there is a 5% chance that the incorrect conclusion is reached. As the alpha value is decreased, there is a less chance of a Type I error but a higher chance of a Type II error resulting in a false negative.

Type II Error (Beta Error): incorrectly accepting the null hypothesis – false negative
- Type II error increases with: variability within the population
- Type II error decreases with: increased difference between control and study sample increasing the number of data points

Evaluation of Diagnostic Tests

True positive: TP
True negative: TN
False positive: FP
False negative: FN

Sensitivity: ability of a test to detect a disease when it is present
- Sensitivity = TP/(TP + FN) = 1 – false negative rate
  Specificity: ability of a test to indicate nondisease when it is not present
- Specificity = TN/(TN + FP) = 1 – false positive rate
  Positive predictive value (PPV): probability that a person with a positive test result actually has the disease
- PPV = TP/(TP + FP)
  Negative Predictive Value (NPV): probability that a person with a negative test actually does not have the disease
- NPV = TN/(FN + TN)

References

1. Curran PJ, Obeidat K, Losardo D. Twelve frequently asked questions about growth curve modeling. *J Cogn Dev* 2010;**11**(2):121–136. doi:10.1080/15248371003699969

2. Rich JT, Neely JG, Paniello RC, et al. A practical guide to understanding Kaplan–Meier curves. *Otolaryngol Head Neck Surg* 2010;**143**(3):331–336. doi:10.1016/j.otohns.2010.05.007.

3. Burt Gerstman B. *Basic Biostatistics: Statistics for Public Health Practice*, 2nd ed. Jones and Bartlett Learning, 2014.

General Pharmacology

David Convissar, Victoria Nguyen, Shaji Faisal, and Ben Toure

One of the core principles essential to an anesthesiologist's fund of knowledge is that of general pharmacology. The understanding of pharmacokinetics and pharmacodynamics is fundamental to providing anesthesia in a safe and effective manner. This chapter aims to provide a foundation of key pharmacological principles necessary for the clinical application of anesthesia.

Pharmacokinetics vs. Pharmacodynamics

- Pharmacokinetics: The relationship between drug administration and drug concentration at various sites of action throughout the body (the effect the body has on the drug)
  - Involves concepts such as absorption, distribution, metabolism, and excretion.
- Pharmacodynamics: The relationship between drug concentration and clinical effect (the effect the drug has on the body)

Potency

- The relationship between amount of *drug required to produce desired clinical effect*
  - That is, if drug A can produce the same clinical effect as drug B at a lower dose, then drug A has greater potency relative to drug B.
  - The half maximal effective concentration (EC_{50}) is the concentration of drug needed to obtain 50% of the intended effect
  - Effective dose$_{50}$ (ED_{50}) is the dose required to produce a desired clinical effect in 50% of individuals
  - Note: ED_{95} is the average dose required to achieve 95% reduction in maximal twitch response from baseline in 50% of the population. In simpler terms, ED_{95} is the ED_{50} for the desired effect of 95% reduction in train of four twitch height.

Efficacy

- A measure of *the maximum clinical effect* of the drug upon binding to the receptor site irrespective of required drug dosage (Figure 8.1)

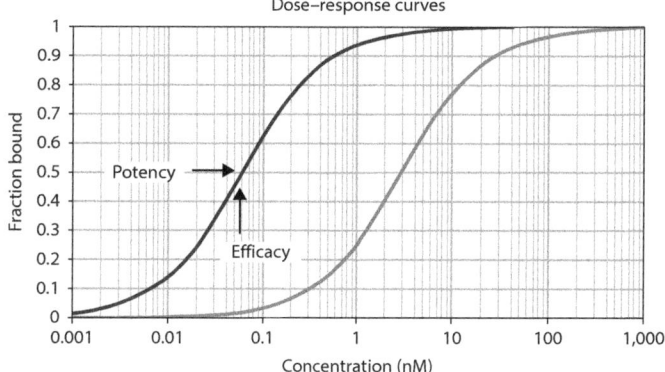

Figure 8.1 Dose–response curve.

Absorption

- Process by which a drug moves from the site of administration to the systemic circulation
  - That is, drugs administered orally must first be absorbed via the gastrointestinal tract before traveling to the liver and finally to systemic circulation (first-pass metabolism)
  - That is, intravenous (IV) drugs completely bypass the process of absorption as they immediately enter systemic circulation.

Volume of Distribution

- Volume of distribution (Vd) is the "container size" accounting for the relationship between a given dose of drug and its measured concentration once sufficient time has passed for thorough mixing to occur.
  Vd = Amount (or Dose)/Concentration
- Vd within the human body is not a fixed volume. When a drug is administered intravenously, some drug stays in the intravascular space, but most of the drug redistributes to peripheral tissues. The volume of peripheral tissues (i.e., adipose tissue, muscle) can add significantly to the overall Vd depending on lipid solubility of the drug.
  - The measured blood concentration of a lipophilic drug (i.e., propofol or thiopental) may be substantially lower than the expected value given the administered IV dose due to peripheral redistribution.

Clearance

- The process of removal of drug from a compartment, either the movement from one compartment to another, or out of the body completely
- Hepatic drug clearance is defined as the plasma volume perfusing the liver that is cleared of the drug per unit time. Three major factors influence hepatic drug clearance:
  - Liver blood flow (Q), which reflects drug delivery to the liver
  - Fraction of drug (f) that exists in the free unbound state vs. protein bound state (not capable of interacting with hepatic enzymes)
  - Hepatic intrinsic enzymatic activity defined as "intrinsic clearance" (Cl_{int}). Intrinsic clearance is the ability of the liver to remove drug in the absence of limitations in hepatic blood flow and protein binding.
- The ratio of the hepatic clearance of a drug to the hepatic blood flow is called the extraction ratio. Extraction ratio can be generally classified as high (> 0.7), intermediate (0.3–0.7) or low (< 0.3) according to the fraction of drug removed during one pass through the liver.
  - High extraction ratio (> 0.7): Hepatic clearance is directly proportional to hepatic blood flow, and clearance is independent of protein binding. These drugs (i.e., propofol, morphine, lidocaine) are rapidly cleared from the plasma after a single liver pass.
  - Intermediate extraction ratio (0.3–0.7): Hepatic clearance is dependent on hepatic blood flow, intrinsic hepatic metabolic capacity and the free drug fraction (i.e., midazolam).
  - Low extraction ratio (< 0.3): Hepatic clearance is flow independent, and more significantly influenced by the intrinsic hepatic enzymatic capacity and the free drug fraction. An increase in the fraction of unbound drug will increase clearance (i.e., alfentanil).
  - If nearly 100% of the drug is extracted by the liver, any decrease in hepatic blood flow due to the vasodilatory effects of anesthetic agents, sepsis, hypovolemia, congestive heart failure, or perioperative bleeding can reduce hepatic drug clearance. However, typically the hepatic metabolic capacity for a drug far exceeds what is required to achieve effective clearance. Thus, moderate changes in hepatic blood flow will have minimal clinical impact.

Context-Sensitive Half-Time

- Time for drug plasma concentration to decline by one-half after discontinuation of a drug infusion.

- Continuous infusions of a variety of agents such as propofol, alfentanil, remifentanil, and more are used commonly in the clinical setting, making context-sensitive half-time an important concept to understand.
- Propofol has a context-sensitive half-time that varies between 3 minutes for a very short infusion to about 18 minutes after a 12-hour infusion. This variation in context-sensitive half-time occurs because excretion is rapid compared with redistribution.
  - Fentanyl, a normally rapid-acting drug with a short half-life becomes a long-acting drug after prolonged infusions because it is very lipophilic and has a large peripheral volume of distribution within fat stores with rapid redistribution. Remifentanil has a relatively constant and a short context-sensitive half-time, as it has a rapid clearance due to plasma ester hydrolysis.

Kinetics

- First-order kinetics: The amount of drug removed is a constant fraction per unit time.
  - Increased concentration of the drug will increase the rate of elimination.
- Zero-order kinetics: A constant amount of drug is eliminated per unit time.
  - Elimination depends on enzymes and membrane transporters, which can become saturated. Once these systems are saturated, elimination reaches a maximum level, and a constant amount of drug is eliminated per unit time as opposed to a constant fraction. It may be encountered at high concentrations with aspirin, ethanol, phenytoin, or thiopental.

Hepatic Metabolism

- Oxidation, reduction, hydrolysis, or conjugation of drugs mostly via the cytochrome P450 system
  - These enzymes are induced by certain drugs (i.e., St. John's wort, rifampin, phenytoin).
  - Other drugs (i.e., erythromycin, cimetidine, amiodarone) or hepatic disease can inhibit these enzymes.
  - The effect of hepatic conjugation is to transform water-insoluble agents into water-soluble agents for subsequent renal excretion.
- All inhalational agents are metabolized to some degree by the liver.
  - Isoflurane is the most commonly used inhalational agent for maintenance of anesthesia in patients with liver disease due to its minimal degree of hepatic metabolism as compared with sevoflurane and desflurane.

Liver Disease

- Has a significant impact on pharmacokinetics by alterations in protein binding (i.e., decreased synthesis of albumin can result in a reduction in protein bound drug), altered volume of distribution due to ascites and volume overload, and reduced hepatocellular metabolism of anesthetic agents.
- The metabolism of drugs with low hepatic extraction ratios, such as benzodiazepines, is influenced mainly by protein binding and hepatocellular enzyme function. In patients with liver disease, reduced plasma albumin levels result in greater free fractions of drug.
  - Highly protein bound agents (i.e., benzodiazepines) will have an increased Vd, which in conjunction with reduced hepatic metabolism will increase drug half-life.
  - The Vd of water-soluble drugs is often higher in advanced liver disease due to the presence of ascites and excess fluid.
- Remifentanil is an ultra-short-acting opioid metabolized by plasma and tissue esterases; its clearance and recovery are independent of liver function.
- Propofol and etomidate have high hepatic extraction ratios. However, clearance of these agents is not significantly prolonged in the setting of cirrhosis. This is due to extrahepatic sites of metabolism.
- Neuromuscular blocking agents, such as vecuronium and rocuronium, are metabolized in the liver and elimination half-lives are prolonged in the setting of liver disease.
- Neuromuscular blocking agents that undergo organ-independent elimination, such as atracurium and cisatracurium, have clinical durations of action unaffected by liver dysfunction. However, renal excretion accounts for approximately 15% of cisatracurium elimination, and renal dysfunction can contribute to the accumulation of the neurotoxic metabolite laudanosine, especially when utilizing atracurium.

Renal Disease

- Most anesthetic drugs (i.e., opioids, barbiturates, ketamine, and local anesthetics) are lipid soluble and are non-ionized. Their duration of action is predominantly dependent on renal excretion rather than hepatic metabolism and/or biotransformation and peripheral redistribution.
- By way of hepatic metabolism, many drugs are converted to inactive forms and excreted in urine as water-soluble molecules.

- There are several drugs (i.e., muscle relaxants, cholinesterase inhibitors, antibiotics) that are lipid insoluble or are highly ionized, and their duration of action will likely be prolonged in the setting of renal failure.

Extrahepatic Metabolism

- Succinylcholine, mivacurium, esmolol, and remifentanil are metabolized via various plasma enzymes.
- Succinylcholine is a depolarizing neuromuscular blocking agent, metabolized by plasma pseudocholinesterase. Pseudocholinesterase is synthesized by the liver. Severe hepatic disease is associated with decreased pseudocholinesterase levels and prolonged neuromuscular blockade due to succinylcholine.
- Cisatracurium and atracurium exhibit Hofmann elimination, a type of chemical reaction in the blood, which relies on temperature and pH and is a base-catalyzed nonenzymatic reaction.

Obesity

- Obesity increases the Vd of lipophilic drugs.
- A larger initial loading dose of lipophilic drug is required in obesity. Decreased maintenance doses of lipophilic drugs are appropriate given the high degree of redistribution of lipophilic drugs from the peripheral compartment to the central plasma compartment over time.
- Substances with high lipophilicity, such as barbiturates and benzodiazepines, have high Vd in obese patients due to a larger peripheral volume of distribution (adipose tissue). Certain lipophilic agents, such as remifentanil, do not demonstrate higher Vd in obese patients due to the rapid enzymatic intravascular metabolism. As such, these drugs should be dosed by ideal body weight and not by total body weight in obese patients. Substances with lower lipophilicity have minimal change in Vd with obesity.
  - Drugs generally dosed on total body weight: succinylcholine, fentanyl, remifentanil
  - Drugs generally dosed on ideal body weight: rocuronium, vecuronium, cisatracurium
  - Drugs generally dosed on lean body weight: propofol
- Desflurane is the inhaled agent of choice in obese patients due to its lower degree of lipid solubility as compared to sevoflurane and isoflurane, providing a more rapid recovery and emergence profile.

Further Reading

Atkinson AJ, Kushner W. Clinical pharmacokinetics. *Annu Rev Pharmacol Toxicol* 1979;**19**(1):105–127.

Bairamian M. Anesthetic considerations for bariatric surgery. *Survey Anesthesiol* 2003;**47**(5):298–299.

Beem H, Manger F, Boxtel C, Bentem N. Etomidate anaesthesia in patients with cirrhosis of the liver: pharmacokinetic data. *Anaesthesia* 1983;**38**(S1):61–62.

Buxton ILO. The dynamics of drug absorption, distribution, metabolism, and elimination. In Goodman L, Brunton L, Gilman A, Chabner B, Knollmann B. *Goodman & Gilman's The Pharmacological Basis of Therapeutics.* McGraw-Hill Medical, 2011; chapter 2, pp 17–41.

Carpenter R, Eger E, Johnson B, Unadkat J, Sheiner L. The extent of metabolism of inhaled anesthetics in humans. *Anesthesiology* 1986;**65**(2):201–205.

Craig RG, Hunter JM. Neuromuscular blocking drugs and their antagonists in patients with organ disease. *Anaesthesia* 2009;**64**:55–65.

Gholson C, Provenza JM, Bacon BR. Hepatologic considerations in patients with parenchymal liver disease undergoing surgery. *Am J Gastroenterol* 1990;**85**:487–496.

Hill S. Pharmacokinetics of drug infusions. *Continuing Educ Anaesthes Crit Care Pain* 2004;**4**(3):76–80.

Ingrande J, Lemmens HJM. Anesthetic pharmacology and the morbidly obese patient. *Curr Anesthesiol Rep* 2012;**3**(1):10–17.

Jensen F, Viby-Mogensen J. Plasma cholinesterase and abnormal reaction to succinylcholine: twenty years' experience with the Danish Cholinesterase Research Unit. *Acta Anaesthesiol Scand* 1995;**39**(2):150–156.

Prescott L. Mechanisms of renal excretion of drugs (with special reference to drugs used by anaesthetists). *BJA* 1972;**44**(3):246–251.

Roberts Freshwater-Turner D. Pharmacokinetics and anaesthesia. *Continuing Educ Anaesthes Crit Care Pain* 2007;**7**(1):25–29.

Servin F, Cockshott ID, Farinotti R, et al. Pharmacokinetics of propofol infusions in patients with cirrhosis. *Br J Anaesth* 1990;**65**(2):177–83.

Tegeder I, Lötsch J, Geisslinger G. Pharmacokinetics of opioids in liver disease. *Clin Pharmacokinet* 1999;**37**:17–40.

Verbeeck R. Pharmacokinetics and dosage adjustment in patients with hepatic dysfunction. *Eur J Clin Pharmacol* 2008;**64**(12):1147–1161.

Wastila W, Maehr R, Turner G, et al. Comparative pharmacology of cisatracurium (51W89), atracurium, and five isomers in cats. *Anesthesiology* 1996;**85**(1):169–177.

Anesthetics: Gases and Vapors

Evida Mars-Holt, Jennifer Mardini, and Christopher R. Cowart

General Pharmacokinetics of Anesthetic Gases and Vapors

There are several important factors that directly affect induction and uptake of inhalational anesthetic agents. Some of these factors (Table 9.1) are modifiable, while others are not. Manipulation of these variables allows for the ability to increase or decrease the rate of induction (Table 9.2).

Physical Properties of Anesthetic Gases

Each anesthetic gas has unique physical properties resulting in different clinical effects. The minimum alveolar concentration (MAC) of each agent is listed below, along with factors affecting MAC (Table 9.3), vapor pressures (Table 9.4) and blood:gas partition coefficients (Table 9.5). (Key Point: Low MAC = High Potency)

- Nitrous oxide (N_2O): MAC 105%
  - Odorless – good for inhalation in awake patients, hence its popularity in dental offices
  - Nitrous oxide is a gas at room temp (unlike volatile agents) because the critical temp > room temp.

Table 9.1 Pharmacokinetic factors affecting inhalational induction[1]

Concept	Factors affecting each
Inspired concentration of anesthetic gas (FI)	Fresh gas flow (FGF) Volume of breathing system Circuit absorption
Alveolar concentration of anesthetic gas (FA)	Uptake Alveolar ventilation/minute ventilation Concentration/second gas effect
Uptake	Blood gas solubility Alveolar blood flow/cardiac output Alveolar–venous partial pressure gradient

Table 9.2 Controlling rate of induction

	Speeds induction	Slows induction
Gas solubility	Low solubility	High solubility
CO	Low cardiac output	High cardiac output
P–P gradient	Low P–P gradient	High P–P gradient
Minute ventilation (MV)	High MV	Low MV
Fi	High Fi	Low Fi

- Very high vapor pressure (much higher than desflurane)[2]
- Desflurane: MAC 6%
  - High saturated vapor pressure (SVP, 669 mmHg) → extremely volatile and vaporizes (boils) significantly at room temp
  - Very low solubility in blood → rapid induction and emergence (FA to FI quicker)
  - Requires special vaporizer to maintain constant output → dual gas blender that delivers a *constant concentration* of vapor output heated to 39°C

Table 9.3 Factors affecting MAC[1–3]

Increase MAC	Decrease MAC
Amphetamines (acute)	Amphetamines (chronic)
Alcohol (chronic)	Alcohol (acute)
Cocaine (acute)	Pregnancy
Hypernatremia	Hyponatremia
Hyperthermia	Hypothermia
Young age	Old age
Monoamine oxidase inhibitors (MAOIs)	IV anesthetics
	Local anesthetics
	Lithium

Table 9.4 Vapor pressures at 20°C[2]

Volatile anesthetics with similar saturated vapor pressures (SVP) = "HI SE"	
Halothane = 243 mmHg	**S**evoflurane = 157 mmHg
Isoflurane = 238 mmHg	**E**nflurane = 175 mmHg

Table 9.5 Blood:gas partition coefficients of anesthetic gases[2]

Inhaled anesthetics	Blood:gas partition coefficient at 37°C
Desflurane	0.42
N2O	0.46
Sevoflurane	0.65
Isoflurane	1.46
Halothane	2.4
Xenon	0.115

- Sevoflurane: MAC 2%
  - Non-pungent: Desirable for inhalational induction[2,3]
  - More soluble in blood than desflurane (slower onset)
  - Requires variable bypass vaporizer to deliver a constant partial pressure that does not change with barometric pressures
- Isoflurane: MAC 1.2%
  - Pungent odor
  - Requires variable bypass vaporizer (Figure 9.1)
- Halothane: MAC 0.75%
  - Halogenated alkane
  - Rare use in the United States[2]
  - Requires variable bypass vaporizer
- Xenon: MAC 71%
  - Noble gas
  - Limited availability, high cost[2]
  - Requires closed loop system for delivery[3]

Key Point: Vapor pressure is the pressure exerted by a gas against the walls of its container at constant equilibrium and temperature. If a vaporizer specific for an agent with high SVP (halothane, isoflurane) is misplaced with an agent with low SVP (sevoflurane, enflurane), the actual output concentration would be lower than what is shown by the dial.

Key Point: Less soluble anesthetics (i.e., lower blood:gas partition coefficients) have a faster rate of rise of FA/FI, making their onset faster. More soluble anesthetics have a slower rate of rise of FA/FI because more anesthetic is required to saturate the blood before equilibrium between the lungs and CNS is reached.[4]

Concentrating Effect: Uptake of gases from alveoli into blood will slow the rate of induction. This effect can be overcome by increasing inspired concentration of the gas being delivered. If a very high concentration of gas is delivered to the patient, gas taken into the blood is rapidly replaced, increasing the alveolar concentration of that gas with each breath.

Second Gas Effect: By the same mechanism discussed above, N_2O can be used to increase the concentration of other gases being delivered into the alveoli as well, although unlikely clinically significant levels.

Concentration Effect: Desflurane is less soluble than nitrous oxide. Despite this, nitrous oxide will have a faster induction because it can be used at such high concentrations, which overcomes the small difference in uptake.[2]

Mechanism of Action of Anesthetic Gases

- *Meyer–Overton Rule:* anesthetic gas potency is directly correlated to lipid solubility.[1]
  - N_2O
    - NMDA antagonist (Xenon also)
  - Volatiles
    - Alter neuronal ion channels
    - Particularly the fast synaptic neurotransmitter receptors:
      - Nicotinic acetylcholine receptors
      - $GABA_A$
      - Glutamate receptors[2]

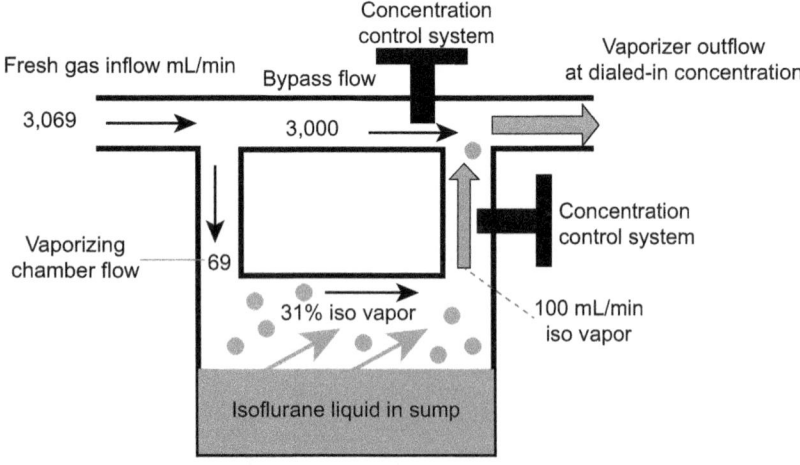

Variable bypass vaporizer delivering 1% iso at 3 L/min

Figure 9.1 Variable bypass vaporizer delivering 1% isoflurane at 3 L/min fresh gas flow at 1 ATM pressure. Note that isoflurane volume is 31% given saturated vapor pressure (SVP) at 760 mmHg.

In the sump, iso is 31% by volume at 20°C.
If sump inflow is 69 mL/min, then outflow is 31 mL iso vapor + 69 mL carrier gas.
To create 1% iso, 31 mL vapor is diluted in total volume of 3,100 mL;
therefore, bypass flow = (3,100 − 69 − 31) = 3,000 mL.
3,069 mL gas entering the vaporizer are split 3,000:69 between bypass and sump.
Splitting ratio = 3,000/69 = 44:1 between bypass and sump *inflow*.

Effects on Major Organ Systems

Physiological changes seen in each major organ system after gases are summarized in Tables 9.6 through 9.10.

Central Nervous System[2,3]

- N_2O
  - Stimulates SNS
  - Increases ICP, increases $CMRO_2$

> Nitrous is
> NOT good
> for Neuro

- Desflurane
  - Increases CBF and ICP
  - Decrease in $CMRO_2$ → vasoconstriction → moderates any increases in ICP
- Sevoflurane
  - Increases CBF and ICP
  - Decreases $CMRO_2$
- Isoflurane
  - Inhibits CSF production, only volatile that increases CSF absorption
  - Increases CBF and ICP > 1 MAC
  - Silent EEG at 2 MAC
- Halothane
  - Dilates cerebral vessels → increases CBF, lowers CVR, reduces $CMRO_2$
  - Blunts autoregulation
- Xenon
  - Decreases CBF
  - Decreases $CMRO_2$
  - Neuroprotective when combined with hypothermia

Table 9.6 CNS effects of anesthetic gases[2,3]

	CBF	ICP	CMRO$_2$
N$_2$O	↑	↑	↑
Desflurane	↑	↑	↓
Sevoflurane	↑	↑	↓
Isoflurane	↑	↑	↓
Halothane	↑	↑	↓
Xenon	↓		↓

Cardiovascular System[1–3]

- N_2O
  - Directly depresses myocardial contractility but BP, CO, and HR are unchanged/elevated due to SNS stimulation
  - Myocardial depression unmasked in CAD or poor volume status
  - Increases pulmonary vascular resistance (PVR) → increased PA pressures
- Desflurane
  - SVR decreases with increasing dose
  - Rapid rise in desflurane concentration → tachycardia, elevated BP
  - QT prolongation[4]
- Sevoflurane
  - Mild decrease in myocardial function
  - CO drops because of lack of rise in HR
  - QT prolongation more than other volatile agents
  - Slows SA node conduction → junctional rhythms or bradycardia
- Isoflurane
  - Minimal LV depression
  - Maintains CO with rise in HR starting at 0.25 MAC (baroreceptors preserved)[2,4]
  - Coronary steal from vasodilation; however, unlikely to be clinically significant
  - QT prolongation[4]
- Halothane
  - Blunts reflex tachycardia
  - Sensitizes heart to catecholamines
  - Slows SA node conduction → junctional rhythms or bradycardia
  - Dose-dependent direct myocardial depression (affects Na+/Ca^{2}+ exchanger and Ca^{2}+ utilization in the cell) → increased right atrial pressure (RAP), central venous pressure (CVP), decreases arterial blood pressure (ABP).
  - Decreases coronary blood flow secondary to a drop in ABP; however, supply/demand is maintained because oxygen demand decreases
- Xenon
  - Minimal decrease in cardiac contractility

Table 9.7 Cardiovascular effects of anesthetic gases[2]

	HR	BP	CO	SVR	Contractility	PAP/RAP/CVP
N$_2$O	–	–	–	–	↓↓	↑
Desflurane	↑	–/↑	–	↓	–	–
Sevoflurane	–	↓	↓	↓	–/↓	–
Isoflurane	↑	↑	–	↓	–/↓	–
Halothane	–	↓	↓	–	↓↓↓	↑
Xenon	–	–	–	–	–	–

Table 9.8 Respiratory effects of anesthetic gases[2,3]

	RR	Vt	MV	PCO_2	Bronchodilation
N_2O	↑	↓	–	–	–
Desflurane	↑	↓↓	↓	↑	+
Sevoflurane	↑	↓↓	↓	↑	+++
Isoflurane	↑	↓↓	↓	↑	+
Halothane	↑	↓↓	↓	↑	+++++

Table 9.9 Volatile anesthetic properties, in order of most to least common[2,3]

Modality affected	Inhaled anesthetics
EEG spike activity	Enflurane > sevoflurane > isoflurane=desflurane
Liver metabolism (CYP2E1)	Halothane (20%) > sevoflurane (2%) > isoflurane (0.2%) > desflurane (0.02%)
Muscle relaxation	Desflurane > sevoflurane > isoflurane > halothane > nitrous oxide
Hepatic blood flow	Sevoflurane > isoflurane > halothane
Fluoride production	Sevoflurane > enflurane > isoflurane > desflurane
Carbon monoxide production	Desflurane > enflurane > isoflurane (desiccated CO_2 absorbers: Barium hydroxide > dry soda lime > wet soda lime)
Respiratory depression	Enflurane > desflurane = isoflurane > sevoflurane = halothane > nitrous oxide
Cerebral blood flow	Isoflurane > desflurane > sevoflurane
Impairment in cerebral autoregulation	Halothane > isoflurane/desflurane > sevoflurane

Table 9.10 Vaporizer output, estimated

Agent	SVP/PP	PP (%)	PP / (ATM – PP)
Sevoflurane	160 mmHg	21%	~ 1/4
Enflurane	175 mmHg	23%	~ 1/3
Isoflurane	238 mmHg	31%	~ 1/2
Halothane	241 mmHg	32%	~ 1/2
Desflurane	669 mmHg	88%	N/A

Pulmonary Function[2]

- All inhaled anesthetics → rapid and shallow breathing
- N_2O
  - Hypoxic drive markedly depressed (mediated by carotid bodies) → must watch closely in recovery room
- Desflurane
  - Highly pungent
  - Airway irritant → manifests as coughing, breath-holding, salivation, and laryngospasm
    - Avoid in asthmatics or hyperreactive airways
- Sevoflurane
  - Lacks pungency (sweet smelling)
  - Rapid shallow breathing
  - Bronchodilator
- Isoflurane
  - Rapid shallow breathing with drop in minute ventilation

- May irritate upper airway; however, remains second-best bronchodilator
- Halothane
  - Drop in minute ventilation → increased $PaCO_2$
  - Apneic threshold increases due to medullary depression and intercostal muscle dysfunction
  - Potent bronchodilator: inhibits intracellular Ca^{2+} mobilization→ reverses bronchoconstriction
  - Depresses mucociliary clearance leading to post-op hypoxia and atelectasis
- Xenon
  - Increases pulmonary resistance → increases work of breathing

Neuromuscular Function[2,3]

- Nitrous oxide
  - Not considered a trigger for MH
  - No significant muscle relaxation on its own in contrast to other inhalational anesthetics
    - Minimally potentiates NMBDs
- Desflurane
  - Dose-dependent decrease in TOF response and tetany
  - Potentiates NMBDs
- Sevoflurane
  - Creates intubating conditions in children when used for inhalation induction

- Isoflurane
  - Relaxes skeletal muscle
  - Potentiates NMBDs
- Halothane
  - Relaxes skeletal muscle
  - Potentiates NMBDs
  - Triggers MH
- Xenon
  - Not believed to trigger MH (tested in animal models)

Renal Function[2,3]

- N_2O
  - Decrease RBF, GFR, UOP
- Desflurane
  - Decrease GFR, RBF, UOP
- Sevoflurane
  - Slightly reduces RBF
  - Can metabolize to Compound A → nephrotoxic in rats, never proven in humans
- Isoflurane
  - Decrease GFR, RBF, and UOP
- Halothane
  - Decrease RBF, GFR and UOP (secondary to drop in ABP and CO)
  - Drop in renal blood flow > drop in GFR → increased filtration fraction
- Xenon
  - Little effect on renal system

Hepatic Function[2]

- N_2O
  - Less drop in hepatic blood flow (HBF) compared to other inhalationals
- Desflurane
  - No major hepatic effects
  - HBF maintained
- Sevoflurane
  - Decreases portal venous flow
  - Increase hepatic artery flow
  - Hepatic blood flow and O_2 delivery are maintained → ideal for patients with liver disease
- Isoflurane
  - Decreased total HBF (both hepatic artery and portal venous flow) but maintained better than halothane
  - Hepatic blood flow and O_2 delivery are maintained → ideal for patients with liver disease
- Halothane
  - Perioperative hepatic dysfunction can be seen with halothane

- Drop in HBF is congruent with drop in cardiac output
- Halothane hepatitis (rare)
  - Multiple halothane anesthetics at short intervals, middle-aged obese women, and persons with a familial predisposition to halothane toxicity or a personal history of toxicity are considered to be at increased risk
- Centrilobular necrosis of hepatic cells
- Xenon
  - No effect on hepatic artery blood flow

Hematologic and Immune Systems[2]

- N_2O
  - Bone marrow depression (megaloblastic anemia) causing peripheral neuropathy
    - Irreversibly inhibits B12-dependent enzymes:
      - Methionine synthetase ⊣ myelin
      - Thymidylate synthase ⊣ DNA
  - May alter immune response to infection → poor chemotaxis and polymorphonucleocyte (PMN) movement

Biotransformation and Toxicity

- N_2O
  - Avoided in pregnant patients (1st and 2nd trimesters) due to possible teratogenic effects
  - Thirty-five times more soluble than nitrogen in blood → escapes into close spaces
- Desflurane
  - Undergoes minimal metabolism
  - Degraded by desiccated CO_2 absorbents more than other volatiles→ carbon monoxide production
  - Associated with emergence delirium in pediatrics
- Sevoflurane
  - Undergoes the most metabolism of three main gases! (Sevoflurane > Isoflurane > Desflurane)
  - Broken down to Compound A
    - Clinically significant renal impairment secondary to fluoride ions and/or Compound A has never been proven with sevoflurane in humans
  - Associated with highest levels of fluoride; can breakdown to hydrogen fluoride → can produce acidic burn on contact with respiratory mucosa
  - Associated with emergence delirium in pediatrics
- Isoflurane
  - Metabolized to trifluoroacetic acid (TFA), unlikely to cause kidney or liver issues even after prolonged exposure
  - When degraded by desiccated CO_2 absorbents → carbon monoxide production

- Halothane
  - Oxidized in liver by CYP2EI to TFA, which can be inhibited with disulfiram
  - "Halothane hepatitis" extremely rare; hepatotoxicity after phenobarbital use, and hypoxia is more likely; however, only seen in rat models
- Xenon
  - Inert → nontoxic, minimal/no metabolites
  - Only non-halogenated inhaled anesthetic other than N_2O
  - Similar to nitrous oxide as it diffuses into air-containing spaces

Note: Fluoride production is directly related to the amount of metabolism a gas undergoes, that is, sevoflurane produces the most fluoride because it undergoes the most extensive metabolism of the anesthetic gases we use today.[2]

Trace Concentrations, Operating Room Pollution, Personnel Hazards[2,3]

- N_2O
  - Colorless and odorless greenhouse gas
    - Alone does not destroy the ozone layer; however, does contribute to ozone destruction as nitric oxide when paired with oxygen
  - Always coupled with oxygen/air in order to avoid hypoxia
  - As capable as oxygen of supporting combustion
- Desflurane
  - Carbon monoxide production with desiccated CO_2 absorbents
- Sevoflurane
  - Broken down into Compound A by CO_2 absorbents
- Isoflurane
  - Nonflammable
- Halothane
  - Broken down into BCDFE by CO_2 absorbents (negligible toxicity compared to Compound A)
- Xenon
  - Environmentally friendly
    - Concerns regarding N_2O safety have led to continuous interest in Xenon as alternative

Volatile Anesthetic Properties

Although not commonly tested, enflurane and halothane have been included.

High-Yield Topics and Concepts[4]

1. Effects of intracardiac shunts on induction
   - R → L (i.e., congenital abnormalities including tetralogy of Fallot, Eisenmenger syndrome)
     - Inhaled anesthetics = slower induction (insoluble > soluble)
     - IV anesthetics = rapid induction
   - L → R (i.e., ventricular septal defect, atrial septal defect):
     - IV and inhaled anesthetics = limited effect
2. Volatiles at different temperatures
   - Critical temperature: highest T at which an agent cannot be liquified regardless of pressure
     - Nitrous oxide critical temp = 36.5°C
       - It is a gas at standard temp and pressure. When stored under pressure in an E-cylinder, exists as both liquid and gas.

Boiling point: occurs at 20°C and 1 ATM, where all inhalational anesthetics exist in liquid form EXCEPT for N_2O:

Desflurane = 24°C | Isoflurane = 49°C | Sevoflurane = 59°C | N_2O = −88°C

3. Vaporizers and altitude
   - Decreased ATM pressure = increased vaporizer output
   - Key point: partial pressure is the SAME
4. Vaporizer output
   - ESTIMATED vaporizer output
   - For sevoflurane, ~ ¼ of the input
   - Ex: if 100 mL/min of inflow O_2 goes through a sevoflurane vaporizer, ~ ¼ of flow will be sevoflurane (25 mL). 25 mL / FGF = __ %
5. Alveolar concentration (FA) to inspired concentration (FI) ratio:
   - Normally related to solubility or blood:gas coefficient
   - Nitrous oxide has the most rapid rate of rise of FA/FI than desflurane, despite blood:gas coefficients, d/t concentration effect

Common Volatile Anesthetic Equations

$$Amount\ of\ liquid\ volatile\ used\ (mL/h)$$
$$= 3 \times FGF\ rate\ (L/min) \times vaporizer\ volume\ (\%)$$

$$Vapor\ concentration\ (\%) = \frac{SVPagent}{ATM} \times 100$$

$$Vaporizer\ output\ (mL) = carrier\ gas\ flow\ (mL/min)$$
$$\times \frac{SVP}{(ATM - SVP)}$$

$$Misfilled\ vaporizers: output\ calculation$$
$$VA = \frac{SVP \times VC}{PT - SVP}$$

- SVP = agent SVP (mmHg)
- P_T = total pressure (barometric P, mmHg)

- V_A = agent vapor volume (%)
- V_C = carrier gas volume (%)

% agent (isoflurane or sevoflurane)/% agent (isoflurane or sevoflurane) = VA/VA

$$\text{Volatile delivered (\%)} = \frac{\text{vaporizer output} \times 100}{\text{FGF} \times \text{vaporizer output}}$$

Volatile needed for a given barometric pressure $(v/v\%)$

Partial pressure of agent $= (v/v\%) \times$ current barometric pressure

$$(v/v\%) = \frac{\text{partial pressure of agent}}{\text{new barometric pressure}}$$

References

1. Bhatt H, Powell KJ, Jean DA. *First Aid for the Anesthesiology Boards*. McGraw-Hill Education, 2011.

2. Butterworth JF IV, Mackey DC, Wasnick JD, editors. *Morgan & Mikhail's Clinical Anesthesiology*, 6th ed. McGraw-Hill Education, 2018.

3. Miller RD. *Miller's Anesthesia*, 7th ed. Churchill Livingstone/Elsevier, 2010.

4. Barash PG, Cullen BF, Stoetling RK, editors. *Clinical Anesthesia*, 8th ed. Lippincott Williams & Wilkins, 2017.

Opioids

Vineet Aggarwal, Kiang Lien Cheung, and Leena Mathew

Opioids are a class of chemically related medications that are the gold standard of analgesia during anesthesia as well as in the perioperative setting and in the treatment of chronic pain associated with malignancy

Indications

- Anesthesia
  - Induction of general anesthesia
  - Adjuvant for total intravenous anesthesia (TIVA) with hypnotic and amnestic agents
  - Postoperative shivering

- Analgesia
  - Acute postoperative pain
  - Chronic pain – severe or refractory chronic nonmalignant pain
  - Pain of malignancy

Classifications

Classification Based on Origin

Natural Opioids/Opiates

- Naturally occurring
- Derived from the latex resin of the poppy (*Papaver somniferum*)
  - Morphine, codeine

Endogenous Opioids

- Synthesized in the brain and spinal cord, occurring naturally
  - Enkephalins, endorphins, dynorphins

Synthetic Opioids

- Laboratory synthesized molecules that act at opioid receptors to produce agonistic effects
  - Semisynthetic (*morphine-based structures with differing functional groups*)
    - Hydrocodone, hydromorphone, oxycodone, oxymorphone
    - buprenorphine, diacetylmorphine (heroin)
  - Fully synthetic
    - Meperidine, fentanyl analogs, methadone

Classification Based on Action at Opioid Receptors: Agonist, Partial Agonist, or Antagonist

- Agonists
  - Bind at the opioid receptor to provide a *full* therapeutic response
    - Examples: morphine, oxycodone, heroin, methadone, hydrocodone

- Partial Agonists
  - Bind at the opioid receptors to provide *less* than a full response
  - Provide a "ceiling effect," producing analgesia with relatively lower risk of respiratory depression as compared to full agonists.
  - Decreased euphoria leading to decreased risk of overdose and abuse[1]
    - Example: Tramadol

  - *If a person with opioid dependence consuming an opioid agonist were to take a partial agonist concurrently, the latter would antagonize the agonist, and potentially lead to opioid withdrawal.*

- Antagonists
  - High affinity for opioid receptors without activating them
    - Naloxone
      - Fast onset opioid antidote
      - Due to its short half-life and rapid metabolism, opioid antagonism wears off prematurely when used for opioid-related respiratory depression.
      - May need redosing/infusion

    - Naltrexone
      - Opioid receptor antagonist used for opioid use disorder and as a therapeutic agent in several chronic pain states such as fibromyalgia[2]
      - Has the potential to precipitate withdrawal symptoms and block opioid analgesia
      - Its derivative, **methylnaltrexone**, cannot cross the blood–brain barrier. As a peripherally acting mu opioid receptor antagonist, it has efficacy in the treatment of opioid-induced constipation without significant decrease in analgesia.[3]

- Mixed Agonist–Antagonist
  - Agonistic and antagonistic effects at opioid receptors
    - Buprenorphine
      - Weak partial agonist of the mu receptor and an antagonist at the kappa and delta receptors
      - Used in the treatment of chronic pain in lower doses and opioid addiction at higher doses
      - Opioid misuse deterrent sublingual formulations of buprenorphine combined with naloxone (Suboxone) are available. Buprenorphine treats the opioid addiction while the naloxone deters the abuse of buprenorphine by inducing opioid withdrawal symptoms.
    - Nalbuphine
      - Primarily used in the treatment of opioid-induced pruritus

Classification Based on Lipophilicity/Hydrophilicity

MOST LIPOPHILIC   Sufentanil

Buprenorphine
Fentanyl
Methadone
Hydromorphone
Hydrocodone
Oxycodone
Morphine
MOST HYDROPHILIC   Codeine

Opioid Receptors

- G protein-coupled receptors
- Locations
  - Spinal – *Rexed's laminae I and II of dorsal horn* both pre- and post-synaptic
  - Supraspinal – brainstem, thalamus, amygdala, and hypothalamus
- Types: three classic opioid receptors
  - Mu (μ) – *endogenously binds to beta-endorphin, endomorphin 1 and 2*
    - Location
      - Distributed throughout the neuraxis
      - Highest μ receptor densities are found in thalamus, caudate putamen, neocortex, nucleus accumbens, amygdala, superficial layers of the dorsal horn of the spinal cord, periaqueductal gray, and raphe nuclei
    - Action
      - (μ)1- analgesia and dependence
      - (μ)2 – euphoria, dependence, respiratory depression, miosis, decreased digestive tract motility/constipation
      - (μ)3 – vasodilation
  - Delta (δ) – *endogenously binds to enkephalins*
    - Action

- Analgesia, modulation of GI motility, mood, and behavior
  - Kappa (κ) – *endogenously binds to dynorphins*
    - Action
      - Analgesia, diuresis, dysphoria, neuroendocrine, immune functions

See Table 10.1.

Mechanism: The Activation of Opioid Receptors (Figure 10.1)

- Prevents the release of **excitatory** neurotransmitters, for example, glutamate, calcitonin gene-related peptide and substance P
- Decreases the formation of cAMP, increasing the efflux of K^+ out of the neuron and inhibiting the influx of Ca^{2+} by voltage-dependent Ca^{2+} channels
- These processes help maintain cell *hyperpolarization*, reducing neuronal depolarization leading to inhibition in the propagation of nociceptive signals.[5]
- Opioids also modulate the transmission of nociceptive stimuli at the level of the brainstem by regulating the ability of the dorsal root ganglion (DRG) to transmit pain signals.

Table 10.1 Summary of the effects of opioid receptor stimulation

	Mu	Delta	Kappa
Sedation	Yes	No	Yes
Respiratory depression	Yes	No	No
Gastrointestinal effects	Yes	No	Yes
Endogenous ligand	Endorphins	Enkephalins	Dynorphin
Inhibit ADH release	No	No	Yes

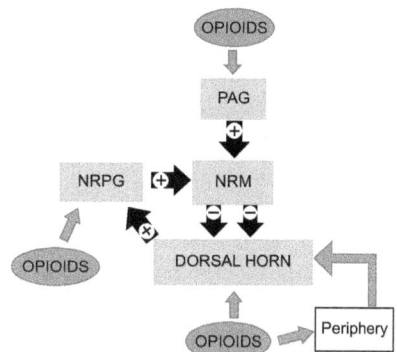

Figure 10.1 Opioid mechanism. Opioid agonists produce analgesia by increasing neuronal activity through descending pathways at NRPG (nucleus reticularis paragigantocellularis) and PAG (periaqueductal gray matter) or directly inhibiting peripheral nociceptive afferents. NRM = nucleus raphe magnus. Adapted from Pathan H, Williams J, Basic opioid pharmacology: an update. *Bri J Pain* 2012;6(1):14.[4]

This is achieved by stimulating descending inhibitory pathways from the brainstem to the DRG.[6]

Routes of Administration

- Oral
- Transmucosal
- Rectal
- Transdermal
- Parenteral: Subcutaneous (SC), intramuscular (IM), intravenous (IV)
- Neuraxial
- Peripheral

Opioid Effects on Different Organ Systems

- **Tolerance:** Larger doses are required to produce the same effect.
- **Dependence:** In situations with prolonged exposure, withdrawal symptoms occur in the absence of the agent.
- **Tachyphylaxis:** Rapid/acute desensitization occurs with initial doses of a drug. **For example,** this can occur with remifentanil infusions during anesthesia.

Cardiovascular System

- *Nucleus tract solitarius* is a part of the brain that processes information from the periphery with regard to arterial blood pressure and carbon dioxide concentrations.[7–9]
  - Mu and delta receptors are located in this region.[9]
  - Stimulation of these receptors results in *hypotension* and *bradycardia*.[9]
- In general, most opioids *enhance parasympathetic tone* and *reduce sympathetic tone*.[8]
  - Often the drugs of choice in cardiac inductions for that reason
- Morphine and meperidine can both lead to *histamine release.*
  - Can have resultant *drop in systemic vascular resistance* and can develop hypotension[10]
  - Can be treated with the use of H1 and H2 blockers[10]
- Opioids have been shown to have vasodilatory effects by direct action on vasculature. These mechanisms work independently of their effect on neurogenic centers.[8]
  - Mu-3 receptors are found on human endothelial cells and may contribute to vasodilation when activated by opioids such as morphine.[8]
  - Sufentanil has a direct vasodilatory impact on vasculature.[8,11]

Respiratory System

- **Mu opioid receptor** is primarily responsible for **respiratory depression.**[12-14]

- Medullary raphe region – area likely involved in the *ventilatory response to hypercapnia*[12,13]
  - Dose response curve to *carbon dioxide is shifted to the right and downward* → decreased alveolar ventilation7 for a given $PaCO_2$.
  - Ultimately leads to an increase in the apneic threshold, which is essentially defined as the highest $PaCO_2$ for which a patient is apneic.[7]
- Opioids impact airway reflexes.
  - Inhibit *lower airway* reflexes as an antitussive agent[15,16]
  - Inhibit upper airway by blunting the body's response to laryngoscopy
- Patients on chronic opioids develop a *central tolerance* to opioids, but they *do not* develop a *tolerance to the peripheral effects.*[17]
  - Leads to the development of abnormal breathing patterns during non-REM sleep[17]
  - Mechanism: During non-REM sleep, peripheral carotid chemoreceptors are responsible for detecting hypoxia and maintaining a breath-by-breath control of the ventilatory pattern.[17,18]
    - Mu receptor activation inhibits peripheral chemoreceptors control of ventilatory pattern → abnormal breathing patterns during non-REM sleep.[19]

Central Nervous System

- Sedation, decreased cognition, fine motor impairment, decreased REM and slow wave sleep, ventilatory depression, and miosis[8]
- Metabolites of hydromorphone, morphine, tramadol, and meperidine can produce central nervous system (CNS) excitation precipitating myoclonus and seizures.[8]

Gastrointestinal

- The enteric nervous system (ENS) – neural network that regulates reflex activities, controls secretory functions, and coordinates peristaltic movements
- Opioid receptors, particularly mu opioid receptors, present throughout the enteric nervous system, especially in myenteric and submucosal plexuses.[20,21]
- The opioid receptors modulate the activity on the ENS by **inhibiting** neurotransmitter release from **excitatory** motor neurons and by **stimulating** the release of neurotransmitters from **inhibitory** neurons.[22]
- Leads to nausea, vomiting, decreased gastric emptying, and inhibited intestinal peristalsis[21]
- Opioids activate the *chemotactic trigger zone* in the area postrema projecting to the vomiting center in the medulla, and may sensitize vestibular neurons.[8]
- Constipation and ileus are common side effects of opioids.
- Tolerance does not develop toward constipation.
- Treated with mu opioid receptor antagonist: Methylnaltrexone, alvimopan[23]

- Opioid agonists also impact biliary duct pressure by increasing tone in the sphincter of Oddi in a dose-dependent manner.[24]

Renal

- Studies involved in measuring levels of plasma renin, ADH, and aldosterone during IV infusions of fentanyl, alfentanil, and remifentanil show that renal function is preserved by opioids.[25]
- Intrathecal morphine and sufentanil decrease bladder function in a dose-dependent manner.[26]
- Intrathecal opioids impact spinal receptors, which cause suppression of detrusor contractility and create a decreased urge to urinate.[27]
- Elderly male patients appear to be most sensitive to these effects.[8]

Endocrine

- Opioids cause suppression in multiple axes of the endocrine system.[28]
  - Decreases: Epinephrine, cortisol, GH, ADH, ACTH, FSH, LH, glucose
  - Increases: Prolactin
- Somatotropic axis
  - In patients on chronic opioids, there is evidence of GH deficiency.[28,29]
- Lactotropic axis
  - Morphine administration *increases serum prolactin* in men and in woman that are postmenopausal.[30]
- Hypothalamic–pituitary–adrenal axis
  - Thought to decrease the pituitary glands response to CRH and subsequently cause a decrease of ACTH and cortisol in plasma.[31]
  - Likely mediated by the kappa opioid receptor[31]
  - Studies have shown a *decrease in adrenal androgen dehydroepiandrosterone sulfate* (DHEAS) during the administration of opioids.[32]
- Hypothalamic–pituitary–gonadal axis
  - Chronic opioid use is associated with *hypogonadism.*[28,33]
  - *Loss of libido, erectile dysfunction, depression and anxiety, fatigue and hot flashes*[28]

Miscellaneous: Opioid-Induced Pruritus

- May occur following parenteral or neuraxial administration
- Unclear mechanism, *not* related to the release of histamine
- Treatment often includes opioid antagonist such as nalbuphine.[34]

Risk Factors for Chronic Opioid Use and Opioid Misuse

- **Opioid use following surgery**
  - Opioid non-naïve patients
  - Use of antidepressants or benzodiazepines preoperatively
  - History of substance abuse[2]
- **Opioid misuse following surgery**
  - Age > 50 years
  - Use of antidepressants or benzodiazepines preoperatively
  - History of substance abuse
  - Mood disorder preoperatively
  - Pain disorder preoperatively
  - Taking greater than 60 mg of morphine milligram equivalents (MMEs) of opioids preoperatively

Opioid-Induced Hyperalgesia

- Paradoxical phenomenon seen with prolonged opioid usage that leads to increased sensitivity to pain and development of tolerance to opioids
- Seen in the treatment of chronic pain as well as in the treatment of postoperative pain
  - Most notable with the use of remifentanil
  - Incidence is reduced with use of multimodal analgesia and opioid rotation tactics.[35]

Equianalgesia

- When changing routes of administration or switching to a different opioid an equianalgesic table may be useful as a guide for initial dose selection.
- The significant first-pass metabolism is the reason relatively larger oral or rectal doses are needed to provide the same degree of analgesia as compared with equivalent parenteral doses of the same opioid.
- The consensus for equianalgesic ratios comes from limited evidence that is mostly anecdotal and usually from single-dose studies in the acute pain setting.
- It's important then to keep in mind that the available equianalgesic guidelines only serve as a "guideline" and dose regimens must be highly individualized based on several patient characteristics.
- Opioid rotation – strategy of switching opioids often to improve clinical outcomes (poor analgesic efficacy, avoidance of side effects)
  - Consider a 25–50% dose reduction from calculated equianalgesic dose to account for incomplete cross tolerance[36]
- Administering intrathecal opioids results in much higher CSF concentrations of opioids compared with epidural and intravenous administration.
  - Onset of analgesia is also fastest with intrathecal injection.
- Approximate conversions between routes of administration:
  - **Morphine:** 10 mg IV = 1 mg epidural = 0.1 mg intrathecal (1/10 conversion ratio)
  - **Hydromorphone:** 1 mg IV = 0.2 mg epidural = 0.04 mg intrathecal (1/5 conversion ratio)

Table 10.2 Morphine milligram equivalents (MMEs)

Opioid	Conversion factor (convert to MMEs)	Duration (hours)	Dose equivalent morphine sulfate (30 mg)
Codeine	0.15	4–6	200 mg
Fentanyl (mcg/hr)	2.4		12.5 mcg/hr
Hydrocodone	1	3–6	30 mg
Hydromorphone	4	4–5	7.5 mg
Morphine	1	3–6	30 mg
Oxycodone	1.5	4–6	20 mg
Oxymorphone	3	3–6	10 mg

www.cdc.gov/drugoverdose/pdf/calculating_total_daily_dose-a.pdf

○ **Fentanyl**: 100 mcg IV = 25 mcg epidural = 6–7 mcg intrathecal (1/4 conversion ratio)

See Table 10.2.

Metabolism

- Liver is the site of metabolism for most opioids.
- Converted to more water-soluble metabolites in order to be excreted from the body
- Two main pathways:
  ○ Phase I metabolism:
    ▪ Cytochrome P450 system = hydrolysis, oxidation, reduction reactions
    ▪ Rate of metabolism of opioids may be altered if the patient is taking other medications that affect the cytochrome P450 system.
  ○ Phase II reaction = glucuronidation

Morphine

- Phase II metabolism → morphine-3-glucuronide (M3G) + morphine-6-glucuronide (M6G)
- M6G
  ○ Full mu opioid receptor agonist
  ○ In patients with renal failure, M6G can accumulate in the plasma causing *respiratory depression* and loss of consciousness.[37]
- M3G has been implicated with inducing *hyperalgesia.*

Piperidines

- Fentanyl, alfentanil, sufentanil
- Lipophilic = cross the blood–brain barrier rapidly and are metabolized by phase I reactions
- Remifentanil is an **exception** to this group because it is not metabolized by the liver. Instead, it is metabolized in the blood by *nonspecific esterases.*

Codeine

- Weak analgesic pro-drug that is bio-transformed to morphine by **CYP-2D6**

- Five to 10 percent of Caucasians are poor metabolizers for codeine and are unable to benefit from analgesia.
- In contrast, also a high prevalence of patients who *rapidly* metabolize codeine
  ○ Rapid generation of morphine, increases risk of respiratory depression
    ▪ **Avoid** in pediatric population for postoperative analgesic, especially with history of obstructive sleep apnea (OSA)/sleep disordered breathing[8]

Meperidine

- Meperidine is an older opioid: many side effects including anticholinergic effects due to its structural *similarity to atropine*
- Metabolized to normeperidine
  ○ Can cause tremors, myoclonus, tachycardia, seizures
    ▪ Increased risk with renal or liver disease
- Commonly used for postoperative shivering as well
- Has weak serotonin reuptake inhibition
  ○ Combining with MAOIs or SSRIs can lead to overstimulation of receptors causing *serotonin syndrome.*
  ○ Phenylpiperidine opioids, methadone, and tramadol also have weak serotonin reuptake inhibition.[38]

Excretion of Opioids

- Ninety percent renal and less than 10% via fecal elimination
- Because many of the metabolites of opioids are active, it is imperative that opioids be used cautiously in the setting of renal insufficiency.
  ○ Not recommended in renal insufficiency: meperidine, morphine, codeine, hydrocodone, and tramadol due to active metabolites
- Use cautiously and with dose reduction: oxycodone and hydromorphone
- Can be safely used in patients with renal insufficiency: fentanyl, sufentanil, remifentanil, and methadone (no active metabolites)

Table 10.3 Acute opioid toxicity symptoms[8]

Toxicity	Symptoms
Lethargy/coma	Cold, clammy skin
Hypoventilation	Seizure
Hypoxia	Decreased muscle tone
Pinpoint pupils	Hypotension
Pulmonary edema	Respiratory failure

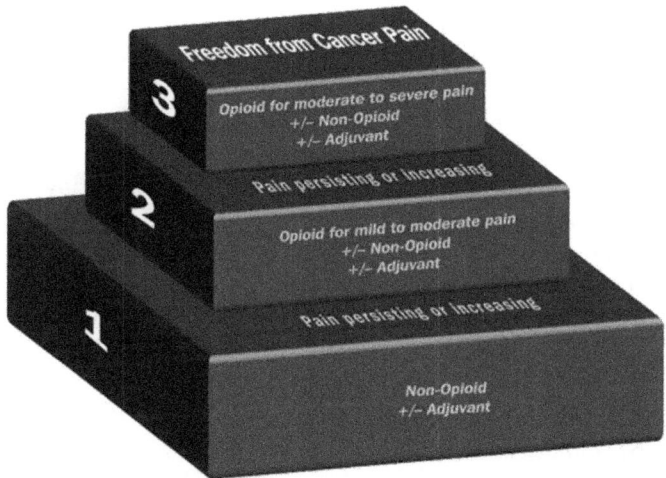

Figure 10.2 World Health Organization Pain Relief Ladder.

Toxicity

See Table 10.3.

- Respiratory failure or the sequela of respiratory depression is the most common cause of death from opioid use.
  - Treatment
    - Establishment of an airway, supplemental oxygen, ventilation, and administration of the opioid antagonist naloxone
    - Naloxone should be titrated to arousal, and return of spontaneous ventilation to prevent precipitation of withdrawal symptoms in opioid-dependent patients
    - Duration of action is shorter than the offending opioid → repeated dosing or a continuous infusion are indicated

Contraindications

- Pregnancy
  - Animal studies have shown adverse fetal effects of opioids, but no controlled human studies exist.
  - Neonatal withdrawal has been observed with opioid use late in pregnancy.[39] Therefore, fetal risk vs. maternal benefit must be considered before administering opioid therapy.
- Renal and hepatic failure
  - Complicated by inadequate clearance of the parent drug and active metabolite(s)[8,37,38]
  - Agents with active metabolites such as codeine, morphine, hydrocodone, and meperidine are avoided secondary to increased risk of respiratory depression and also worsening hepatic encephalopathy in patients with hepatic failure.
  - Consider lower doses and less frequent dosing intervals.
- Adrenal insufficiency
  - Inhibit the pituitary-adrenal axis resulting in decreases in plasma epinephrine, cortisol, GH, ADH, ACTH, FSH, LH, and glucose, which may precipitate adrenal insufficiency in at risk populations or worsen established adrenal insufficiency[28]

Role of Opioids in Postoperative Pain Control

- World Health Organization (WHO) Analgesic Ladder:
  - Three-step ladder initially developed for the treatment of cancer pain, also has been extended clinically in the treatment of acute non-cancer pain[28] (Figure 10.2)
    - Step 1 – Mild Pain
      - Nonopioid analgesics (acetaminophen, NSAIDs)
      - +/– Adjuvant analgesics (TCAs, anticonvulsants)
    - Step 2 – Moderate Pain
      - Short-acting/weak opioids (tramadol, codeine, hydrocodone)
      - +/– Nonopioid and adjuvant analgesics
    - Step – Severe Pain
      - Potent opioids (oxycodone, hydromorphone, morphine, methadone)
      - +/– Nonopioid and adjuvant analgesics
- CDC Clinical Practice Guidelines for Prescribing Opioids for Pain:[40]
  - Set of recommendations released by CDC for clinician providing pain care:
1. Nonopioid therapies are at least as effective as opioids – maximize use of nonpharmacological and nonopioid pharmacological therapies.
2. Nonopioid therapies are preferred for subacute and chronic pain.
3. When starting opioid therapy, immediate-release instead of extended-release or long-acting opioids should be used.
4. Lowest effective dose of opioids should be used for opioid-naïve patients.
5. For those already receiving opioid therapy, risk and benefits should be weighed when changing dosage.

6. No greater quantity should be prescribed than needed for expected duration of pain.

7. Benefits and risk of continuing opioid therapy should be evaluated regularly.

8. Before starting and periodically during continuation of opioid therapy, risks and management of risks should be discussed with patients (includes offering naloxone).

9. History of controlled substance prescriptions should be reviewed prior to prescribing and periodically.

10. Consider toxicology testing before prescribing opioids.

11. Use caution when prescribing opioids with benzodiazepines and other CNS depressants.

12. Treatment for opioid use disorder should be offered or arranged.

Special Note on Neuraxial Opioid Administration (Epidural and Intrathecal)

• Hydrophilic opioids: delayed onset (30–50 minutes), longer duration (5–24 hours), **extensive CSF spread**, site of action primarily spinal

• Lipophilic opioids: rapid onset (5–10 min), shorter duration (2–4 hours), **minimal CSF spread**, site of action primarily spinal ± systemic

• **Higher incidence** of nausea, vomiting, pruritus and delayed respiratory depression with hydrophilic opioids. Late respiratory depression due to rostral migration of medication affecting respiratory centers in the brain

Enhanced Recovery after Surgery (ERAS) Protocols[41]

○ Protocols originally developed to speed recovery time, decrease length of stay and morbidity (Figure 10.3)

○ Opioids should be limited to reduced side effects, which include ileus, respiratory depression, nausea, vomiting.

  ▪ Multimodal analgesia should be used to minimize these opioid-related side effects (Figure 10.4).

Opioid Risk Tool

• Office-based screening tool designed to help predict likelihood of opioid abuse when prescribed opioids for chronic pain[42]

• Patients are categorized as low, moderate, or high risk based on number of known risk factors associated with abuse (Table 10.4).

Table 10.4 Opioid Risk Tool*

Mark each box that applies	Female	Male
Family history of substance abuse		
Alcohol	1	3
Illegal drugs	2	3
Rx drugs	4	4
Personal history of substance abuse		
Alcohol	3	3
Illegal drugs	4	4
Rx drugs	5	5
Age between 16 and 45 years	1	1
History of preadolescent sexual abuse	3	0
Psychological disease		
ADD, OCD, bipolar, schizophrenia	2	2
Depression	1	1
Scoring totals	26	26

*Note differences in scoring with certain risk factors between genders.

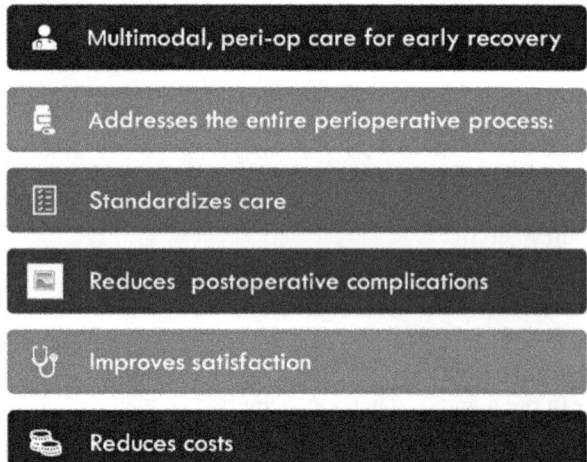

Figure 10.3 ERAS protocol.

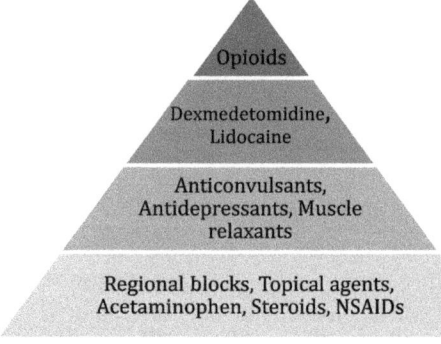

Figure 10.4 ERAS analgesic escalation pyramid.

References

1. Dahan A, Yassen A, Romberg R, et al. Buprenorphine induces ceiling in respiratory depression but not in analgesia. *Br J Anaesth* May 2006;**96**(5):627–632. doi:10.1093/bja/ael051

2. Younger J, Parkitny L, McLain D. The use of low-dose naltrexone (LDN) as a novel anti-inflammatory treatment for chronic pain. *Clin Rheumatol* Apr 2014;**33**(4):451–459. doi:10.1007/s100 67-014-2517-2

3. Greenwood-Van Meerveld B, Standifer KM. Methylnaltrexone in the treatment of opioid-induced constipation. *Clin Exp Gastroenterol* 2008;**1**:49–58. doi:10.2147/ceg.s3889

4. Pathan H, Williams J. Basic opioid pharmacology: an update. *Br J Pain* Feb 2012;**6**(1):11–16. doi:10.1177/2049463712438493

5. Chieng B, Christie MJ. Hyperpolarization by opioids acting on mu-receptors of a sub-population of rat periaqueductal gray neurones in vitro. *Br J Pharmacol* Sep 1994;**113**(1):121–128. doi:10.1111/j.1476-5381.1994.tb16183.x

6. Dubin AE, Patapoutian A. Nociceptors: the sensors of the pain pathway. *J Clin Invest* Nov 2010;**120**(11):3760–3772. doi:10.1172/JCI42843

7. Morgan GE, Mikhail MS, Larson CP, editors. *Clinical Anesthesiology*, 3rd ed. McGraw-Hill, 2002.

8. Miller RD, editor. *Miller's Anesthesia*, 8th ed. Churchill Livingstone/Saunders, 2015.

9. Feldman PD, Parveen N, Sezen S. Cardiovascular effects of Leu-enkephalin in the nucleus tractus solitarius of the rat. *Brain Res* Feb 19 1996;**709**(2):331–336. doi:10.1016/000 6-8993(95)01434-9

10. Blunk JA, Schmelz M, Zeck S, et al. Opioid-induced mast cell activation and vascular responses is not mediated by mu-opioid receptors: an in vivo microdialysis study in human skin. *Anesth Analg* Feb 2004;**98**(2):364–370. doi:10.1213/01.ANE.0000097168.32472.0D

11. Ebert TJ, Ficke DJ, Arain SR, Holtz MN, Shankar H. Vasodilation from sufentanil in humans. *Anesth Analg* Dec 2005;**101**(6):1677–1680. doi:10.1213/01.ANE.0000184119.85400.0E

12. Freye E, Latasch L, Portoghese PS. The delta receptor is involved in sufentanil-induced respiratory depression–opioid subreceptors mediate different effects. *Eur J Anaesthesiol* Nov 1992;**9**(6):457–462.

13. Dahan A, Sarton E, Teppema L, et al. Anesthetic potency and influence of morphine and sevoflurane on respiration in mu-opioid receptor knockout mice. *Anesthesiology* May 2001;**94**(5):824–832. doi:10.1097/0000 0542-200105000-00021

14. Zhang Z, Xu F, Zhang C, Liang X. Activation of opioid mu receptors in caudal medullary raphe region inhibits the ventilatory response to hypercapnia in anesthetized rats. *Anesthesiology* Aug 2007;**107**(2):288–297. doi:10.1097/01.anes.0000270760.46821.67

15. Erb T. Fentanyl does not reduce the incidence of laryngospasm in children anesthetized with sevoflurane *Anesthesiology* 2010;**113**(1):41–47.

16. Bennett JA, Abrams JT, Van Riper DF, Horrow JC. Difficult or impossible ventilation after sufentanil-induced anesthesia is caused primarily by vocal cord closure. *Anesthesiology* Nov 1997;**87**(5):1070–1074. doi:10.1097/00000542-199711000-00010

17. Walker JM, Farney RJ, Rhondeau SM, et al. Chronic opioid use is a risk factor for the development of central sleep apnea and ataxic breathing. *J Clin Sleep Med* Aug 15 2007;**3**(5):455–461.

18. Santiago TV, Goldblatt K, Winters K, Pugliese AC, Edelman NH. Respiratory consequences of methadone: the response to added resistance to breathing. *Am Rev Respir Dis* Oct 1980;**122**(4):623–628. doi:10.1164/arrd.1980.122.4.623

19. Santiago TV, Pugliese AC, Edelman NH. Control of breathing during methadone addiction. *Am J Med* Mar 1977;**62**(3):347–354. doi:10.1016/0002-9343(77)90831-2

20. Kurz A, Sessler DI. Opioid-induced bowel dysfunction: pathophysiology and potential new therapies. *Drugs* 2003;**63**(7):649–671. doi:10.2165/0000 3495-200363070-00003

21. Wood JD, Galligan JJ. Function of opioids in the enteric nervous system. *Neurogastroenterol Motil* Oct 2004;**16** (Suppl 2):17–28. doi:10.1111/j.1743-3 150.2004.00554.x

22. Sternini C, Patierno S, Selmer IS, Kirchgessner A. The opioid system in the gastrointestinal tract. *Neurogastroenterol Motil* Oct 2004;**16** Suppl 2:3–16. doi:10.1111/j.1743-3150.2004.00553.x

23. Cassel JA, Daubert JD, DeHaven RN. [(3)H]Alvimopan binding to the micro opioid receptor: comparative binding kinetics of opioid antagonists. *Eur J Pharmacol* Sep 27 2005;**520**(1–3):29–36. doi:10.1016/j.ejphar.2005.08.008

24. Fragen RJ, Vilich F, Spies SM, Erwin WD. The effect of remifentanil on biliary tract drainage into the duodenum. *Anesth Analg* Dec 1999;**89**(6):1561–1564. doi:10.1097/00000539-199912000-00047

25. Yuan CS, Foss JF, O'Connor M, et al. Methylnaltrexone prevents morphine-induced delay in oral-cecal transit time without affecting analgesia: a double-blind randomized placebo-controlled trial. *Clin Pharmacol Ther* Apr 1996;**59**(4):469–475. doi:10.1016/S0009-9236(96)90117-4

26. Kamphuis ET, Kuipers PW, van Venrooij GE, Kalkman CJ. The effects of spinal anesthesia with lidocaine and sufentanil on lower urinary tract functions. *Anesth Analg* Dec 2008;**107**(6):2073–2078. doi:10.1213/ane.0b013e318187bc0e

27. Kuipers PW, Kamphuis ET, van Venrooij GE, et al. Intrathecal opioids and lower urinary tract function: a urodynamic evaluation. *Anesthesiology* Jun 2004;**100**(6):1497–1503. doi:10.1097/00000542-200406000-00023

28. Buss T, Leppert W. Opioid-induced endocrinopathy in cancer patients: an underestimated clinical problem. *Adv Ther* Feb 2014;**31**(2):153–167. doi:10.1007/s12325-014-0096-x

29. Abs R, Verhelst J, Maeyaert J, et al. Endocrine consequences of long-term intrathecal administration of opioids. *J Clin Endocrinol Metab* Jun 2000;**85**(6):2215–2222. doi:10.1210/jcem.85.6.6615

30. Hemmings R, Fox G, Tolis G. Effect of morphine on the hypothalamic–pituitary axis in postmenopausal women. *Fertil Steril* Mar 1982;**37**(3):389–391. doi:10.1016/s0015-0282(16)46101-7

31. Howlett TA, Rees LH. Endogenous opioid peptides and hypothalamo-pituitary function. *Annu Rev Physiol* 1986;**48**:527–536. doi:10.1146/annurev.ph.48.030186.002523

32. Grossman A, Moult PJ, Cunnah D, Besser M. Different opioid mechanisms are involved in the modulation of ACTH and gonadotrophin release in man. *Neuroendocrinology* 1986;**42**(4):357–360. doi:10.1159/000124463

33. Daniell HW. Hypogonadism in men consuming sustained-action oral opioids. *J Pain* Oct 2002;**3**(5):377–384. doi:10.1054/jpai.2002.126790

34. Szarvas S, Harmon D, Murphy D. Neuraxial opioid-induced pruritus: a review. *J Clin Anesth* May 2003;**15**(3):234–239. doi:10.1016/s0952-8180(02)00501-9

35. Amano H, Ito Y, Suzuki T, et al. Roles of a prostaglandin E-type receptor, EP3, in upregulation of matrix metalloproteinase-9 and vascular endothelial growth factor during enhancement of tumor metastasis. *Cancer Sci* Dec 2009;**100**(12):2318–2324. doi:10.1111/j.1349-7006.2009.01322.x

36. Fine PG, Portenoy RK, Ad Hoc Expert Panel on Evidence R, Guidelines for Opioid R. Establishing "best practices" for opioid rotation: conclusions of an expert panel. *J Pain Symptom Manage* Sep 2009;**38**(3):418–425. doi:10.1016/j.jpainsymman.2009.06.002

37. Barash PG, Cullen BF, Stoetling RK, editors. *Clinical Anesthesia*, 7th ed. Lippincott Williams & Wilkins, 2013.

38. Goodman LS, Brunton LL, Chabner B, Knollmann BC. *Goodman & Gilman's The Pharmacological Basis of Therapeutics*, 12th ed. McGraw-Hill, 2011; p xvi.

39. Babb M, Koren G, Einarson A. Treating pain during pregnancy. *Can Fam Physician* Jan 2010;**56**(1):25, 27.

40. Dowell D, Ragan KR, Jones CM, Baldwin GT, Chou R. CDC Clinical Practice Guideline for Prescribing Opioids for Pain – United States, 2022. *MMWR Recomm Rep* Nov 4 2022;**71**(3):1–95. doi:10.15585/mmwr.rr7103a1

41. Simpson JC, Bao X, Agarwala A. Pain management in Enhanced Recovery after Surgery (ERAS) protocols. *Clin Colon Rectal Surg* Mar 2019;**32**(2):121–128. doi:10.1055/s-0038-1676477

42. Webster LR, Webster RM. Predicting aberrant behaviors in opioid-treated patients: preliminary validation of the Opioid Risk Tool. *Pain Med* Nov-Dec 2005;**6**(6):432–442. doi:10.1111/j.1526-4637.2005.00072.x

Intravenous Anesthetics

Chapter 11

Chris Sikorski

Overview of Pharmacology

See Table 11.1 for a summary of the pharmacodynamics of intravenous (IV) anesthetics.

Pharmacokinetics of IV Anesthetics

- After induction dose:
  - Rapid onset due to lipophilicity and relatively high cerebral blood flow
  - Offset via redistribution from brain (highly perfused) to muscle and fat (less perfused)
- Time to offset after discontinuation of infusion depends on context-sensitive half-time (CSHT): time for drug plasma level to drop 50% after cessation of infusion for certain duration (Figure 11.1).
- In general, IV anesthetics are eliminated via hepatic metabolism followed by renal excretion of metabolites, which may be inactive (majority) or active (minority).

- Active metabolites (dose cautiously in setting of renal insufficiency): Diazepam, midazolam, ketamine
- Inactive metabolites: All other IV anesthetics
- Plasma protein binding (PPB) impedes diffusion across membranes, which opposes its action but also slows its elimination.
  - Decreased PPB (e.g., hepatic or renal disease) may prolong IV anesthetic duration of action as well as its elimination.
- Hepatic clearance of IV anesthetics depends on hepatic blood flow (HBF) and function (i.e., enzymatic activity and protein production).
  - Reduced HBF (e.g., congestive heart failure [CHF], ↓CO, ↑systemic vascular resistance [SVR]) impairs hepatic clearance.
  - Cirrhosis has unpredictable effect on hepatic clearance because of enzyme hypoactivity.

Propofol

Pharmacodynamics of Propofol

- Acts via agonism of neuroinhibitory $GABA_A$ receptors
  - Both directly activates $GABA_A$-R and potentiates its activation by GABA
- Effects: sedative-hypnotic, amnestic, anxiolytic, anticonvulsant, antiemetic, antipruritic
  - Antiemetic mechanism unclear (possibly antidopaminergic and/or antiserotonergic activity causing depression of chemoreceptor trigger zone in area postrema)

Table 11.1 Pharmacodynamics of IV Anesthetics

Sedative-hypnotic:	All IV anesthetics
Amnestic:	Benzodiazepines > others
Anxiolytic:	Benzodiazepines > others
Analgesic:	Ketamine > dexmedetomidine
Antiemetic:	Midazolam, propofol
Anticonvulsant:	Barbiturates,* benzodiazepines, etomidate, propofol

* Exception: methohexital is epileptogenic.

Figure 11.1 Context-sensitive half-time (longest → shortest).

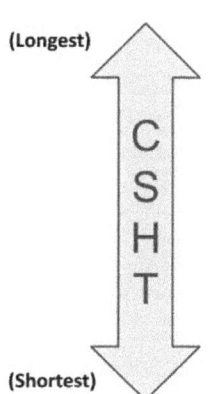

(Longest)

C S H T

Diazepam: CSHT ~50 min after 10 min infusion, >150 min after 30 min

Thiopental: CSHT ~45 min after 10 min infusion, >150 min after 5 hrs

Dexmedetomidine: CSHT ~4 min after 10 min infusion, 250 min after 8 hrs

Midazolam: CSHT ~20 min after 10 min infusion, ~75 min after 8 hrs

Ketamine: CSHT ~30 min after 4 hrs infusion, ~40 min after 8 hrs

Propofol: CSHT ~25 min after 4 hrs infusion, ~40 min after 8 hrs

Etomidate: CSHT ~12.5 min after 4 hrs infusion, ~25 min after 8 hrs

Remimazolam: CSHT 5–9 min after 4 hrs infusion

(Shortest)

Pharmacokinetics of Propofol

- Rapid onset and offset after boluses or brief infusions
  - Relatively short CSHT even after prolonged infusions
- Undergoes rapid hepatic *and extrahepatic* metabolism to renally excreted inactive metabolites
  - Hepatic: CYP450 (phase I), glucuronidation (phase II)
  - Extrahepatic: Lungs, kidneys, small intestine

Cerebrovascular Effects of Propofol

- Reduces cerebral metabolic rate of oxygen ($CMRO_2$), cerebral blood flow (CBF), and intracranial pressure (ICP)

Cardiovascular Effects of Propofol

- Substantial dose-dependent hypotension via vasodilation (both venodilation/↓preload and arterodilation/↓afterload) +/− direct myocardial depression
- Inhibition of baroreceptor reflex which blunts compensatory tachycardia and exacerbates hypotension
  - Lack of reflex tachycardia accounts for more profound hypotension than from all other IV anesthetics.
- Hemodynamic effect lags significantly behind hypnotic effect.

Respiratory Effects of Propofol

- Significant dose-dependent respiratory depression through reduction in minute ventilation and suppression of ventilatory response to hypercarbia and hypoxemia
- Induces bronchodilation
- Suppresses airway reflexes

Other Physiological and Adverse Effects of Propofol

- Pain on injection common but can be attenuated by injection into larger veins, premedication with fentanyl, pre-injection of lidocaine, or admixture with lidocaine or normal saline/lactated Ringers (NS/LR)
- Propofol infusion syndrome: Lipemia, metabolic acidosis, rhabdomyolysis, renal failure, refractory bradycardia, cardiovascular collapse
  - Usually infusions > 48 hr at > 67 mcg/kg/min, particularly pediatric and critically ill patients, but may occur with high-dose short-term infusions
- Lipid emulsion (soybean oil, glycerol, egg lecithin) supports bacterial growth so it should be drawn up with aseptic technique and used within 12 hours.
- Concern for allergy cross-reactivity in patients allergic to egg or soy is unsubstantiated.

Indications and Contraindications of Propofol

- Primarily used for induction of general anesthetic (GA) and sedation for surgeries under local/regional anesthesia, endoscopic procedures, or mechanical ventilation in ICU
- Superior for supraglottic airway (SGA) placement or esophagogastroduodenoscopy (EGD) (suppresses upper airway reflexes more than other IV anesthetics)
- Advantageous in patients with asthma or bronchospasm (bronchodilatory)
- Total intravenous anesthesia (TIVA) with propofol or subanesthetic boluses/infusion can prevent postoperative nausea and vomiting (PONV).
- TIVA with propofol possibly improves long-term outcomes after cancer surgery (antitumor properties).
- Avoid or reduce dose in patients with advanced age, hypovolemia, or cardiac disease (profound hypotension without reflex tachycardia)

Dosing of Propofol

- Induction of GA: 1–2.5 mg/kg (older age 1–1.5 mg/kg; hypovolemia/hypotension ≤ 1 mg/kg)
- Maintenance of GA: 50–200 mcg/kg/min
- Sedation: 25–75 mcg/kg/min
- PONV prevention: 10–20 mcg/kg/min

Barbiturates: Methohexital, Thiopental*

Pharmacodynamics of Barbiturates

- Act via agonism of neuroinhibitory $GABA_A$ receptors
  - Lower doses: Impede dissociation of GABA, increasing *duration* of chloride channel opening
  - Higher doses: Activate $GABA_A$-R chloride channels directly
- Effects: Sedative-hypnotic, amnestic, anticonvulsant*
  - *Exception: Methohexital is epileptogenic

Pharmacokinetics of Barbiturates

- Rapid onset and offset after single bolus, but delayed offset with repeated boluses or infusion
- Undergo hepatic metabolism (oxidation, N-dealkylation, desulfuration) to inactive metabolites that undergo renal or biliary excretion

Cerebrovascular Effects of Barbiturates

- Reduce $CMRO_2$, CBF, and ICP

Cardiovascular Effects of Barbiturates

- Substantial hypotension via vasodilation and direct myocardial depression with consequent baroreceptor-mediated reflex tachycardia

---

* Note: Thiopental no longer available in the United States.

Respiratory Effects of Barbiturates

- Significant dose-dependent respiratory depression through reduction in minute ventilation and suppression of ventilatory response to hypercarbia and hypoxemia
- Suppress airway reflexes (but less effectively than propofol)

Other Physiological and Adverse Effects of Barbiturates

- Promote production of porphyrins and may precipitate acute porphyria in predisposed patients
- Reconstituted in NS or water to produce alkaline solution so mixture with acidic solutions (e.g., LR, midazolam, neuromuscular blockers) results in precipitation and vascular occlusion
- Extravasation causes local tissue irritation
- Intra-arterial injection causes painful severe vasoconstriction and tissue ischemia.
  - Treatment: Intra-arterial injection of papaverine or lidocaine, heparinization, stellate ganglion block (i.e., sympathectomy)
- Methohexital may cause coughing, hiccupping, twitching, and tremors.

Indications and Contraindications of Barbiturates

- Methohexital (epileptogenic) is primarily used for induction for electroconvulsive therapy (ECT) (but should be avoided for non-ECT anesthetics in patients with epilepsy).
- Contraindicated in patients with porphyria
- Use cautiously in patients with advanced age, hypovolemia, or cardiac disease

Dosing of Barbiturates

- Induction of GA:
  - Methohexital: 1–1.5 mg/kg

Benzodiazepines: Diazepam, Lorazepam, Midazolam, Remimazolam

Pharmacodynamics of Benzodiazepines

- Act via agonism of neuroinhibitory $GABA_A$ receptors
  - Enhance coupling of GABA, increasing *frequency* of chloride channel opening
- Effects: Sedative-hypnotic, amnestic, anxiolytic, anticonvulsant, antiemetic[†]
  - Particularly potent for anxiolysis and amnesia (anterograde, not retrograde)

Pharmacokinetics of Benzodiazepines

- Quick onset but offset relatively slow[‡] even after single bolus and substantially protracted after infusion
- Undergo metabolism to renally excreted metabolites
  - Diazepam and midazolam are metabolized by hepatic CYP450 to *active* metabolites (dose cautiously in patients with acute kidney injury/chronic kidney disease (AKI/CKD) or on medications that are CYP3A4 inhibitors).
  - Lorazepam is metabolized by hepatic glucuronidation to inactive metabolites.
  - Remimazolam is metabolized by tissue esterases to inactive metabolites.
- Metabolism is increased with habitual alcohol consumption, but decreased with cirrhosis.

Cerebrovascular Effects of Benzodiazepines

- Reduce $CMRO_2$ and CBF, but less than barbiturates and propofol, and negligible effect on ICP

Cardiovascular Effects of Benzodiazepines

- Relatively modest BP reduction via mild arterodilation (↓ SVR) without affecting HR or cardiac contractility.
  - Hypotensive effect potentiated by coadministration with opioid.

Respiratory Effects of Benzodiazepines

- Relatively minimal dose-dependent respiratory depression and rarely apnea
  - Hypoventilatory effect potentiated by coadministration with opioid
- Predispose to upper airway obstruction by reduction of oropharyngeal tone

Other Physiological and Adverse Effects of Benzodiazepines

- Promote postoperative delirium in patients with critical illness or advanced age
- Prolonged sedation from midazolam and diazepam can occur with AKI/CKD or coadministration of CYP3A4 inhibitors (e.g., antifungals, antiretrovirals)
- Propylene glycol in diazepam and lorazepam makes IV injection painful and has potential for toxicity with prolonged infusions
  - Propylene glycol toxicity: skin and soft tissue necrosis (from extravasation), hemolysis, dysrhythmias, hypotension, lactic acidosis, seizure, coma, multi-organ failure

---

[†] Antiemetic: Midazolam (mechanism unclear).

[‡] Exception: Remimazolam has fast offset even with prolonged infusion.

Indications and Contraindications of Benzodiazepines

- Typically used as premedication before general or regional anesthesia
  - Midazolam can also be administered IM or PO (i.e., pediatric patients)
- May be used as adjunct for intraoperative sedation or induction/maintenance of GA
  - Can reduce minimum alveolar concentration (MAC) of volatile anesthetics
- Seizure suppression (e.g., local anesthetic systemic toxicity, alcohol withdrawal, status epilepticus)
- Midazolam: PONV prevention
- Avoid benzodiazepines in critically ill or elderly patients (more sensitive to cognitive effects)
- Use midazolam and diazepam cautiously in patients with AKI/CKD (active, renally excreted metabolites)

New Benzodiazepine: Remimazolam

- Ultrashort-acting benzodiazepine approved by FDA in 2020 for induction/maintenance of sedation in adults undergoing procedures lasting ≤ 30 min
- Rapidly metabolized by tissue esterases to an inactive metabolite
- Moderate hemodynamic effects ($\downarrow$BP or $\uparrow$BP) and minimal respiratory depression
- Promising sedative for brief procedures (e.g., endoscopies): Faster recovery than midazolam (< 15 min vs. < 2 hr), less respiratory depression than propofol

Reversal of Benzodiazepines: Flumazenil

- Competitive antagonist at benzodiazepine receptors that rapidly reverses their sedative effect
- May be used for benzodiazepine-related delayed awakening or overt benzodiazepine overdose
- May have shorter duration of action than benzodiazepine so re-sedation may occur, requiring redosing
- Unlike reversal of opioids by naloxone, reversal of benzodiazepines by flumazenil has negligible CV effects.

Dosing of Benzodiazepines

- Sedation:
  - Midazolam: 0.5–2 mg Q2–5 min PRN up to 5 mg
  - Remimazolam: 2.5–5 mg followed by 1.25–2.5 mg Q ≥ 2 min PRN

Dexmedetomidine

Pharmacodynamics of Dexmedetomidine

- Selective central α_2-adrenergic receptor agonist that induces endogenous sleep pathways
- Effects: sedative-hypnotic, amnestic, anxiolytic, analgesic
  - Unique cooperative-sedative state allowing smooth arousal from sleep
  - Analgesic, opioid-sparing properties (but less than ketamine)

Pharmacokinetics of Dexmedetomidine

- Relatively slow onset (~ 15 min) and protracted offset after long infusions
- Undergoes hepatic metabolism (glucuronidation and CYP450) to renally excreted inactive metabolites
  - Dose cautiously in patients on medications that are CYP2A6 inhibitors

Cerebrovascular Effects of Dexmedetomidine

- Reduces CBF but does not affect $CMRO_2$ or ICP

Cardiovascular Effects of Dexmedetomidine

- Sympatholysis: bradycardia, vasodilation ($\downarrow$SVR), hypotension
- However, "loading" bolus may cause transient hypotension or *hypertension*, depending on whether central α_2-mediated vasodilation or peripheral α_2-mediated vasoconstriction predominates.

Respiratory Effects of Dexmedetomidine

- Generally preserves respiratory drive; may cause slight reduction in tidal volume (TV) and response to hypoxia, but respiratory rate (RR) and ventilatory response to hypercarbia are unchanged

Other Physiological and Adverse Effects of Dexmedetomidine

- Blunts surgical stress response via inhibition of cortisol, catecholamines, and proinflammatory cytokines.
- Prolonged (> 24 hr) infusion may cause α_2-R upregulation and consequent withdrawal if abruptly discontinued (i.e., tachycardia, hypertension, agitation).

Indications and Contraindications of Dexmedetomidine

- Generally used for sedation or as an adjunct to GA
- Useful for awake fiberoptic intubation and intraoperative sedation (relative preservation of respiratory drive)
- Useful for minimizing opioid in patients prone to postoperative hypoventilation/apnea (e.g., obstructive sleep apnea [OSA])
- Useful for reduction of emergence agitation and postoperative delirium
- Useful for conscious sedation of mechanically ventilated patients in ICU

- May improve outcomes in patients with cardiovascular (CV), endocrine, metabolic, immune, or infectious disorders (suppression of surgical stress response)
- Use with caution in patients with baseline bradycardia or hypotension (sympatholytic)
- Does not induce sedation deep enough for neuromuscular blockade

Dosing of Dexmedetomidine

- Induction of sedation: 0.5–1 mcg/kg over 10 min (if hemodynamically stable)
- Maintenance of sedation: 0.2–1 mcg/kg/hr

Etomidate

Pharmacodynamics of Etomidate

- Acts via agonism of neuroinhibitory $GABA_A$ receptors
  - Lower (clinical) doses: reduces amount of GABA necessary to activate $GABA_A$-R
  - Higher (supraclinical) doses: directly activates $GABA_A$-R
- Effects: sedative-hypnotic, amnestic, anticonvulsant*
  - *May activate epileptic foci on EEG without causing convulsions

Pharmacokinetics of Etomidate

- Rapid onset and offset after boluses or even prolonged infusions
- Hydrolyzed by hepatic and plasma esterases to inactive metabolites that undergo renal or biliary excretion

Cerebrovascular Effects of Etomidate

- Reduces $CMRO_2$, CBF, and ICP

Cardiovascular Effects of Etomidate

- Relatively minimal CV effects (slight ↓ in SVR, slight ↑ in HR and CO) allowing hemodynamic stability on induction
- Does not blunt sympathetic response to laryngoscopy so opioid should be co-administered

Respiratory Effects of Etomidate

- Relatively minor dose-dependent respiratory depression; unlikely to cause apnea when used alone

Other Physiological and Adverse Effects of Etomidate

- Even a single induction dose can induce adrenocortical suppression for several hours, blocking normal stress-induced increase in cortisol production
  - Mechanism: inhibition of 11β-hydroxylase, which aids in biosynthesis of cortisol

- Its use in critically ill patients (e.g., septic shock) has been associated with increased mortality
  - Thus, despite its excellent CSHT, it is inadvisable for continuous infusion.
- Formulated with propylene glycol, which makes IV injection painful and has potential for propylene glycol toxicity with prolonged infusion
- Associated with myoclonic movements, hiccups, and PONV
  - Myoclonic activity is due to subcortical disinhibition, not cortical seizure activity, and may be attenuated by preadministration of benzodiazepine or opioid.

Indications and Contraindications of Etomidate

- Generally reserved for induction of GA in patients who cannot tolerate hypotension
- Advantageous for induction in patients with cardiac disease and/or hemodynamic instability (minimal CV effects)
- Use with caution for induction in patients with sepsis, other critical illness, or adrenal insufficiency, and should not be used as a continuous infusion (adrenocortical suppression)
- Avoid in patients at high risk for PONV (emetogenic)

Dosing of Etomidate

- Induction of GA: 0.2–0.3 mg/kg

Ketamine

Pharmacodynamics of Ketamine

- Acts primarily via antagonism of neuroexcitatory NMDA receptors and, to a lesser extent, via agonism of opioid and monoamine (serotonin, norepinephrine, dopamine) receptors
  - Produces functional dissociation between thalamocortical system (depressed) and limbic system (stimulated)
- Effects: Sedative-hypnotic, amnestic, anticonvulsant, analgesic
  - "Dissociative anesthesia," a unique cataleptic trance-like state with preservation of brainstem reflexes, spontaneous breathing, and possibly consciousness, but profound analgesia and amnesia
  - Potent analgesic properties with potential opioid-sparing effects and inhibition of central sensitization
- Racemic mixture of R(–) and S(+) isomers, latter of which has 3–4× more anesthetic and analgesic potency with faster offset and fewer psychomimetic effects

Pharmacokinetics of Ketamine

- Rapid onset and offset after boluses or brief infusions

- Undergoes hepatic CYP450 metabolism to multiple renally excreted metabolites, including *active* metabolite norketamine ($\leq$ ⅓ as potent as parent compound)
  - Dose cautiously in patients with AKI/CKD or on medications that are CYP2B6/CYP3A4 inhibitors

Cerebrovascular Effects of Ketamine

- Unlike other IV anesthetics, raises $CMRO_2$, CBF, +/– ICP, as well as intraocular pressure (IOP)

Cardiovascular Effects of Ketamine

- Sympathetic nervous system stimulation increases plasma catecholamine levels, which increases cardiac contractility, HR, CO, and BP
  - Hyperdynamic effects can be attenuated with benzodiazepine or opioid
- Direct myocardial depressant effect (normally counteracted and outweighed by sympathomimetic effects)

Respiratory Effects of Ketamine

- Generally preserves respiratory drive; apnea unlikely even after induction doses
- Induces bronchodilation
- Preserves upper airway reflexes, though airway protection not guaranteed

Other Physiological and Adverse Effects of Ketamine

- May cause psychomimetic emergence reactions: Vivid dreams, extracorporeal experiences, and hallucinations, which may be euphoric or dysphoric
  - Less common in children than in adults
  - Premedication with benzodiazepine can attenuate this.
- Causes sialorrhea, which may provoke laryngospasm
  - Premedication with glycopyrrolate can attenuate this.
- May cause lacrimation, nystagmus, and myoclonic movements

Indications and Contraindications of Ketamine

- Used for sedation, induction of GA, or as anesthetic adjunct for preventive analgesia
  - May also be given IM or PO (i.e., uncooperative patients, pediatric patients)
- Advantageous in patients with asthma or bronchospasm (bronchodilatory)
- Useful in patients prone to hypoventilation/apnea (preservation of respiratory drive and airway reflexes)
- Useful in patients with chronic pain, hyperalgesia, or opioid tolerance (analgesic and opioid-sparing effects)
- Subanesthetic infusions used to treat refractory chronic pain and refractory major depression

- Advantageous in patients with hypovolemia, hemorrhage, sepsis, or cardiac tamponade (sympathomimetic)
- Disadvantageous in patients with coronary artery disease (CAD), uncontrolled hypertension (HTN), tachyarrhythmia, aneurysms, or pheochromocytoma (sympathomimetic)
- Avoid in patients with chronic HF or cardiogenic/hypovolemic/septic shock (myocardial depressant effect in setting of depleted catecholamine reserves)
- Avoid in patients with head trauma or cerebral space-occupying lesions (potential to increase CBF and ICP)
- Avoid in patients with open eye injuries (potential to increase IOP)
- Avoid in patients with schizophrenia (psychomimetic)
- Use cautiously in patients on SSRIs, SNRIs, or MAOIs (monoaminergic)
- Avoid in patients with cocaine use, either acute (potentiation of CV toxicity) or chronic (myocardial depression in setting of catecholamine depletion)

Dosing of Ketamine

- Induction of GA: 1–2 mg/kg IV or 4–6 mg/kg IM
- Maintenance of GA: 30–90 mcg/kg/min
- Sedation: 0.25–0.5 mg/kg or 2.5–15 mcg/kg/min

Summary of Key Points

Context-Sensitive Half-Times

- Short CSHT (optimal for infusion):
  - Etomidate (however, avoided due to adrenocortical suppression)
  - Ketamine
  - Propofol
  - Remimazolam
- Intermediate CSHT (suboptimal for prolonged infusion):
  - Dexmedetomidine
  - Midazolam
- Long CSHT (unsuitable for infusion):
  - Diazepam
  - Lorazepam
  - Thiopental

Mechanism of Action

- $GABA_A$-R agonism: Barbiturates, benzodiazepines, etomidate, propofol
- NMDA-R antagonism: Ketamine
- α2-adrenoR agonism: Dexmedetomidine

Cerebrovascular Effects

- Significant $\downarrow$ $CMRO_2$, CBF, and ICP: Barbiturates, etomidate, propofol

- Modest ↓ $CMRO_2$ and CBF but unchanged ICP: Benzodiazepines
- ↓ CBF but unchanged $CMRO_2$ and ICP: Dexmedetomidine
- ↑ $CMRO_2$, CBF, +/− ICP: Ketamine

Cardiovascular Effects

- Hypotension: Barbiturates (↓BP, ↑HR), dexmedetomidine (↓BP, ↓HR), propofol (↓↓BP, stable HR)
- Stability: Benzodiazepines (stable or mild ↓BP, stable HR), etomidate (mild ↓BP, stable HR)
- Hypertension: Ketamine (↑BP, ↑HR)

Respiratory Effects

- Substantial, dose-dependent hypoventilation: Barbiturates, propofol
- Minimal, dose-dependent hypoventilation: Benzodiazepines, dexmedetomidine, etomidate, ketamine

Other Physiological and Adverse Effects

- Adrenocortical Suppression: etomidate
- Bronchodilation: Ketamine, propofol
- Emetogenic: Etomidate
- Epileptogenic: Methohexital
- Myoclonic activity: Etomidate, ketamine

- Painful injection: Diazepam, lorazepam, etomidate, propofol
- Porphyrogenic: Barbiturates
- Propylene glycol toxicity: Diazepam, lorazepam, etomidate
- Psychomimetic: Ketamine
- Sialorrhea: Ketamine

Indications

- Premedication: Midazolam
- Sedation: Midazolam, remimazolam, dexmedetomidine, ketamine, propofol
- Induction of GA: Barbiturates, etomidate, ketamine, propofol
  - Propofol: Patients able to tolerate hypotension; asthma/bronchospasm
  - Ketamine: Patients requiring hemodynamic augmentation; asthma/bronchospasm
  - Etomidate: Patients requiring hemodynamic stability
  - Methohexital: Patients undergoing ECT
- TIVA: Propofol (primary anesthetic); dexmedetomidine, ketamine, midazolam (adjuncts)
- Preventive analgesia: Ketamine > dexmedetomidine
- PONV reduction: Midazolam, propofol

Further Reading

Bokoch MP, Su PP. Intravenous anesthetics. In Pardro MC, editor. *Miller's Basics of Anesthesia*, 8th ed. Elsevier, 2022; pp 107–124.

Bravenec B. General anesthesia: intravenous induction agents. In Nussmeier NA, editor. *UpToDate*. UpToDate Inc., 2022. Available at: https://medilib.ir/uptodate/show/94533

Butterworth JF, Mackey DC, Wasnick, JD. Intravenous anesthetics. In Butterworth JF, Mackey DC, Wasnick JD, editors. *Morgan & Mikhail's Clinical Anesthesiology*, 7th ed. McGraw-Hill, 2022; pp 165–180.

Puskas F, Howie MB, Graviee GP. Induction of anesthesia. In Hensley FA,

Martin DE, Gravlee GP, editors. *A Practical Approach to Cardiac Anesthesia*, 5th ed. Lippincott Williams & Wilkins, 2013; pp 180–191.

Rosero E. Monitored anesthesia care in adults. In Crowley M, editor. *UpToDate*. UpToDate Inc., 2023. Available at: https://medilib.ir/uptodate/show/94529

Schüttler J, Eisenried A, Lerch M, et al. Pharmacokinetics and pharmacodynamics of remimazolam (CNS 7056) after continuous infusion in healthy male volunteers: part I. Pharmacokinetics and clinical pharmacodynamics. *Anesthesiology* 2020;**132**:636–651.

Tietze KJ, Fuchs B. Sedative-analgesic medications in critically ill adults: properties, dosage regimens, and adverse effects. In Finlay G, editor. *UpToDate*. UpToDate Inc., 2023. Available at: https://medilib.ir/uptodate/show/1616

Vuyk J, Sitsen E, Reekers M. Intravenous anesthetics. In Gropper MA, Cohen NH, Eriksson LI, et al., editors. *Miller's Anesthesia*, 9th ed. Elsevier, 2020; pp 638–679.

White PF, Eng MR. Intravenous anesthetics. In Barash PG, Cullen BF, Stoelting RK, et al., editors. *Clinical Anesthesia*, 7th ed. Lippincott Williams & Wilkins, 2013; pp 478–500.

Local Anesthetics

Christopher X. Muñoz and Christina L. Jeng

General Characteristics

Structure
There are three major structural components of local anesthetics (Figure 12.1):
1. Lipophilic benzene ring
2. Hydrophilic tertiary amine (responsible for weak base properties)
3. Amide or ester linkage connects above components – determines class of local anesthetic

Amide vs. Ester Local Anesthetics
- Esters (chloroprocaine, tetracaine, procaine, cocaine, benzocaine) are metabolized by pseudocholinesterase in plasma.
- Amides (lidocaine, ropivacaine, bupivacaine, mepivacaine, etidocaine, prilocaine – have the letter "i" before "-caine") are metabolized by hepatic microsomal enzymes and are affected by liver dysfunction such as cirrhosis.

Function and Mechanism of Action
- Local anesthetics are placed in proximity to nerve membranes to produce reversible blockade of conduction. Systemic absorption progressively reduces their effect.
- Uncharged form of local anesthetics readily cross cell membranes. Charged form of local anesthetics bind to intracellular sodium channels to keep them closed → Prevents increase in permeability of nerve membrane to sodium ions → Slows rate of depolarization. Threshold potential is not reached → Action potential is not propagated.
- Three successive nodes of Ranvier have to be blocked in order to have predictable conduction blockade.

Nerve Fibers' Susceptibility to Blockade:
- Order of blockade (fastest to slowest): Autonomic > Sensory > Motor

–Small diameter nerves	More easily blocked than	Large diameter nerves
–Myelinated nerves	More easily blocked than	Non-myelinated nerves
–Active nerves	More easily blocked than	Non-active nerves

See Table 12.1 for characteristics of nerve fibers.

Pharmacological Properties
See Table 12.2 for a summary of pharmacological properties of select local anesthetics.
- Potency: Proportional to *lipid solubility*.
- Speed of onset: Largely dependent *on pKa* (pH at which 50% of molecules exist in unionized form and 50% in ionized form). Lower pKa = higher percentage in unionized form (because uncharged form of local anesthetics readily cross cell membranes) → faster onset. Onset time is also proportional to dose and concentration.
- Duration of action: Dependent on *protein binding*: higher affinity for protein leads to longer duration.
- Termination of action: Diffusion away from site of action.

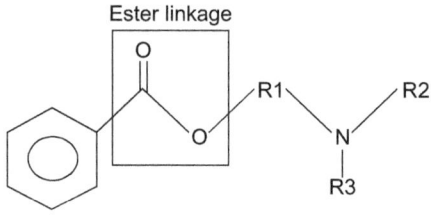
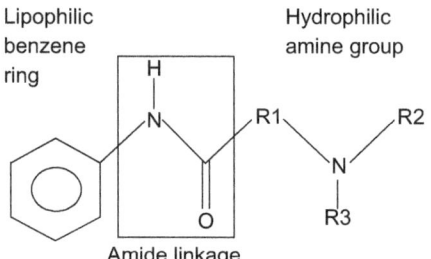

Figure 12.1 Structural components of amide and ester local anesthetics.

Table 12.1 Characteristics of nerve fibers

Fiber	Myelinated?	Diameter (μm)	Function/comments
Aα	Yes	12–20	Motor
Aβ	Yes	5–15	Tactile, proprioception
Aγ	Yes	3–8	Muscle tone/most susceptible to block by local anesthetic
Aδ	Yes	2–5	Pain, cold temperature, touch
B	Yes	3	Preganglionic sympathetic
C	No	0.3–1.5	Dull pain, warm temperature, touch/least susceptible to block by local anesthetic

Table 12.2 Pharmacological properties of various local anesthetics

Agent	pKa	Relative potency	Duration (min)	Maximum dose (mg/kg)
Procaine	8.9	1	45–60	12
Chloroprocaine	8.7	2	30–60	12
Tetracaine	8.5	8		3
Lidocaine	7.9	2	60–120	4.5; 7 w/ epinephrine
Mepivacaine	7.6	2	90–180	4.5; 7 w/ epinephrine
Prilocaine	7.9	2	60–120	8
Bupivacaine	8.1	8	240–480	3
Ropivacaine	8.1	6	240–480	3

Agents That Prolong Duration of Local Anesthetics

- Epinephrine: (1) Causes local tissue vasoconstriction, (2) Limits systemic absorption, (3) Keeps contact with nerve fibers, (4) Prolongs duration of action, little effect on onset
- Most common epinephrine dilution – 1:200,000 = 5 mcg/mL
- Other agents: Buprenorphine, clonidine, dexmedetomidine, dexamethasone, tramadol

Systemic Absorption of Local Anesthetics

Systemic absorption of local anesthetics depends upon various factors, including:

- Site of local anesthetic delivery (from greatest to least systemic absorption): Intravenous > Trachea > Intercostal > Caudal > Epidural > Brachial Plexus > Sciatic > Spinal > Skin infiltration.
- Choice of local anesthetic: High degree of tissue binding (e.g., etidocaine, bupivacaine) or large volume of distribution (e.g., prilocaine) will have lower blood levels.
- Dose: Higher dose → higher blood levels. 1% solution = 1,000 mg/100 mL = 10 mg/mL
- Addition of vasoconstrictors: Lowers blood level and increases time to peak blood level
- Metabolism: Need absorption and delivery to site of metabolism.
- *Metabolism*: Esters are metabolized by *pseudocholinesterase in plasma*; amides are metabolized by *hepatic microsomal enzymes.*
- *Excretion*: Both ester and amide local anesthetics undergo renal excretion.

Characteristics of Individual Local Anesthetics

Which local anesthetic to use for which anesthetic technique:

- Spinal: Tetracaine (hyperbaric), bupivacaine (isobaric, hyperbaric, hypobaric), mepivacaine (isobaric)
- Epidural: Chloroprocaine, lidocaine, bupivacaine, ropivacaine
- Peripheral nerve blocks: Lidocaine, mepivacaine, bupivacaine, ropivacaine

- Lidocaine – Most common offending agent for transient neurological symptoms
- Chloroprocaine – Undergoes rapid ester linkage hydrolysis by pseudocholinesterase. It is used commonly in obstetrics because of its rapid onset and decreased risk of fetal exposure due to rapid metabolism in bloodstream. Chloroprocaine has a fast speed of onset mostly due to its high concentration rather than its pKa.
- Cocaine – Only local anesthetic with vasoconstricting properties. Used as topical anesthetic for ENT procedures. Side effects include tachycardia, hypertension, and dysrhythmias.
- Bupivacaine – Poses the greatest risk for cardiotoxicity. Severe cardiovascular collapse can be seen with toxic doses. Bupivacaine toxicity is more likely to contribute to ventricular arrhythmias and is more resistant to cardiopulmonary resuscitation than lidocaine. The reasons for this are believed to be due to:
  1. Stronger binding to resting and inactivated sodium channels
  2. Slower disassociation from sodium channels.
- Ropivacaine – Is an enantiomer of bupivacaine, but has reduced systemic toxicity than bupivacaine due to increased vasoconstriction and decreased lipid solubility.
- Eutectic mixture of local anesthetics (EMLA) cream = Lidocaine 2.5% + Prilocaine 2.5%
  - EMLA cream provides dermal anesthesia. It is commonly used for pediatric IV placement.
  - Applied to intact skin and covered with occlusive dressing. Onset takes 45–60 minutes and reaches peak effect in 2–3 hours.
  - Precautions and contraindications include: Patients with allergy to amide anesthetics Patients with congenital methemoglobinemia; or infants < 1 year old receiving treatment with methemoglobin-inducing agents because prilocaine metabolite o-toluidine can cause methemoglobinemia Patients undergoing treatment with class I or class III antiarrhythmic drugs due to potential additive or synergistic cardiotoxic effects

Complications of Local Anesthetics

- Allergies – True allergies to local anesthetics are rare. Allergic-type reactions to PABA (para-aminobenzoic acid) metabolite are more common. PABA is an *ester metabolite* that can cause allergic-type reactions in small percentage of people. Most reactions that appear allergic are more likely due to epinephrine, systemic toxicity, or vasovagal reaction.
  - Signs: Urticaria, flushing, edema, dyspnea, hypoxia, wheezing, hypotension, tachycardia
  - Treatment: Stop suspected offending agent. Epinephrine, intravenous fluids, oxygen, bronchodilators, H1 and H2 blockers, steroids.

- Cauda equina syndrome (CES) – Neurotoxicity of sacral nerves. Anesthesia-related causes of CES include maldistribution of local anesthetic, direct needle-induced trauma, or intraneural injection during spinal anesthetic; spinal cord hematoma, ischemia, or infection; and improper patient positioning. Lidocaine is the most common LA associated with CES, but there are case reports of bupivacaine as the offending agent.
  - Signs: Saddle anesthesia, pain, bladder/bowel dysfunction
  - Treatment: Immediate MRI; discussion with surgeon regarding possible decompression
- Transient neurological symptoms (TNS) – A pain disorder after receiving a spinal anesthetic with local anesthetic, especially lidocaine. Onset typically occurs 12–24 hours after surgery. Risk factors include lithotomy position.
  - Signs: Pain and dysesthesia in lower back, buttocks, and lower extremities. No neurological dysfunction is noted, and MRI and other diagnostic modalities are normal.
  - Treatment: Symptoms are usually transient. Treatment consists of NSAIDs. Symptoms usually resolve within 3 days and rarely last more than a week.
- *Methemoglobinemia* – Excess of certain local anesthetic agents have been known to oxidize normal hemoglobin to methemoglobin; methemoglobinemia decreases oxygen delivery to tissues. Classic offending agents are prilocaine (hepatically metabolized to ortho-toluidine, which can induce methemoglobinemia) and benzocaine. Lidocaine and tetracaine have been implicated but rare.
  - Signs: Fatigue, headache, cyanosis, dyspnea, mental status changes; can progress to dysrhythmias, coma, and death (> 50% of total hemoglobin levels). Classically described as chocolate brown appearance of blood. Decreased SaO_2 despite satisfactory PaO_2 (requires co-oximetry for accurate diagnosis and treatment).
  - Treatment: Methylene blue (reduces methemoglobin to normal hemoglobin). G6PD-deficient patients treated with ascorbic acid.
- Local anesthetic systemic toxicity (LAST): Toxicity of the central nervous system (CNS) and cardiovascular system (CVS) due to excessive plasma concentrations of local anesthetic. Initial signs of excitation are typically seen and eventually lead to signs of depression with increasing blood levels of local anesthetics for both CNS and CVS.
  - Light-headedness/dizziness, vertigo, tinnitus, perioral numbness, metallic taste in mouth
  - Slurred speech, changes in mental status, agitation
  - Tonic–clonic seizures
  - Coma and apnea
  - Death

- Signs of CVS toxicity (note that CVS is more resistant to local anesthetic adverse effects than CNS):
  - Hypertension, tachycardia initially possible – likely due to sympathetic activity and vasoconstriction
  - Bradycardia and hypotension from arteriolar vasodilation
  - ECG changes: PR prolongation & widening of QRS complex
  - Dysrhythmias, complete heart block
  - CVS collapse, death
- Treatment (as outlined by American Society of Regional Anesthesia's Checklist for Treatment of LAST):
  - Call for help.
  - Secure airway if not already done so and ventilate with 100% oxygen. Hyperventilate to normalize pH and increase oxygenation.
  - Treat seizures with benzodiazepine or barbiturates. Avoid propofol in setting of cardiovascular instability.
  - ACLS: Chest compressions, defibrillation, vasopressors – adjustment of medications and prolonged effort may be required. Since epinephrine can exacerbate dysrhythmias caused by local anesthetics and reduce the efficacy of lipid emulsion therapy, reduced doses of epinephrine are recommended (< 1 mcg/kg). Also avoid vasopressin, calcium channel blockers, beta blockers, or local anesthetic.
- Lipid emulsion – 20% lipid emulsion bolus of 1.5 mL/kg over 1 minute, repeat every 3–5 minutes as needed. After sinus rhythm is restored, start 20% lipid emulsion at 0.25 mL/kg/min until hemodynamically stable. Recommended upper limit of lipid emulsion is approximately 10 mL/kg over the first 30 minutes.
  - Proposed mechanisms of lipid emulsion:
    1. Increases clearance of local anesthetic from plasma or tissue to decrease effective plasma concentration (lipid sink)
    2. Reverses the inhibition of myocardial fatty acid oxidation caused by local anesthetic.
  - Alert nearest facility having cardiopulmonary bypass capability.

Clinical Uses

Neuraxial Anesthesia

Local anesthetic can be injected into the subarachnoid space for a spinal anesthetic or through ligamentum flavum into the epidural space.

- Spinal anesthesia: Local anesthetic baricity and patient position affects dermatomal spread. Duration is proportional to dose.

- Epidural anesthesia: Local anesthetic volume is proportional to dermatomal spread and density of block is proportional to dose.

Peripheral Nerve Block

Type of local anesthetic, concentration, and volume can change characteristic of block depending on goals for surgery. Higher concentration will provide more motor blockade, lower concentration will provide more sensory blockade.

Intravenous Regional Anesthesia (Bier Block)

Intravenous regional anesthesia is most commonly used in upper limb surgery. Tourniquet is applied and local anesthetic diffuses from peripheral vascular bed to nonvascular tissue where axons and nerve endings reside. Prilocaine or Lidocaine are the most frequently used agents.

Topical Anesthesia

Applications can include skin (see EMLA as described above) or for awake intubation with nebulized, atomized, liquid, or gel local anesthetic.

- Awake fiberoptic cranial nerve blocks: Lidocaine can be used to block nasopharynx innervated by CN V, oropharynx innervated by CN IX and hypopharynx innervated by internal branch of the superior laryngeal nerve (branch of CN X), larynx innervated by internal and external branch of the superior laryngeal nerve and recurrent laryngeal nerve – branch of CN X.

Tumescent Anesthesia

Large volumes of dilute local anesthetic injected into subcutaneous tissue. Used during liposuction procedures. Dose of Lidocaine is 35–55 mg/kg. Levels can peak after 20 hours. Beware of CNS and cardiotoxicity.

Further Reading

Berde CB, Strichartz. GR. Local anesthetics. In Miller R, editor. *Miller's Anesthesia*, 8th ed. Churchill Livingstone/Elsevier, 2016; chapter 10, pp 1028–1054.

Brummett CM, Williams BA Additives to local anesthetics for peripheral nerve blockade. *Int Anesthesiol Clin* 2011;49 (4):104–116.

Neal JM, Bernards CM, Butterworth JF, et al. ASRA practice advisory on local anesthetic systemic toxicity. *Reg Anesth Pain Med* 2010;35:152–161.

Rosenblatt MA, Abel M, Fischer GW, et al. Successful use of a 20% lipid emulsion to resuscitate a patient after a presumed bupivacaine-related cardiac arrest. *Anesthesiology* 2006;105 (1):217–218.

Weinberg G, Ripper R, Feinstein DL, et al. Lipid emulsion infusion rescues dogs from bupivacaine-induced cardiac toxicity. *Reg Anesth Pain Med* 2003;28 (3):198–202.

Muscle Relaxants (Depolarizing, Non-Depolarizing)

Katherine Loftus and Palak Patel

Depolarizing Muscle Relaxants: Succinylcholine

Mechanism of Action

- Succinylcholine is an acetylcholine (ACh) receptor agonist. Its structure is two linked ACh molecules.
- Binds alpha subunits of ACh receptors and generates a prolonged action potential because it is not metabolized as rapidly as ACh.
- Voltage-gated Na+ channels become inactivated. Can't reopen until succinylcholine unbinds the acetylcholine receptor (AChR) (Phase I block)
- A prolonged period of end-plate depolarization → conformational changes in AChR that cause Phase II block (mimics a non-depolarizing block)
  - Seen with large single dose, repeated doses, or continuous infusion

Pharmacokinetics and Metabolism

See Tables 13.1 and 13.2.

Prolongation of Action

Can be due to *decreased amount or decreased activity of pseudocholinesterase*

- Decreased amount (levels must be reduced > 75% for significant prolongation of blockade)
  - Decreased production of enzyme in liver
    - Dilution of enzyme seen in pregnancy, cirrhosis, malnutrition
- Decreased activity
  - Atypical pseudocholinesterase prolongs the duration of action of succinylcholine
    - Genetics: Autosomal recessive pattern of inheritance
    - Dibucaine number: Dibucaine is an amino amide local anesthetic. It is capable of inhibiting the plasma cholinesterase enzyme.
    - In normal patients, dibucaine will inhibit 80% of enzyme activity which corresponds to dibucaine number of 80. Heterozygous atypical pseudocholinesterase corresponds to a dibucaine number between 30 and 65 (Table 13.3).
- Cholinesterase Inhibitors
  - Increase the ACh concentration at nerve terminals and intensify depolarization
  - Reduce the hydrolysis of succinylcholine by inhibiting pseudocholinesterase
  - Common example: echothiophate eye drops used for glaucoma (an organophosphate that causes irreversible inhibition of pseudocholinesterase)
  - Edrophonium is an exception. Has no effect on pseudocholinesterase
- Other drugs can also decrease the activity of pseudocholinesterase (Table 13.4).

Table 13.1 Pharmacokinetic properties of succinylcholine

Rapid onset (30–60 s)
Duration of action < 10 min
$ED_{95} = 0.3$ mg/kg
Intubating dose 1.0–1.5 mg/kg IV
Low lipid solubility → small volume of distribution

ED_{95} = dose that produces 95% twitch suppression in 50% of individuals.

Table 13.2 Metabolism/termination of action of succinylcholine

- Termination of action when succinylcholine molecules diffuse away from neuromuscular junction (NMJ)
- Subsequent rapid metabolism by pseudocholinesterase (also called plasma cholinesterase or butyrylcholinesterase) in plasma

Table 13.3 Dibucaine number

	Inhibition by dibucaine	Duration of action of succinylcholine
Normal pseudocholinesterase	80%	5–10 min
Heterozygote for atypical pseudocholinesterase	40–60%	20–30 min
Homozygote for atypical pseudocholinesterase	20%	4–8 hr

Table 13.4 Drugs that decrease pseudocholinesterase activity

Cholinesterase inhibitors	Cyclophosphamide
Esmolol	Metoclopramide
Pancuronium	Oral contraceptives
Phenelzine	

Side Effects

- Bradycardia and nodal rhythms (after a 2nd dose in adults or initial dose in children)
- Fasciculations
- Myalgias
- ↑ Intragastric pressure (but also ↑ lower esophageal sphincter tone so no ↑ aspiration risk)
- ↑ Intraocular pressure
- Masseter muscle rigidity (a marked increase in tone that prevents laryngoscopy is abnormal and may be a sign of malignant hyperthermia [MH])
- Malignant hyperthermia trigger
- ↑ intracranial pressure. Can be attenuated by hyperventilation. Can be prevented with a defasciculating dose of a non-depolarizer (10–15% of usual intubating dose given about 5 minutes prior to succinylcholine)
- Histamine release (usually no adverse effect beyond a transient rash)
- Hyperkalemia. Typically increases K+ by 0.5 mEq/L.
  ○ K+ release is much more extensive after denervation injuries (see Table 13.5), which lead to up-regulation of extra-junctional ACh receptors
  ○ Risk is increased with increased amount of tissue affected
  ○ Period of risk starts 48 hours after injury, peaks at 7–10 days, unknown duration of risk (at least 60 days)

Absolute contraindications to succinylcholine are listed in Table 13.6.

Which side effects can be prevented by pre-treatment with a defasciculating dose of a non-depolarizer?
- Prevents fasciculations, which prevents increased abdominal pressure and ICP
- Decreases incidence of myalgias
- *Does not* prevent increased intraocular pressure

Non-Depolarizing Muscle Relaxants

Mechanism of Action

- Competitive antagonists at the ACh receptor

Table 13.5 Conditions causing susceptibility to succinylcholine-induced hyperkalemia

Burns
Crush injury/massive trauma
Spinal cord injury
Stroke
Guillain–Barré syndrome
Severe Parkinson's disease
Prolonged immobilization
Prolonged sepsis
Myopathies (e.g., Duchenne's)

Table 13.6 Contraindications to succinylcholine

- Hyperkalemia or susceptibility to succinylcholine-induced hyperkalemia
- Susceptibility to MH
- Open eye injuries
- Avoid routine use in children due to risk of undiagnosed myopathies

- Bind to ACh receptors but cannot induce necessary conformational change for channel opening and resultant ion flow.[1]
- Prevents ACh from binding to its receptor and generating an end-plate potential
- Neuromuscular blockade can occur with only one subunit blocked.

Pharmacokinetics

- Highly ionized and water-soluble due to quaternary ammonium groups, therefore they do not easily cross blood–brain barrier, placenta, or other lipid membranes.
- Classified by chemical structure as benzylisoquinoline or steroidal compounds
- Pharmacokinetic properties of individual drugs are listed in Table 13.7

Priming Dose

- Administering 10%–15% of the intubating dose 5 minutes before induction. Enough receptors are occupied to speed the onset of paralysis when the full dose is given. Rarely this can cause dyspnea, diplopia, dysphagia, or respiratory compromise.

Potentiation of Blockade

- Neuromuscular blockade can be augmented by a variety of factors (Table 13.8).

Antagonism of Blockade

Cholinesterase inhibitors (neostigmine, pyridostigmine, edrophonium, physostigmine)
- Cause increased levels of ACh at the NMJ. ACh competes with non-depolarizing agents to reestablish normal neuromuscular transmission.
- Ceiling effect: Once acetylcholinesterase is maximally inhibited, additional drug will not further increase block recovery. Therefore, neuromuscular blockade cannot be adequately reversed if high concentrations of muscle relaxant are still present at the NMJ.
- There should be evidence of spontaneous recovery (TOF count ≥ 2) prior to administration of cholinesterase inhibitors to avoid prolonged recovery times.
- Side effects: Bradycardia that can progress to sinus arrest, bronchospasm, nausea and vomiting, fecal incontinence, salivation, increased bladder tone, miosis
  ○ Physostigmine can cause diffuse cerebral excitation (the only cholinesterase inhibitor that is a tertiary amine and crosses the blood–brain barrier)

Table 13.7 Properties of non-depolarizing muscle relaxants

Drug name & chemical structure	Ed$_{95}$ (mg/kg)	Intubating dose (mg/kg)	Onset of action (min)	Duration of action (min)	Metabolism	Side effects & other clinically relevant facts
Atracurium (benzylisoquinoline)	0.2	0.5	2.5–3	30–45	Primarily by non-specific esterase hydrolysis (NOT pseudocholinesterase) Also by Hofmann elimination in plasma	• *Laudanosine* is a breakdown product of Hofmann elimination that is associated with CNS excitation and seizures. Laudanosine is metabolized by the liver and excreted renally • *Dose-dependent histamine release* • Can cause hypotension, tachycardia, bronchospasm, or anaphylaxis
Cisatracurium (benzyliso-quinoline)	0.05	0.15–0.2	2–3	40–75	Hofmann elimination (This process is slowed in hypothermia)	• Tends to produce less laudanosine than atracurium due to greater potency and therefore lower doses administered • *Not associated with histamine release, no autonomic effects*
Mivacurium (benzyliso-quinoline)	0.08	0.15–0.3	0.5–1	15–20	Pseudocholinesterase	• Block can last hours in patients homozygous for atypical pseudocholinesterase • Not available in the United States
Pancuronium (steroid)	0.07	0.08–0.12	2–3	60–120	Primarily by the liver, 40% renal excretion,10% bile excretion (Reduced clearance in renal and liver failure)	• Vagal blockade and sympathetic stimulation (increased catecholamine release and decreased catecholamine reuptake) • Dose-dependent tachycardia and hypertension • Increased likelihood of ventricular arrhythmias in predisposed patients
Vecuronium (steroid)	0.05	0.1–0.2	2–3	45–90	Minimal metabolism by liver, 75% bile excretion, 25% renal excretion (Duration of action somewhat prolonged in renal failure)	• No significant cardiovascular effects • Long-term administration in ICU patients can cause prolonged neuromuscular blockade possibly due to accumulation of its active 3-hydroxy metabolite and can lead to polyneuropathy in some patients
Rocuronium (steroid)	0.3	0.6	1.5	35–75	Almost no metabolism by liver. 10% renal excretion Primarily cleared by bile (Duration of action somewhat prolonged in severe hepatic failure)	• No active metabolites. No significant cardiovascular effects • Rapid onset (60–90 seconds) at higher dose (1.2 mg/kg) makes it a suitable alternative to succinylcholine for rapid sequence inductions

Table 13.8 Factors that potentiate neuromuscular blockade

Volatile agents	Decrease non-depolarizer dosage requirements by at least 15%. Desflurane > sevoflurane > isoflurane >N_2O
Combinations of non-depolarizers	Mixtures of structurally similar compounds produce additive effects; mixtures of structurally dissimilar compounds (ex. steroid + benzylisoquinoline) produce synergistic effects
Hypothermia	Decreases drug metabolism
Extremes of age	Neonates are more sensitive to non-depolarizers due to immature NMJs (though dosage requirements not significantly changed due to a larger volume of distribution) Reduced drug clearance in elderly populations
Electrolyte abnormalities	Acidosis, hypokalemia, hypocalcemia, hypermagnesemia augment blockade
Drug interactions	Antibiotics: aminoglycosides (streptomycin, gentamicin, tobramycin), tetracycline, polymyxin, clindamycin
Calcium channel blockers	Dantrolene, lithium, high-dose local anesthetics, furosemide
	Note: Chronic use of anti-epileptic drugs has an opposite effect and can increase resistance to non-depolarizers.

Anticholinergic Drugs (Glycopyrrolate, Atropine, Scopolamine)

- Paired with cholinesterase inhibitors to minimize unwanted muscarinic side effects
- Glycopyrrolate: Given with neostigmine based on similar time to onset of action
  - Quaternary amine. Does not cross blood–brain barrier. No effect on pupils or CNS
  - Does not cross placenta (although neostigmine does). Atropine should be used instead of glycopyrrolate when utilizing neostigmine for neuromuscular reversal in pregnancy.
- Atropine: Given with edrophonium based on more rapid onset of action
- Atropine and scopolamine are tertiary amines and cross the blood–brain barrier. Cause mydriasis, disorientation, and delirium.

Sugammadex

- Gamma-cyclodextrin that encapsulates steroidal muscle relaxants (rocuronium, vecuronium) and transports them away from the NMJ, thus preventing them from being competitive at ACh receptors.[2]
- Rapid and complete reversal of neuromuscular blockade within 2–3 minutes, even with profound neuromuscular blockade.[2]
- Dosing: 2 mg/kg if 2/twitches present on TOF; 4 mg/kg if 1/4 twitches present on TOF or one to two post tetanic; 16 mg/kg if 1.2 mg/kg dose of rocuronium used for rapid sequence intubation[2]

- If a patient requires paralysis after receiving a sugammadex dose, a non-steroidal muscle relaxant should be used.[2]
- Female patients using hormonal contraceptives should be counseled on reduced effectiveness after sugammadex administration due to unwanted encapsulation of steroidal structure drugs and the need for use of additional non-hormonal contraception method for 7 days.[2]
- Elimination of sugammadex and the sugammadex-rocuronium complex is primarily via renal excretion. Therefore, sugammadex use is currently not recommended for patients with severe renal impairment.[2]

Monitoring of Blockade

- Degree of neuromuscular blockade is commonly monitored with train-of-four (TOF) stimulation (four supramaximal stimuli at 2 Hz frequency).[1-4]
  - TOF ratio < 0.9 residual neuromuscular blockade
  - 1/4 twitches present: 90%–95% ACh receptors remain blocked
  - 2/4 twitches present: 80%–90% ACh receptors remain blocked
  - 3/4 twitches present: 70%–80% ACh receptors remain blocked
  - 4/4 twitches present: 65%–75% ACh receptors remain blocked

- Tetany is a sustained stimulus of 50–100 Hz usually lasting 5 seconds. Sustained tetanus corresponds to a TOF likely > 0.7. With non-depolarizing neuromuscular blockade there is potentiation of subsequent twitch responses after tetany due to increased availability of ACh. Post-tetanic potentiation is not seen with succinylcholine Phase I block.[2,3]
- The occurrence of fade indicates a non-depolarizing block or a Phase II block with succinylcholine (Figure 13.1).
  - Fade is likely explained by the prejunctional effect of non-depolarizing neuromuscular blockade decreasing the amount of ACh available for release in the pre-synaptic nerve terminal into the NMJ during stimulation.[2,3]
  - Phase II block with succinylcholine occurs when the repolarized post junctional membrane still does not respond normally to ACh stimulation.[2,3]

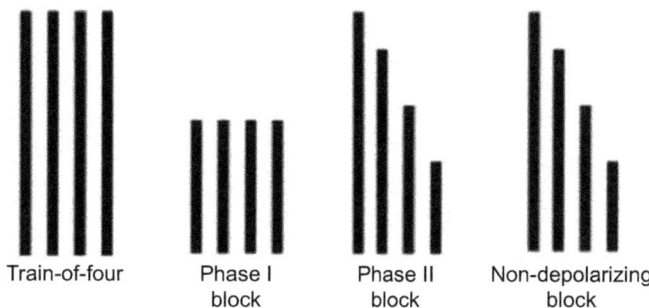

Figure 13.1 Train-of-four evoked responses to muscle relaxants.

Table 13.9 Response to muscle relaxants in myasthenia gravis and myasthenic syndrome

	Succinylcholine	Non-depolarizers
Myasthenia gravis Antibodies to acetylcholine receptors on skeletal muscle cause a decreased number of available Ach receptors.	Resistance: Exposure to a normal dose may not activate enough ACh receptors to result in perijunctional depolarization	Hypersensitivity (There are less receptors to block, so competitive inhibitors can cause a block at lower doses)
Eaton–Lambert (myasthenic syndrome) Antibodies to calcium channels causing reduced amount of presynaptic ACh release.	Hypersensitivity There are usually increased numbers of post-synaptic ACh receptors	Hypersensitivity (There is less ACh to compete with, so competitive inhibitors can cause a block at lower doses)

- Variable sensitivity of muscle groups to muscle relaxants
  - Diaphragm, muscles of larynx, and facial muscles are most resistant and recover the fastest. Good intubating conditions and surgical conditions associated with loss of eyebrow twitch response of the orbicularis oculi from stimulation of the facial nerve
  - Adductor pollicis and muscles of upper airway patency are more sensitive. Return of twitch response at thumb associated with good extubating conditions

Diseases with altered responses to muscle relaxants (Tables 13.9 and 13.10).

Table 13.10 Diseases with altered responses to non-depolarizing muscle relaxants

Hypersensitivity	Resistance
Myasthenia gravis	Burns
Eaton–Lambert	Stroke
ALS	Spinal cord injury
Lupus	Prolonged immobility
Familial periodic paralysis	Cerebral palsy
Guillain–Barré syndrome	Tetanus or botulism
Muscular dystrophy	
Myotonia	
Peripheral neuropathies	

References

1. Butterworth JF, Mackey DC, Wasnick JD. *Morgan & Mikhail's Clinical Anesthesiology*, 7th ed. McGraw-Hill Medical, 2022.

2. Gropper, MA, Eriksson LI, Fleisher LA, et al., editors. *Miller's Anesthesia*, 9th ed. Elsevier, 2020.

3. Pardo MC Jr. *Miller's Basics of Anesthesia*, 8th ed. Elsevier, 2023.

4. Barash, PC, Cahalan MK, Cullen BF, et al. *Clinical Anesthesia*, 8th ed. Lippincott Williams & Wilkins, 2017.

Understanding the Role of the Anesthesia Preop Evaluation

Barbara Orlando

Introduction

This chapter reviews the role and importance of preoperative assessment and evaluation. Preoperative assessments are designed to prepare patients to undergo anesthesia and surgery while incurring as little risk as possible.[1] The preoperative assessment gives the opportunity to collect patient information (through patient and/or family interviews centered on medical and anesthesia histories and medication list), and identify and stratify the risk in the hope of mitigating it by optimization of the patient's conditions. Assessing the patient's medical and surgical risks in the context of evidence-based guidelines is used to implement rational decision making when ordering appropriate additional workup (such as lab work or cardiac or pulmonary testing). Education regarding what to expect and how to prepare for anesthesia and surgery may also reduce the patient's and family's anxiety.

The goal of the preoperative assessment clinic is to allow for a standardized, evidence-based workup in preparation for the anesthesia and the surgery procedure. This has been shown to decrease morbidity and mortality. Those goals include:

- Evidence-based testing
  - Test only when clinically indicated and if the results will change your management (see this chapter's Appendix, part 1),[2] which will reduce excessive and unnecessary testing
  - Use national and international guidelines using the levels of evidence and classification of recommendations shown in this chapter's Appendix, part 2 and part 3.
- Communicating the risks to the patient and the other providers
  - Surgeon
  - Anesthesiologist
  - Medicine services
  - Social services, when indicated
  - Ultimately, the American Society of Anesthesiologists (ASA) classification is a way of assessing and communicating a patient's pre-anesthesia comorbidities (see this chapter's Appendix, part 4)
- Ensuring patient's optimization through
  - Consistent manner of assessment
  - Common systems and diseases to optimize

  - Cardiac
  - Pulmonary
  - Anemia
  - Obstructive sleep apnea
  - Smoking cessation
  - Physical reserve
  - Preventive vaccination status
  - Medication management
  - Opioid reduction
  - Treatment of depression or anxiety
  - Selective consultation with cardiology, pulmonary, hematology
  - Care pathways in place to streamline referrals or facilitate specific optimization goals
  - Adequate time left before scheduling surgery, allowing for optimization efforts (when possible)
  - Initiate appropriate medication which may reduce patient's risks such as
    - Statins
    - Beta blockers
- Minimizing reasons for surgical delays and cancellations due to
  - Inadequate preoperative workup
  - Change in patient's medical condition
  - Misunderstanding of recommendations made by non-anesthesiologist providers
- Contributing to the "triple aim" of the Affordable Care Act (ACA):
  - Improve patient experience
  - Improve population health
  - Reduce per capita cost
- Increasing satisfaction for patient and surgeon
  - Facilitating continuity of care from when surgery is scheduled through procedure and discharge
  - Facilitating communication among providers
  - Increasing patient's sense of trust by creating patient/anesthesia provider relationship prior to the day of the procedure
  - Educating patients
    - Communication regarding patient's risks
    - Communication regarding potential opportunities for health improvement and optimization
    - Anesthesia education

- Preoperative needs
  ○ Fasting/NPO guidelines
  ○ Perioperative anticoagulation guidelines
- Anesthetic technique options

Exceptions to the Rule

The level of urgency often dictates the degree of workup and/or optimization possible:

- Emergent: Threat to life or limb if no surgery < 6 hours
- Urgent: Life or limb threat if no surgery within 6–24 hours
- Time Sensitive: Delay of surgery for > 6 weeks will negatively affect outcome
- Elective: Surgery could be delayed up to 1 year without harm
- Surgery performed under emergency conditions will allow to proceed to the operating room with little or no further workup

THE NEED FOR PERIOPERATIVE INVASIVE MONITORING MAY BE INCREASED IN EMERGENCY SURGERIES.

- The most recent American College of Cardiology (ACC) and American Heart Association (AHA) Guidelines for Perioperative Cardiovascular Evaluation were updated in 2014.[3] For patients with coronary artery disease, the decision to delay surgery for additional workup can be made based on the following:
  1. If it is an emergency, proceed to surgery even if the patient has known cardiac risk factors.
  2. If the procedure is not an emergency and the patient is having acute coronary syndrome (ACS), patient should be referred to or the case should be discussed with a cardiologist for management of ACS prior to surgery.
  3. Estimate the risk of having a major adverse cardiac event (MACE) using risk calculators such as the American College of Surgeons National Surgery Quality Improvement Program (NSQIP) or the Revised Cardiac Risk Index (RCRI).
     a. NSQIP risk calculator includes: age, sex, BMI, functional status, ASA score, emergent case or not, and variables with patients who have a history of hypertension, diabetes, congestive heart failure (CHF), respiratory comorbidities and so on.
     b. RCRI calculator includes less data than the NSQIP: High-risk surgery (i.e., intraperitoneal, intrathoracic, supra-inguinal vascular), history of ischemic heart disease, history of CHF, history of cerebrovascular disease, insulin-dependent diabetes, and preoperative creatinine of > 2 mg/dL
  4. If MACE risk is < 1%, the patient is deemed as low risk and can proceed with surgery without any additional testing.

5. If MACE risk is > 1%, their functional capacity needs to be determined.
   a. If metabolic equivalents (METS) > 4, proceed with surgery without any further testing
   b. If METS < 4 or functional capacity cannot be determined, the team needs to determine whether further testing will impact the decision making or perioperative care.
      i. If further testing is recommended, obtain stress test followed by coronary revascularization if the stress test is abnormal

- Risk identification and mitigation is important in determining how best to manage patient and proceed with surgery.[4] It may be necessary to delay surgery for:
  ○ Cardiac or pulmonary comorbidities requiring additional information to assess risk of surgery vs benefit of procedure
  ○ To allow for preoperative risk mitigation and patient optimization
- Workup is necessary in patients with:
  ○ High-grade Mobitz type II or 3rd degree block
  ○ Symptomatic ventricular arrhythmias
  ○ Severe/symptomatic aortic or mitral valve stenosis
  ○ Pulmonary hypertension
  ○ Severe respiratory pathology
  ○ Stable angina
- Preoperative laboratory testing
  ○ No tests required in healthy patients undergoing surgery with low risk of complications. However, a urine pregnancy or blood HCG test should be ordered for all women of childbearing age unless they have had a hysterectomy.
  ○ Order tests based on
    ▪ History
    ▪ Physical exam
    ▪ Medications
    ▪ Type of surgery
  ○ Do not test based on "someone might want it"
  ○ Predictive value
    ▪ Normal test values are defined as results that are within 2 standard deviations of the mean
      • Five percent of patients receiving a test will have an abnormal result
    ▪ Test results in healthy patients have a low predictive value for disease
    ▪ False positives
      • Increase the likelihood of further testing
      • May delay surgery
      • May lead to medico-legal issues when not acted upon
      • May refer to NICE clinical guidelines[5] from the National Institute for Health and Care Excellence in England and Wales (www.nice.org.uk)

Appendix

1. **Common Preoperative Evaluations and Their Levels of Evidence**
   - EKG: Level B evidence, no Class I recommendation for acquiring an EKG
   - Echocardiogram: No Class I recommendation
   - Balloon Angioplasty: Class I recommendation to wait 14 days after a balloon angioplasty before proceeding with non-cardiac surgery, 30 days after bare metal stent and 6 months after drug eluting stent
   - Beta Blockers: Class I recommendation to continue beta blockers in patients on chronic beta blocker therapy
     - In patients with more than three RCRI risk factors, it is reasonable to start beta-blocker therapy BUT not on the day of the surgery

2. **Classification of Recommendations**
   - Class I: Benefit ≫ Risk, no additional studies needed
     - Proceed with procedure/treatment
   - Class IIa: Benefit ≫ Risk, additional studies with focused objectives needed
     - It is reasonable to proceed with procedure/treatment
   - Class IIb: Benefit × Risk, additional studies with broad objectives needed
     - It is unreasonable to proceed with procedure/treatment
   - Class III: Risk > Benefit, no additional studies needed
     - Do not proceed with procedure/treatment

3. **Level of Evidence**
   - Level A: Multiple populations evaluated with general consistency of direction and magnitude of effect with robust evidence to recommend a procedure/treatment
   - Level B: Limited populations evaluated with a balance of evidence and procedure/treatment is recommended with caution
   - Level C: Very limited populations evaluated with inadequate evidence and a procedure/treatment is recommended based on consensus opinion.

4. **American Society of Anesthesiologists (ASA) Physical Status Classification**
   1. Normal, healthy patient
   2. Patient with mild systemic disease
   3. Patient with severe systemic disease but the disease is not a threat to life
   4. Patient with severe systemic disease that is a constant threat to life
   5. Moribund patient not expected to survive without the surgery
   6. Brain dead patient for organ donation

References

1. Forkin, KT, Nemergut EC. Anesthesiology. In Miller R, editor. *Miller's Anesthesia*, 8th ed. Churchill Livingstone/Elsevier, 2016; pp 977–978.

2. Committee on Standard and Practice Parameters, et al. Practice Advisory for Preanesthesia Evaluation: an updated report by the American Society of Anesthesiologists Task Force on Preanesthesia Evaluation. *Anesthesiology* 2012;**116** (3):522–538.

3. Fleisher LA, Fleischmann KE, Auerbach AD, et al. American College of Cardiology; American Heart Association. 2014 ACC/AHA guideline on perioperative cardiovascular evaluation and management of patients undergoing noncardiac surgery: a report of the American College of Cardiology/American Heart Association Task Force on practice guidelines. *J Am Coll Cardiol* 2014 Dec 9;**64**(22):e77–137.

4. Moonesinghe SR, Mythen MG, Das P, Rowan KM, Grocott MP. Risk stratification tools for predicting morbidity and mortality in adult patients undergoing major surgery: qualitative systematic review. *Anesthesiology* 2013 Oct;**119**(4):959–981.

5. National Guideline Centre (UK). *Preoperative Tests (Update): Routine Preoperative Tests for Elective Surgery.* London: National Institute for Health and Care Excellence (NICE), 2016 Apr. (NICE Guideline No. 45), p 1, Guideline summary.

Preparation for General Anesthesia and Premedication

John Yin, Daniel G. Springer, and Theresa A. Gelzinis

Before taking a patient to the operating room, premedication is frequently administered to alleviate anxiety, to treat current or to ameliorate postoperative pain, or to prevent postoperative nausea and vomiting. The most common anxiolytic drug class is the benzodiazepines with midazolam being the most widely used. Analgesic premedication is more varied and, depending on the type of anesthetic used, can consist of opioids, most commonly fentanyl, anti-inflammatory medications, such as ibuprofen, ketorolac, or acetaminophen, gabapentinoids, and other sedative-hypnotics with analgesic properties, such as ketamine and dexmedetomidine. Similarly, antiemetic agents are varied in their pharmacodynamics and include ondansetron, aprepitant, and transdermal scopolamine. The choice of agent depends on the number of risk factors for postoperative nausea and vomiting (PONV) the patient has, previous episodes of PONV, and patient tolerance to the drug. When administering these medications to patients, it is important to know their mechanism of action, physiological effects, and metabolism under the influence of various patient comorbidities or chronic preoperative medications.

Interactions with Chronic Medications and General Anesthetics

Benzodiazepines

- GABA$_A$ receptor agonist
- Midazolam 0.5 mg/kg PO or 0.1 mg/kg IV in children has been shown to reduce preoperative anxiety.
  - Onset of PO 10 minutes, peak effect in 20–30 minutes
  - Onset of IV 60 seconds, peak effect in 10 minutes
- Midazolam adult dosing often between 1 and 4 mg as an IV bolus
  - Avoidance of administration in elderly patients (age > 65) given concerns for postoperative delirium and cognitive dysfunction
  - Can administer to an elderly patient on chronic benzodiazepine therapy, but dose reduction may be required
- Combination with other agents, such as the opioids can lead to significant respiratory depression and hypotension due to synergism (e.g., fentanyl and midazolam) and can reduce propofol dose and volatile MAC in a dose-dependent fashion. This is helpful in the patient who has hemodynamic instability and is unable to tolerate large doses of propofol and volatile agents.

- Hepatic metabolism of midazolam and diazepam via CYP3A makes them vulnerable to interactions with other agents that induce and inhibit the CYP family of enzymes (see Table 15.1).

Ketamine

- NMDA antagonist
- Premedication dosing
  - Adult
    - 1–2mg/kg IV
    - 4–5mg/kg IM as single dose
    - Geriatric dosing as above
  - Pediatric
    - IV and IM same as adults
    - 6–10 mg/kg PO as single dose
- Often co-administration of a benzodiazepine to reduce hallucinogenic effects
- Low-dose ketamine can be used as a preemptive analgesic
- Side effects: Increased secretions, hallucinations, nausea/vomiting, myoclonus, and possible intraocular pressure

Dexmedetomidine

- Selective alpha-2 agonist with analgesic and sedative effects in the locus ceruleus and spinal cord with minimal amnestic properties
- Same class as clonidine but more selective for alpha-2 vs. alpha-1 adrenergic receptors
- Premedication dosing
  - Adult and pediatric
    - 0.5–1 mcg/kg bolus
    - Dose reduction in geriatric patients
- Induces sedation via sleep promoting pathways unlike propofol or other GABA agonists
- Side effects: Bradycardia, hypertension, when bloused, via vasoconstriction of peripheral alpha-2 receptors, hypotension

Fentanyl

- Opioid analgesic mu-receptor agonist
- Premedication dosing
  - Adult
    - 50–100 mcg IV/IM 60 minutes prior to surgery or 25–50 mcg IV immediately before induction
    - Dose reduction in geriatric patients
  - Pediatric
    - 1–2 mcg/kg IV prior to surgery

Table 15.1 Significant cytochrome P450 enzymes and their inhibitors, inducers, and substrates

Enzyme	Potent inhibitors	Potent inducers	Substrates
CYP1A2	Cimetidine, ciprofloxacin, fluvoxamine, rucaparib, vemurafenib	Carbamazepine, omeprazole rifampin, tobacco	Caffeine, clozapine, estradiol, naproxen, ondansetron, ropivacaine, theophylline
CYP2B6	Clopidogrel, ticlopidine, voriconazole	Carbamazepine, efavirenz, phenobarbital, phenytoin, rifampin	Ketamine, meperidine, methadone, propofol, tramadol
CYP2C9	Amiodarone, fluconazole, metronidazole, ritonavir, sulfamethoxazole, sulfaphenazole	Carbamazepine, phenobarbital, phenytoin, rifampin	Amitriptyline, celecoxib, clopidogrel, glipizide, ibuprofen, irbesartan, losartan, meloxicam, naproxen, warfarin, valproic acid
CYP2C19	Cimetidine, esomeprazole, fluconazole, fluoxetine, fluvoxamine, isoniazid, ketoconazole, omeprazole, ticlopidine	Carbamazepine, phenytoin, prednisone, rifampin, ritonavir, St. John's wort	Amitriptyline, clopidogrel, diazepam, labetalol, omeprazole, phenobarbital, phenytoin, warfarin
CYP2D6	Amiodarone, bupropion, cimetidine, diphenhydramine, duloxetine, fluoxetine, paroxetine, quinidine, ritonavir, terbinafine	No significant inducers	Amitriptyline, carvedilol, clonidine, codeine, donepezil, flecainide, haloperidol, metoprolol, paroxetine, risperidone, tramadol
CYP3A4 CYP3A5 CYP3A7	Aprepitant, ciprofloxacin, clarithromycin, diltiazem, fluconazole, erythromycin, grapefruit juice, imatinib, itraconazole, ketoconazole, nefazodone, ritonavir, telithromycin, verapamil, voriconazole	Barbiturates, carbamazepine, St. John's wort, glucocorticoids, phenytoin, rifampin	Alfentanil, Alprazolam, amlodipine, apixaban, aprepitant, atorvastatin, clopidogrel, dexamethasone, cyclosporine, fentanyl, lidocaine, methadone, midazolam, ondansetron, sildenafil, verapamil, zolpidem

Table adapted from Flockhart DA, Thacker, D., McDonald, C., Desta, Z. The Flockhart Cytochrome P450 Drug-Drug Interaction Table. Division of Clinical Pharmacology, Indiana University School of Medicine (updated 2021). https://drug-interactions.medicine.iu.edu. Accessed [12/05/2022].

- Chronic pain patients may present with transdermal fentanyl patches
- Side effects: Respiratory depression, itching, chest wall rigidity, cough

Postoperative Nausea and Vomiting Treatments

- Risk factors for PONV in adults per Apfel score include female sex, history of PONV and/or motion sickness, nonsmoking status, gastroparesis, opioid and cannabis use.
  - Incidence of PONV within 24-hour postoperative period with the presence of four risk factors is approximately 80%
  - Other factors include general vs. regional anesthesia, use of volatile gases and nitrous oxide (use over duration of 1 hour), and type of and duration of surgery. Surgeries that are known to contribute to PONV include laparoscopic, gynecological, eye, ENT, and intracranial.
  - Pediatric PONV have slightly different risk factors including age > 3, history and family history of PONV, post-pubertal female, surgical risk factors including duration greater than 30 minutes, strabismus surgery, adenotonsillectomy, otoplasty and use of volatile anesthetics, anticholinesterases, and opioids
- PONV prophylaxis given before induction include:
  - Ondansetron
    - 5-HT$_3$ receptor antagonist
    - Considered gold standard in PONV management. Other generation of 5-HT$_3$ antagonists such as granisetron or palonosetron may be more effective.
      - Premedication dose at 4 mg IV although usually given at end of surgery
  - Amisulpride
    - Dopamine D2, D3 receptor antagonist
    - Side effects include mildly elevated prolactin level
  - Aprepitant
    - NK1 receptor antagonist
    - Has half-life of 40 hours with more reduction of vomiting than nausea.
  - Dexamethsasone
    - Does not have significant mineralocorticoid effect. PONV dosing of 4–8 mg IV with no increased risk of bleeding, infection, or significant increase in blood glucose
  - Antihistamines dimenhydrinate, diphenhydramine, and promethazine can all be used for PONV prophylaxis
  - Scopolamine patch onset of action is around 2–4 hours with mild side effects including visual hallucinations, dry mouth, and dizziness.
- In general, combination therapy is recommended over single drug therapy as the effects of antiemetics are additive if acting on different receptors (exception is metoclopramide).

Concerns with Specific Disease States

Thyroid Dysfunction (Hypothyroidism and Hyperthyroidism)

- Hyperthyroidism
  - Patients with increased metabolism due to elevated thyroid hormone levels
  - Thionamide medications (e.g., PTU), nonspecific beta blockers, such as propranolol and glucocorticoids should be administered to decrease hormone release in emergent cases.
  - May require higher doses of medications to achieve same level of sedation
  - Avoid drugs that stimulate the sympathetic nervous system (e.g., ketamine).
  - Opioid premedication safe in these patients
- Hypothyroidism
  - Patients may be extremely sensitive to any sedative medication
  - Limit the dose or administration of preoperative sedatives
  - Delayed gastric emptying may increase the risk of emesis and aspiration

Uremia

- Extreme levels of urea can lead to sedation and neurological changes; therefore, avoidance of further sedation is advised.

Increased Intracranial Pressure

- Minimize sedative medications as any increase in $PaCO_2$ from hypoventilation may lead to increased cerebral vasodilation, cerebral blood flow, and further increases in ICP.

Chronic Steroids

- Will likely require stress-doses of steroids to prevent perioperative hypotension from deficient cortisol levels
- Guidelines differ on the management and dosing of preoperative glucocorticoid coverage but recommend individualized approach.
  - Stress dose steroid recommendations:
    - Non-suppressed hypothalamic–pituitary–adrenal (HPA) axis: patients taking < 5 mg prednisone for < 3 weeks or taking < 10 mg every other day
      - Continue with routine glucocorticoid regimen
    - Suppressed HPA axis: patients taking > 20 mg prednisone for > 3 weeks or have Cushingoid appearance with likely have HPA suppression
      - For minor stress procedures: continue routine glucocorticoid regimen with no extra supplementation
      - For moderate stress procedures (e.g., joint replacement): continue routine glucocorticoid regimen + 50 mg hydrocortisone IV at induction + 25 mg IV q 8 hr for 24 hr
      - For major stress procedures (e.g., large abdominal cases, open heart surgery): continue routine glucocorticoid regimen + 100 mg hydrocortisone IV at induction + 50 mg IV q 8 hr for 24 hr
  - Note: Taper dose by half per day to routine maintenance level.

Obesity

- Often associated with obstructive sleep apnea, hypertension
- More sensitive to sedatives; use sedatives with caution using lean body weight and titrating to effect
- Can use any of the commonly utilized sedative if patient is monitored closely

Obstructive Sleep Apnea

- Often avoidance of sedative medications advised given concern for airway obstruction
- Dexmedetomidine can be a useful anxiolytic for the extremely anxious patient, as it can preserve respiratory drive better than the other sedatives.

Depression

- May require increased doses of premedication due to alterations in baseline catecholamine levels from antidepressant therapy in the CNS
- Current antidepressant regimen must be known, as there may be potential for interactions between antidepressants and anesthetic medications that can lead to serious adverse reactions such as:
  - Serotonin syndrome: Can occur with the selective serotonin reuptake inhibitors, such as citalopram, fluoxetine, paroxetine, sertraline, venlafaxine, dextromethorphan, tramadol, and trazodone
    - Management: Stop offending agent, support hemodynamics, control hyperthermia
  - Neuroleptic malignant syndrome: Can occur with the antipsychotic agents haloperidol, perphenazine, risperidone, and thioridazine, the antiemetic agents droperidol, metoclopramide, prochlorperazine, and promethazine, and with the withdrawal of anti-Parkinson medications
    - Management: Stop offending agent, support hemodynamics, control hyperthermia, dantrolene for muscle rigidity or dopamine agonist such as bromocriptine
  - Tardive dyskinesia: Involuntary, repetitive movements caused from use of high-dose antipsychotics
    - Management: Stop offending agent, support hemodynamics, symptomatic control, medications for treatment include reserpine, ondansetron, donepezil, clonidine, baclofen
- In patients who are taking monoamine oxidase inhibitors (MAOIs), the use of meperidine can result in serotonin syndrome and hyperpyrexia. Due to its mechanism of

action, hypotension should be treated with direct acting agents, such as phenylephrine.

- Patients taking cyclic antidepressants may have exaggerated response to anticholinergic medications such as scopolamine. leading to postoperative confusion.
- The evidence between SSRI and risk of bleeding is not well established and current recommendation is to continue antidepressants.

Chronic Obstructive Pulmonary Disease (COPD)

- Attempt to minimize sedation given concerns for reduction in respiratory drive leading to development of worsening hypercapnia and hypoxia
- Preinduction anticholinergic and/or beta agonist inhalers may be useful in preventing perioperative bronchospasm and postoperative pulmonary complications
- Patients using long-term steroid inhalers or taking oral steroid medications may require intraoperative stress dose steroids. The risk of wound infections is low.

Hypertension

- Avoid sedative medications that can increase blood pressure (e.g., ketamine) in the immediate preoperative period.
- Depending on antihypertensive agents, patients may have exaggerated blood pressure responses to sedatives.

NPO and Full Stomach Status

- Table 15.2 shows updated guidelines from the American Society of Anesthesiologists published March 2017.
- Note in Table 15.2 the recommendations for the use of medications to modify gastric pH, volume, and sphincter tone.
- Patients that have violated these NPO guidelines for elective surgery should be postponed until NPO appropriate.
- General endotracheal anesthesia can be used to help minimize the risk of pulmonary aspiration. It is prudent to avoid all anesthetics compromising the airway and laryngeal mask airways.
- Airway management for a patient with a full stomach should include a rapid sequence induction (RSI). The utility of cricoid pressure remains controversial but is considered standard of care.
- In addition to NPO status, patients must be evaluated for any underlying medical condition that may lead to decreased gastric emptying or increased gastrointestinal transit time such as diabetes, GERD, morbid obesity, small bowel obstruction.

Continuation vs. Discontinuation of Chronic Medications

- Antihypertensives
  - Beta blockers: should be continued in the perioperative period.
  - Discontinuation of ACE Inhibitors and ARBs (24 hours) prior to surgery is encouraged to minimize

Table 15.2 Fasting and pharmacological recommendations

A. Fasting recommendations[*]

Ingested material	Minimum fasting period[†]
• Clear liquids[‡]	2 hr
• Breast milk	4 hr
• Infant formula	6 hr
• Nonhuman milk[§]	6 hr
• Light meal[**]	6 hr
• Fried foods, fatty foods, or meat	Additional fasting time (e.g., 8 or more hr) may be needed

B. Pharmacological recommendations

Medication type and common examples	Recommendations
Gastrointestinal stimulants:	
• Metoclopramide	May be used/no routine use
Gastric acid secretion blockers:	
• Cimetidine	May be used/no routine use
• Famotidine	May be used/no routine use
• Ranitidine	May be used/no routine use
• Omeprazole	May be used/no routine use
• Lansoprazole	May be used/no routine use
Antacids:	
• Sodium citrate	May be used/no routine use
• Sodium bicarbonate	May be used/no routine use
	May be used/no routine use
• Magnesium silicate	
Antiemetics:	
• Ondansetron	May be used/no routine use
Anticholinergics:	
• Atropine	No use
• Scopolamine	No use
• Glycopyrrolate	No use
Combinations of the medications above:	No routine use

[*] These recommendations apply to healthy patients who are undergoing elective procedures. They are not intended for women in labor. Following the guidelines does not guarantee complete gastric emptying.

[†] The fasting periods noted above apply to all ages.

[‡] Examples of clear liquids include water, fruit juices without pulp, carbonated beverages, clear tea, and black coffee.

[§] Since nonhuman milk is similar to solids in gastric emptying time, the amount Ingested must be considered when determining an appropriate fasting period.

[**] A light meal typically consists of toast and clear liquids. Meals that include fried or fatty foods or meat may prolong gastric emptying time. Additional fasting time (e.g., 8 or more hr) may be needed in these cases. Both the amount and type of foods ingested must be considered when determining an appropriate fasting period.

hypotension from vasodilation and effective hypovolemia.
  - Calcium channel blockers can be continued in the perioperative period, especially if the patient has pulmonary hypertension.
  - Diuretics: no consensus on continuation vs. discontinuation
  - Clonidine: should be continued to avoid rebound hypertension.

- Antihyperglycemics
  - All PO agents should be held prior to surgery to prevent perioperative hypoglycemia.
  - Long-acting insulin dosages should be reduced prior to patient being made NPO.
- Psychotropic Medications
  - SSRIs/SNRIs: Can be continued into the perioperative period (limited data for SNRIs)
  - TCAs: Can be continued
  - Buproprion: No data available
  - MAOIs: Can be continued
  - Valproate and lithium: Should be continued, close monitoring of patient on lithium
  - Antipsychotics: Can be continued but may potentiate effects of sedative/opioids
  - Antianxiety: Can be continued
  - Psychostimulants (e.g., methylphenidate): Can safely be discontinued
- Anticoagulants
  - Each has a specific time frame for discontinuation to allow full coagulation.
  - Warfarin: Discontinue 5 days before surgery if deemed appropriate
  - Dabigatran: Discontinue 2–3 days before surgery
  - Rivaroxaban: Discontinue 2–3 days before surgery
  - Apixaban: Discontinue 2–3 days before surgery
  - Edoxaban: Discontinue 2–3 days before surgery
  - Herbal medications such as garlic may increase bleeding and should be discontinued a week prior to surgery.
- Antiplatelet Agents
  - If deemed appropriate based on indication for initiation and type of surgery being performed, these may or may not be discontinued
  - Aspirin: Discontinue 7–10 days before surgery
  - Clopidogrel and ticagrelor: Discontinue at least 5 days before surgery
  - Prasugrel: Discontinue at least 7 days before surgery
- Digoxin
  - Can continue before surgery. Obtaining drug level preoperatively is not usually needed.
- Opioids and Opioid Agonists–Antagonists
  - Methadone: Continue normal PO dose on the morning of surgery; if unable to take PO, IV methadone can be dosed parenterally at one-half to two-thirds the maintenance dose divided into 2–4 equal doses a day.
  - Buprenorphine: There are no clear guidelines but there is a recommendation that buprenorphine can be continued into the perioperative period.

Prophylactic Cardiac Risk Reduction
- All patients should be evaluated for cardiac risk prior to surgery

- Preoperative revascularization.
  - Except in setting of acute coronary syndrome, not recommended as has not been shown to improve outcomes
- Preoperative Beta Blockade
  - Numerous trials have supported the continuation of chronic beta blockade therapy in patients on these agents for specific indications (e.g., prior MI, atrial fibrillation rate control, heart failure).
    - No outcomes have been shown to be better for one agent over another.
  - Initiation of beta blockade is not recommended for prevention in non-cardiac surgery due to increase stroke and 30-day mortality.
- Antiplatelet Therapy
  - Recommendation to hold prophylactic aspirin 5–7 days before surgery and to not initiate an aspirin regimen prior to noncardiac surgery
  - Other antiplatelet agents as indicated above
- Statin Therapy
  - Continuation of statins in the perioperative period encouraged
  - May initiate statin therapy in patients prior to surgery if indicated
- ACE Inhibitors and ARBs
  - Discontinuation for at least 24 hours prior to surgery encouraged
  - Initiation in the immediate perioperative period not recommended
  - Chronic therapy may be continued if indicated by clinical conditions.
- Nitrate Therapy
  - Prophylactic administration/initiation is not recommended.

Prophylactic Antibiotics
- Goal is prevention of surgical site infections (SSI).
- Cefazolin is drug of choice for many procedures due to study-proven efficacy and spectrum of coverage although other agents may be chosen based on specific microorganism risks associated with a specific procedure.
- Repeat administration timing specific to each antimicrobial drug but generally done when procedure length is greater than 2.5 half-lives of drug and/or blood loss greater than 1,500 mL
- Greatest risk with administration of antimicrobial drugs is allergic reaction
  - Concern for cross-reactive reaction between penicillin and cephalosporins
    - Safe to administer a cephalosporin if no history of reaction to other cephalosporins and reaction to penicillin is not anaphylaxis.
    - There is < 2% cross reactivity between the two classes.

Further Reading

Anderson DJ. Antimicrobial prophylaxis for prevention of surgical site infection in adults. In Hall KK, editor. *UpToDate.* UpToDate Inc., 2022. Available at: www .uptodate.com/contents/antimicrobial-pro phylaxis-for-prevention-of-surgical-site-inf ection-in-adults

Devereaux PJ, Cohn SL, Eagle KA. Management of cardiac risk for noncardiac surgery. In Yeon SB, editor. *UpToDate.* UpToDate Inc., 2023. Available at: www.uptodate.com/con tents/management-of-cardiac-risk-for-n oncardiac-surgery

Hemmings HC, Egan TD. *Pharmacology and Physiology for Anesthesia: Foundations and Clinical Application.* Elsevier/Saunders, 2013.

Hines RL, Jones SB, editors. *Stoelting's Anesthesia and Co-Existing Disease*, 8th ed. Elsevier, 2021.

Muluk V, Cohn SL, Whinney C. Perioperative medication management. In Givens J, editor. *UpToDate.* UpToDate Inc., 2024. Available at: www.uptodate.com/con tents/perioperative-medication-management.

Practice guidelines for preoperative fasting and the use of pharmacologic agents to reduce the risk of pulmonary aspiration: application to healthy patients undergoing elective procedures: an updated report by the American Society of Anesthesiologists Task Force on Preoperative Fasting and the Use of Pharmacologic Agents to Reduce the Risk of Pulmonary Aspiration. *Anesthesiology* 2017;**126**(3):376–393.

Regional Anesthesia

Ali Shariat and Poonam Pai

Preparation for Neuraxial and Regional Blocks

Confirm three "must's" before proceeding: Informed consent, resuscitation equipment, intravenous (IV) access

- **Premedication and Sedation:** Provide anxiolytic with short-acting benzodiazepine and as needed analgesic with short-acting opioid during performance of the block, while maintaining meaningful communication with the patient.
- **Monitoring:** Place standard American Society of Anesthesiologists (ASA) monitors including pulse oximetry and noninvasive blood pressure before each block. Electrocardiography and end-tidal CO_2 should be available along with supplemental oxygen. A thermometer may be placed in the operating room.
- **Position:** For regional blocks, position patients comfortably with maximizing block site exposure. Operator should stand in a position comfortable for ultrasound use and needle placement. For neuraxial blocks, patients can be in sitting, lateral decubitus, or prone position.
- **Equipment:** For regional blocks: Chlorhexidine prep, ultrasound with gel and probe cover, +/− nerve stimulator, block needle (+catheter kit if continuous block), local anesthetic (LA) syringes, additives/sedatives/rescue drugs, standardized checklist

For neuraxial blocks: Chlorhexidine prep, sterile spinal needles or epidural kits, local anesthetic (LA)/additives/sedatives/rescue drugs, sterile gloves, mask, ultrasound if needed

Neuraxial Blocks (Spinal, Epidural, Caudal, Combined Spinal/Epidural)

Indications

- Anesthesia for procedures involving the lower limbs, lower abdomen, pelvis and perineum, long-lasting analgesia for labor and delivery, laparotomy and thoracotomy, chronic pain treatments – Particularly useful in patients with severe respiratory disease, difficult airway, obstetrics

Contraindications

- Absolute: Patient refusal, infection at site of injection, allergy to any drug to be administered, inability to maintain stillness, increased intracranial pressure
- Relative: Preexisting central or peripheral neuropathy (double crush phenomenon), structural issues with spine, multiple sclerosis, aortic stenosis, refractory hypovolemia, coagulopathy, patients on antithrombotic and thrombolytic therapies, active systemic infection

Mechanism and Sites of Action

- Combination of blockade of sympathetic, sensory and/or motor systems, along with compensatory reflexes and unopposed parasympathetic activity
- Progression happens in following order → small B fibers → C fibers (cold temperature) → A delta fibers (pinprick sensation) → A beta fibers (touch) → A alpha fibers (motor)
- Regression follows reverse order.

Physiological Effects

- Cardiovascular: Reduction in SVR, CO, BP, and HR is seen
  - Extent of hemodynamic changes is determined by block height and baseline sympathetic tone.
  - Block below T4: Sympathetic fibers from T5–L1 maintain vasomotor tone. Arterial and venous vasodilation lead to ↓ SVR (afterload) and ↓ preload (preload). ↓ venous return leads to ↓ right atrial pressure, ↓ stroke volume and ↓ cardiac output. Initial ↑ HR due to hypotension.
  - Block above T4: Blockade of cardiac accelerator fibers (T1–T4). Results in ↓ cardiac contractility, ↓ BP and ↓ HR.
  - Sympathectomy extends 2–6 dermatomes cephalad to the sensory block with spinal, both levels are same with epidural
  - In hypovolemic patients, Bezold–Jarisch reflex can cause profound bradycardia and circulatory collapse
- Central Nervous System
  - Spinal can cause significant sedation by itself due to decreased afferent stimulation of reticular activating system, may need to reduce dose of hypnotics and anxiolytics.
  - Though cerebral perfusion may drop, no study has shown postoperative cognitive changes.
- Respiratory
  - ↓ vital capacity from paralysis of abdominal muscles but sparing of diaphragm, pronounced in patients with severe respiratory disease or obesity

○ Still preferred for analgesic effects after thoracoabdominal surgery as it renders improvement in respiratory function

- Gastrointestinal
  ○ Unopposed parasympathetic effects include ↑ gut mucosal blood flow barring systemic hypotension, may ↑ gut peristalsis, ↑ secretions, sphincters relax, bowel constriction, slight reduction of hepatic blood flow
  ○ Effects on anastomotic healing and postoperative ileus are areas of ongoing research.
  ○ Nausea and vomiting risk increases with hypotension and concomitant opioid administration.
- Renal
  ○ Urinary retention from weak detrusor due to S2, S3, and S4 blockade

Technique (Midline)

- Spinal anesthesia: LA placement between L2 and L4 levels
  ○ Needle trajectory from posterior to anterior: Skin →subcutaneous tissue → supraspinous ligament → interspinous ligament → ligamentum flavum → dura mater → arachnoid mater → subarachnoid space (Table 16.1)
  ○ Indication: Cesarean deliveries, surgeries involving lower abdomen, lower limbs, and pelvic organs
- Epidural anesthesia: LA placement in epidural space
  ○ Needle trajectory from posterior to anterior: Skin → subcutaneous tissue → supraspinous ligament → interspinous ligament → ligamentum flavum → epidural space
  ○ Indication: Labor analgesia, acute pain management after major abdominal/thoracic surgery (Table 16.2)
- Caudal anesthesia: LA placement in sacral portion of *epidural space*
  ○ Needle trajectory from posterior to anterior: skin→ subcutaneous tissue → sacrococcygeal ligament → caudal space

Table 16.1 Factors influencing spinal block height

Factors	More Important	Less Important	Not Important
Drug factors	Dose baricity	Volume Concentration Temperature of injection Viscosity	Additives other than opioids
Patient factors	CSF volume Advanced age pregnancy	Weight Height Spinal anatomy Intra-abdominal pressure	Menopause Gender
Procedure factors	Patient position Epidural following spinal	Level of injection Fluid currents Needle orifice direction Needle type	

Table 16.2 Factors influencing epidural block height

Factors	More important	Less important	Not important
Drug factors	Volume dose	Concentration	Additives
Patient factors	Elderly pregnancy	Weight Height Pressure in adjacent cavities	
Procedure factors	Level of injection	Position	Speed of injection Needle orifice direction

○ Indication: Surgery and acute analgesia in children, chronic analgesia in adults

- Combined spinal epidural (CSE): Combination of spinal and epidural
  ○ Same trajectory as spinal, can be performed with "needle-through-through" technique or separate needle insertions in same or different interspace
  ○ Spinal provides rapid onset of predictable block and epidural catheter provides *possibility for long-lasting analgesia with dose titration.*

Pharmacology

- Local Anesthetics
  ○ Short- and intermediate-acting: Procaine, chloroprocaine, lidocaine, prilocaine, mepivacaine are rarely used due to associated side effects like transient neurological symptoms
  ○ Long-acting: Bupivacaine most commonly used, rarely cause TNS, ropivacaine gives slightly less motor block, tetracaine provides unreliable duration
- Additives
  ○ **Opioids**: Hydrophilic preservative-free morphine can last up to 24 hours, lipophilic fentanyl and sufentanil are commonly used in obstetrics.
  ○ **Factors Influencing Onset of Action**
    ▪ Bicarbonate: Increases non-ionized form of the drug, allowing it to penetrate nerve cell membranes and speed the process of intraneural diffusion
  ○ **Factors Influencing Duration**
    ▪ Epinephrine: Increases duration by decreasing systemic absorption
    ▪ Alpha-2 agonist: Hyperpolarization at the ventral horn of spinal cord
    ▪ Side effects of neuraxial clonidine: Hypotension, bradycardia, dry mouth, and sedation

Test dose: A small test dose of LA with epinephrine (3 mL of lidocaine 1.5% with epinephrine 1:200,000) is injected into the epidural catheter to reduce the risk of keeping a catheter in a place that is intravascular or intrathecal.

- Positive test dose: ↑ HR by 20% or greater, tinnitus, dysgeusia, perioral numbness/tingling indicates intravascular injection. Significant motor block within 5 minutes of administering test dose indicates intrathecal injection.

Termination of Action

- Blood flow to spinal cord: Elimination is by vascular absorption through subarachnoid and epidural blood vessels.

Complications

- Neurological
- Paraplegia
  - Mechanism: Direct needle trauma, vertebral canal hematoma, epidural abscess, periprocedural hypotension, adhesive arachnoiditis, neurotoxic drug administration
- Epidural/Spinal Hematoma
  - Risk factors: Coagulopathy, traumatic needle insertion, large needles, increased age, female gender, insertion/removal of epidural catheter
  - Presentation: Radicular back pain, prolonged motor and sensory blockade, possible bowel/bladder incontinence
  - Treatment: Magnetic resonance image (MRI) should be obtained urgently followed by immediate surgical decompression, if necessary
- Epidural Abscess
  - Relatively uncommon. Risk factors: Prolonged indwelling epidural catheter, diabetic or immunocompromised patients.
  - Presentation: Fever, insidious back pain and tenderness, radicular pain, progressive neurological deficits, and systemic signs of infection. Delay in diagnosis and treatment leads to poor recovery.
  - Organism: Staphylococci from patient skin
  - Prevention: Aseptic technique, chlorhexidine in alcohol for prep, bacterial micropore filter usage, epidural catheter removal within 4 days, minimal catheter manipulations
  - Treatment: Imaging, antibiotics, surgical decompression
- Post-Dural Puncture Headache
  - Mechanism: Thought to result from loss of cerebrospinal fluid (CSF) through dural puncture thereby lowering CSF pressure causing traction on cranial nerves and roots.
  - Risk factors: Young, female, pregnancy, use of Quincke needle, cutting, and/or large bore needle. Obesity is protective.
  - Presentation: Bilateral, fronto-occipital or retro-orbital headache relieved by lying flat, worsened by upright posture. Cranial nerve signs include diplopia, tinnitus, nystagmus, and hearing loss.
  - Onset: 12–72 hours

- Duration: Typically, 5 days with a range of 1–12 days.
  - Treatment: Conservative treatment first with bedrest, oral and IV hydration, oral or IV caffeine, and analgesics. Invasive treatment with epidural blood patch with 15–20 mL of autologous blood in severe cases
- Transient Neurological Symptoms (TNS)
  - Risk factors: Intrathecal lidocaine or mepivacaine, lithotomy position, obesity, young female, ambulatory surgery
  - Presentation: Unilateral or bilateral buttock pain with radiation to legs without sensory/motor deficits within 24 hours of resolution of spinal
  - Treatment: Spontaneous resolution usually within 7 days, NSAIDS, opioids
- Total/High Spinal
  - Mechanism: Occurs when local anesthetic spreads high enough to block the entire spinal cord and possibly even brainstem. Cervical roots and cardioaccelerator fibers are affected.
  - Presentation: Rapid ↓ BP and ↓ HR due to cephalad spread of local anesthetic. ↓ expiratory reserve volume (ERV), ↓ peak expiratory flow, ↓ maximum minute ventilation, apnea, and unconsciousness
  - Treatment: Airway management with intubation and 100% oxygen. Hemodynamic support with fluids and vasopressors
- Cauda Equina Syndrome
  - Risk factors: Disk herniation, disk stenosis spinal lesion, spinal infection leading to compression and/or injury of nerve roots from L1 to L5 and S1 to S5
  - Presentation: Bowel and bladder incontinence, patchy sensory deficits, pain and paresis of the lower extremities
  - Treatment: Urgent MRI followed by surgical decompression, if necessary
- Adhesive Arachnoiditis
  - Mechanism: Introduction of intrathecal irritant into subarachnoid space leading to inflammation and scarring of the subarachnoid space with collagen deposition and nerve root adherence. Collagen deposits encapsulate spinal nerves resulting in nerve root atrophy as a result of the interruption of blood supply.
  - Risk factors: Trauma, infections, surgery, contaminants, tumors, or subarachnoid administration of medications
  - Presentation: Back pain that increases on exertion, bilateral leg pain, hyporeflexia, decreased truncal range of motion, sensory abnormalities and urinary sphincter dysfunction. Neurological symptoms may progress to permanent disability.
  - Treatment: Physical therapy and opioid analgesics +/− antidepressants

Cardiovascular

- Hypotension
  - Risk factors: High spinal, age 40 years and above, HTN, low baseline BP, combined spinal and general anesthesia, use of phenylephrine as additive, urgent surgeries
  - Treatment: Fluids and pressors
- Bezold–Jarisch Reflex
  - Mechanism: Cardioinhibitory reflex secondary to parasympathetic discharge due to noxious stimuli as sensed by chemo- and mechano-receptors within the left ventricle
  - Presentation: ↓ BP, ↓ HR, coronary artery dilation and cardiovascular collapse

Respiratory

- Respiratory depression from rostral spread of opioids, especially in patients with sleep apnea

Infection

- Bacterial meningitis from oral bacteria viridans streptococci

Nausea and Vomiting

- Mechanism: Exposure of CTZ to opioids, hypotension from spinal, gastrointestinal hyperperistalsis from unopposed parasympathetic activity
- Risk factors: Vasopressors or opioids as additives, T5 and higher block, history of motion sickness

Pruritus

- Risk factors: Parturient, intrathecal opioids
- Treatment: Naloxone, naltrexone, nalbuphine, ondansetron, propofol

Shivering

- Risk factors: Cold epidural injectate
- Prevention: Prewarming patients, neuraxial opioids, avoiding cold injectate

Local Anesthetic Systemic Toxicity (LAST)

- Mechanism: LA blocks the fast sodium channels in the Purkinje fibers and ventricles leading to decreased rate of depolarization
- Presentation: Tinnitus, perioral numbness, blurred vision, muscle twitching, syncope, seizures, bradycardia, junctional rhythms, ventricular fibrillation, cardiac arrest
- Treatment: 100% oxygen, hyperventilation, benzodiazepines, propofol, succinylcholine followed by tracheal intubation. Epinephrine and intralipid 20% therapy –1.5 mL/kg IV bolus, with 0.25 mL/kg/min infusion for at least 10 min after attaining circulatory stability.

IV Regional Anesthesia/Bier Block

- Technique: Double pneumatic tourniquet placed on extremity (arm or leg) being blocked → IV catheter placed on distal portion of extremity → extremity is exsanguinated by elevation and Esmarch bandage from distal to proximal to achieve reliable anesthesia → proximal tourniquet is inflated to 250–275 mmHg → 40–50 mL of plain 0.5% lidocaine injected through IV and IV removed → surgery starts → after 45 minutes, when patient feels tourniquet pain, distal one is inflated and proximal one is deflated. Tourniquets should not be released before 20 minutes but can be safely released after 40 minutes.
- Agents: Lidocaine is most commonly used; mepivacaine, prilocaine, 2-chloroprocaine have also been used. Bupivacaine is not used due to its cardiotoxic profile.

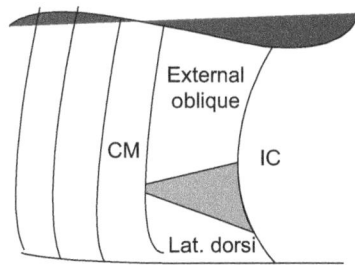

Figure 16.1 Lumbar triangle of Petit: iliac crest (IC), costal margin (CM).

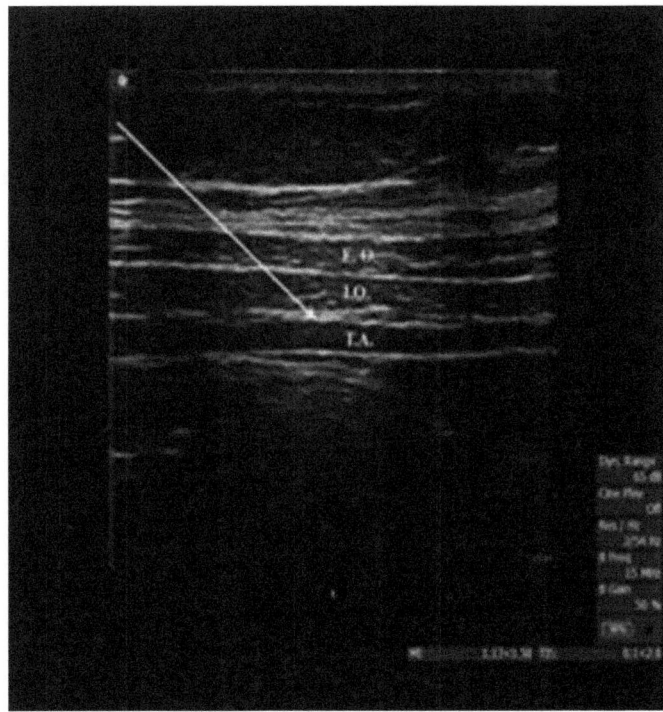

Figure 16.2 Transversus abdominis plane block (TAP). E.O.: external oblique; I.O.: internal oblique; T.A.: transversus abdominis.

- Duration: Limited by maximum allowable tourniquet time and tourniquet pain
- Indications: Limb procedures with minimal postoperative pain or last less than 2 hours
- Contraindications: Crush injury, compound fracture, peripheral vascular disease, A-V shunts, sickle cell disease, infection
- Complications: LAST, bleeding, neurologic complications

Transversus Abdominis Plane Block (TAP)

- Technique: Single entry point, three muscle layers visualized at the mid-axillary line: external oblique (EO), internal oblique (IO), and transversus abdominis (TA).

Local anesthetic is deposited in the plane between the IO and TA muscles (Figures 16.1 and 16.2).

- Nerves: Anterior rami of T6–T12, ilioinguinal and iliohypogastric nerves of L1
- Innervation: Abdominal skin, muscles and parietal peritoneum will be blocked. Dull visceral pain will not be blocked.
- Indications: Lower abdominal surgeries involving T6 to L1 distribution such as an appendectomy, hernia repair, abdominal hysterectomy, cesarean section, open prostatectomy. Bilateral blocks are performed for midline incisions.
- Complications: LAST, visceral injury to bowel, liver, spleen, kidney, or femoral nerve

Chapter 17

General Anesthesia

Petrus Paulus Steyn and Jeffrey Derham

- Definition: A complex drug-induced state of unconsciousness, amnesia, analgesia, and immobility. General anesthesia causes significant physiological changes, most notably cardiovascular and respiratory depression.
- The depth of anesthesia is the probability of unresponsiveness in the face of a stimulus with a given strength.
- **The presence of an endotracheal tube does not define general anesthesia.**
  General anesthesia is clinically differentiated from sedation by the following parameters:
  - ○ *Responsiveness:* Unarousable even with painful stimulation
  - ○ *Airway:* **May** require intervention to keep open. Pharyngeal muscle tone decreases under anesthesia and may lead to upper airway obstruction.
  - ○ *Spontaneous ventilation:* frequently inadequate, thus requiring some form of positive pressure ventilation.
  - ○ *Cardiovascular function:* Possible impairment depending on disease state, function.
- The four stages of ether anesthesia:
  1. **Awake and analgesic:** Awake but cortical processing impaired. Euphoria and/or disinhibition may be present. The threshold of pain perception decreases.
  2. **Delirium:** Loss of consciousness. Eyelid reflex disappears but other reflexes intact. Noxious stimulation can lead to agitated movements, hypertension, tachycardia, vomiting, and laryngospasm. Breath holding and gaze divergence may occur. At the conclusion of this stage respirations are regular and muscle tone diminishes.
  3. **Surgical anesthesia:** Central gaze, pupillary reflexes diminished, respirations regular, airway muscle tone diminished. At this stage somatic movement and deleterious autonomic responses do not occur with noxious stimulation.
  4. **Respiratory paralysis/overdose:** Shallow, insufficient breathing, hypotension, and eventual circulatory collapse.
- In modern anesthesia practice, these stages are rarely seen in the setting of rapid intravenous induction with modern agents. However, they are still relevant with mask inductions. In most clinical settings the estimation of the depth of anesthesia depends on patient outputs, such as somatic movement and hemodynamic responses, which serve as surrogate, albeit often unreliable, markers. The use of *electroencephalogram bispectral index* (BIS) monitoring can be a helpful estimation of anesthetic depth.
- Techniques for general anesthesia:
  - ○ **Inhalational** – accomplished using a potent volatile agent with or without nitrous oxide. Most common agents are isoflurane, sevoflurane, and desflurane. These agents are "complete" anesthetics as they achieve amnesia, analgesia, and immobility. MAC is the minimum alveolar concentration of volatile anesthetic at which 50% of patients will not move in response to skin incision. The end-tidal concentration of agent is used as a surrogate for brain concentrations and thus MAC levels.
  - ○ **Total intravenous anesthesia (TIVA)** – combination of hypnotic (usually propofol), and opioid with or without paralytic. Clinical situations where TIVA may be necessary include malignant hyperthermia, the presence of neuromonitoring utilizing evoked potentials (SSEPs), and where ventilation is often interrupted, as in bronchoscopy. One potential disadvantage is the lack of an end-tidal anesthetic "monitor" possibly leaving the patient more susceptible to light anesthesia and awareness.
  - ○ **Combined** – mixture of techniques using a lower concentration of volatile agents with IV analgesics (opioids, ketamine) with muscle relaxation. Relies on the synergistic interactions between the agents that decreases the likelihood of medication toxicity. The MACs of different volatile anesthetics are additive.
- *Intraoperative awareness with recall* is the consequence of inadequate anesthesia depth. Incidence is estimated at 0.1–0.2%. Risk factors include:
  - ○ Cardiac surgery
  - ○ Trauma surgery
  - ○ Cesarean section
  - ○ Airway endoscopy surgery
  - ○ Pediatric surgery
  - ○ Difficult airway
  - ○ Chronic alcohol, opioid, or amphetamine abuse
- Awareness with recall often occurs with inadequate depth of anesthesia in the setting of hemodynamic instability.

- Anesthetic Plan for Induction and Maintenance of General Anesthesia
  - Considerations include airway assessment, patient physiology/comorbidities, and surgical needs.
  - Any anesthetic plan must consider three basic management decision:
    - *The need for an awake intubation* – Does the administration of general anesthesia pose an unacceptable risk to the airway?
    - *The need for a percutaneous (surgical) airway* – Is ventilation and/or intubation via noninvasive means not possible? Notable examples include severe facial trauma or burns.
    - *The need to maintain spontaneous ventilation* – Pontibus ne perreni tua (do not burn your bridges). Spontaneous ventilation is a security blanket and avoids the very dangerous cannot ventilate/intubate clinical scenario.
  - If the answer to the above is no, then induction with an IV hypnotic agent plus muscle relaxant is the most common technique. Management decision depends heavily on the airway evaluation (see below).
  - The increasing availability of sugammadex, a cyclodextrin synthesized to antagonize rocuronium, may allow for the more liberal use of muscle relaxants.
- Airway Evaluation
  - History:
    - Old anesthesia records are helpful but not foolproof.
    - Appreciation of concomitant disease states that could potentially impact the airway (e.g., rheumatoid arthritis, anterior mediastinal mass). Imaging studies can be helpful.
  - Physical exam– Effective mask ventilation requires **a proper mask/tissue seal** as well as sufficient pressure to **overcome upper airway resistance**. Noninvasive endotracheal intubation requires an unobstructed path from the nasal/oral cavities to the trachea. Gross pathology of the face, neck, and pharynx (facial trauma/burns, neck masses, tonsillar abscesses, etc.) are usually obvious from the history and physical. More important and challenging is identifying potential difficulty in apparently "normal" patients.
    - Predictive factors for difficult facemask ventilation; use the mnemonic OBESE:
      1. Body Mass Index > 26 kg/m^2 (**airway resistance**): **O**verweight
      2. Presence of Beard (**poor seal**): **B**eard
      3. Edentulous (**poor seal**): **E**dentulous
      4. History of snoring (**airway resistance**): **S**noring
      5. Age > 55 years: **E**lderly
    - Other criteria that suggest difficulty:
      a. History of difficult mask ventilation
      b. History of obstructive sleep apnea (**airway resistance**)
      c. Macroglossia (**airway resistance**)
      d. Poor atlanto-occipital extension (**airway resistance**)
      e. Limited mandibular protrusion (**airway resistance**)
  - Risk factors for difficult Intubation:
    1. History of difficult intubation
    2. Poor atlanto-occipital extension
    3. Limited mouth opening: inter-incisor distance less than 3 cm (or two finger breadths)
    4. Overbite/increased length of maxillary incisors-decreases the effective inter-incisor distance and hinders oral/laryngeal alignment
    5. Micrognathia-posterior displacement of tongue leading to poor alignment
    6. Thyromental distance less than 6 cm (three finger breadths) in length
    7. Short neck
    8. Limited mandibular protrusion (inability of mandibular incisors to touch vermillion).
    9. Mallampati/Samsoon classification of III or IV
  - **Mallampati/Samsoon classification:** Based on visible structures when patient opens mouth. A measure of relative tongue size for a given oral cavity.
    - Class I: Soft palate, fauces, uvula, and tonsillar pillars are visible
    - Class II: The soft palate, fauces, and uvular are visible.
    - Class III: The soft palate and base of the uvula are visible.
    - Class IV: The soft palate is not visible.
  - Each of the above risk factors by itself has a very poor sensitivity/specificity for difficulty in ventilation and intubation. Thus, in many cases, the difficult airway will be unanticipated. The more risk factors present, the higher the probability for difficulty. Roughly 15% of difficult intubations will be difficult mask ventilations.
- General Anesthesia Induction Techniques
  - Preparation and optimization–whatever the anesthetic plan, one should adhere to the following principles of endotracheal intubation:
    - Inform the patient of the plan.
    - Coordinate availability of assistance if necessary.
    - Contingency plan/equipment in case primary plan fails.
    - Optimize patient positioning:
      - **Sniffing Position:** Cervical neck flexion with atlanto-occipital extension. Normal atlanto-occipital extension is 35 degrees. Goal is to align the oral/pharyngeal, and laryngeal axes so the laryngoscopist has a straight line of site to the larynx. Best position for most techniques.

- **Head-Elevated Laryngoscopy Position (HELP)** – helpful for obese patients. Sniffing position plus alignment of the external auditory meatus with the sternal notch. Most often achieved via a pile of blankets underneath the shoulders and upper back (ramp) or with reverse Trendelenburg
  - Preoxygenate liberally, meaning 3 minutes of 100% oxygen or four full vital capacity breaths in 30 seconds.
  - Ensure that supplemental oxygen can be delivered throughout the process.
  - High flow nasal oxygenation with heated, humidified oxygen at flows up to 70 L/min shows promise as a supplemental oxygen modality. The high rate of oxygen flow in the nasal/pharyngeal cavities creates a pressure gradient that moves oxygen into alveoli even during apnea. Oxygen delivery need not be interrupted while the airway is secured.
  - Minimize intubation attempts and thus airway trauma. Often the best look is the first.
  - Ensure the presence of end-tidal carbon dioxide monitoring for tracheal intubation confirmation.
- **Inhalational Induction:**
  - Mask induction with a volatile agent at high flow and concentration
  - Sevoflurane is commonly used secondary to low blood-gas partition coefficient and lack of pungency.
  - High levels of end-tidal gas needed for laryngoscopy and intubation. Supplementation with topical lidocaine can be helpful.
  - Requires good facemask technique.
  - Advantages:
    - Spontaneous ventilation maintained. Potential alternative to awake intubation for uncooperative patient.
    - Depth of anesthesia titrated slowly. Respiratory and cardiovascular depression come on more gradually.
    - Excellent alternative if preoperative intravenous unattainable, as in pediatrics.
  - Disadvantages:
    - Longer time required to secure airway. Not optimal for aspiration risk.
    - Longer time spent in stage 2 with possibility of laryngospasm. Antisialagogue can be helpful.
    - Intubating conditions may be suboptimal without the use of muscle relaxants.
- Intravenous Induction:
  - Most often accompanied with hypnotic (propofol, etomidate, midazolam) for amnesia/unconsciousness, opioid (fentanyl) to blunt the hemodynamic effects of laryngoscopy, and muscle relaxant (rocuronium, vecuronium).

- Advantages:
  - Rapid induction that bypasses the dangerous reflexes of stage 2 anesthesia
  - Optimal intubating conditions that minimize airway trauma
  - Technique of choice is setting of aspiration risk and anticipated uncomplicated airway (RSI technique).
- Disadvantages:
  - Spontaneous ventilation lost (even without the use of muscle relaxants) leaving the potential for the cannot ventilate/cannot intubate scenario.
  - Hemodynamic instability secondary to the sudden onset of hypnotics and narcotics.
- Awake intubation with local anesthesia:
  - Successful 80–100% of the time
  - Safe technique for the difficult ventilation/intubation or for potentially difficult intubation with aspiration risk.
  - Requires patient cooperation and blockade of sensory nerves of airway
    - Trigeminal – sensory innervation to the nasal mucosa and nasal cavity
    - Glossopharyngeal – sensory innervation to posterior third of tongue, pharynx, and superior side of epiglottis
    - Vagal branches:
      - Superior laryngeal nerve internal branch – sensory to epiglottis, base of tongue, and supraglottic mucosa up to the false cords
      - Recurrent laryngeal nerve – sensory to the subglottic mucosa including the trachea and motor innervation to the muscles of the larynx except the cricothyroid muscle
  - Local anesthesia can be accomplished via a variety of techniques:
    - Nebulizers/aerosol techniques–will cover entire airway but often needs supplementation with other techniques.
    - Topical sprays and gels–will cover the nose, mouth, and pharynx.
    - Superior laryngeal nerve blocks through the thyrohyoid membrane.
    - "Spray as you go" – topicalizes the larynx and proximal trachea. Can be facilitated by an epidural catheter threaded through the working channel of a flexible fiberoptic scope. This technique may elicit copious coughing from the patient.
    - Transtracheal injection through cricothyroid membrane – tracheal topicalization.
    - Lidocaine 4% for topicalization and 2% for nerve blocks is typically used for efficacy and safety profile.

- Antisialagogue (glycopyrrolate) helpful for visualization and to mitigate dilution of the topicalized anesthetic.
- Sedation (midazolam, fentanyl, dexmedetomidine) helpful but can potentially compromise airway.
- Intubation accomplished via a variety of techniques and devices (rigid direct/indirect laryngoscopes, retrograde wire technique, blind techniques, flexible fiberoptic laryngoscope – see below).

○ Techniques and Devices for Unanticipated Difficult Ventilation (ASA Difficult Airway Algorithm a Good Guide)

- Oral or nasopharyngeal airways – serve to displace the tongue anteriorly
- Two-handed/two-person mask ventilation – improves facemask seal and reduces airway resistance
- Endotracheal intubation
- Insertion of supraglottic airway – can serve as a conduit for endotracheal intubation
- Ventilating rigid bronchoscope
- Intratracheal jet stylet
- Cricothyroid puncture and transtracheal jet ventilation-risks barotrauma if air trapped in lungs

○ Techniques and Devices for Intubation

- No single device or technique perfect for every scenario. Several technique attempts may be necessary in the easy to ventilate but cannot intubate situation.
- **Direct Visualization** – requires line of sight from the maxillary teeth to the larynx. Most commonly employed technique. Accomplished with rigid laryngoscopes. Most common two:
  - Macintosh-curved blade with distal end placed in the vallecular. Accomplishes laryngeal exposure via tension on the hyoepiglottic ligament. Epiglottis "flips up" to expose the cords. The blade's curvature secures tongue anteriorly and creates space in the oral cavity for endotracheal tube manipulation and placement. Chief disadvantage is its reliance on indirect exposure via tension on the ligament. "Floppy epiglottis" refers to insufficient traction to lift the tissue.
  - Miller-straight blade with distal end placed on posterior surface of the epiglottis. This direct elevation exposes the larynx more reliably than the Macintosh does and the view is often superior. Disadvantages include the potential of traumatizing the larynx as the blade's tip is narrow as well as impedance of tube passage given the straight blade's profile.
- **Indirect visualization** – relies on the transmission of optical information from the distal to proximal

ends of the device. Attainment of optimal sniffing position not as important. A major limitation of any indirect technique is camera soiling from blood and/or secretions.

- Video laryngoscopy (e.g., Glidescope)
  ○ Rigid, plastic laryngoscope that provides indirect visualization via a fog resistant distal-end camera.
  ○ Blade angle more acute, thus improving views in anterior airways
  ○ Good view does not guarantee successful intubation. Small mouths and oral cavities may hinder or preclude tube maneuverability into the larynx. Oral/pharyngeal trauma can occur "off camera."

- Flexible fiberoptic laryngoscope:
  ○ Nasal or oral approach
  ○ Flexibility and greater freedom of movement as compared to rigid laryngoscopes gives it superior versatility. Tolerated especially well in the awake technique because it does not forcibly displace pharyngeal structures.
  ○ Sniffing position not necessary. In an asleep patient, better to have cervical spine extended and head flat, thus making it a good choice in cervical spine instability. Assistant may need to pull tongue anteriorly in the asleep patient to expose larynx.
  ○ Once trachea is entered, loaded endotracheal tube can pass over the scope
  ○ Visual confirmation of endotracheal tube position in the trachea.
  ○ Can be used in combination with other devices (LMA, retrograde wire) to secure airway.

- **Blind Techniques (rarely used with the advent of indirect techniques):**
  - Blind nasal intubation
    ○ Awake or asleep/spontaneously breathing technique.
    ○ Nasal mucosa treated with topical lidocaine and vasoconstrictor (usually phenylephrine). The tube is pushed through the nares and guided towards the airway by listening to the distal end of the tube for breath sounds.
    ○ Alternatively, the tube can be connected to a breathing circuit and expired carbon dioxide levels can be used.
    ○ While oral passage is also possible, the nasal route tends to align the tube with the larynx better.

- **Retrograde Wire:**
  - More invasive technique involving needle through cricothyroid membrane with cephalad

passage of wire exiting from the mouth. The endotracheal tube is then passed over the wire and into the airway.

- To facilitate passage of the tube, the wire can be threaded through one of the ports of a flexible fiberoptic scope. Some kits have a catheter that fits over the wire and can function as a stylet to pass the tube.
- Particularly appropriate in the setting of airway bleeding, poor mouth opening, or cervical neck immobility.
- Contraindicated in presence of following:
  ○ Cricothyroid membrane cannot be identified
  ○ Coagulopathy
  ○ Anterior neck lesion (tumors, abscess)

■ **Transillumination (Light Wand):**
- Any device that uses light at the tip as a guide to intubation
- Light is transmitted through the skin and the position of the trachea is approximated by centering the light at midline.
- With tracheal intubation, the transmitted light remains localized. With esophageal intubation, the light is dimmed and more diffuse.
- A proven technique in the setting of difficult airway, although a requires a steep learning curve.
- Does not work well if patient is not paralyzed or cricoid pressure is used.
- Like all blind techniques, damage to the larynx is higher than with direct visualization.

- Surgical Airway
  ○ A surgical airway is indicated in the event of a true "can't intubate, can't ventilate scenario" where all noninvasive options have been exhausted.
  ○ The options include:
  1. Needle cricothyrotomy
  2. Jet ventilation with a transtracheal catheter
  3. Surgical cricothyrotomy:
     - Surgical cricothyrotomy involves an incision through the cricothyroid membrane where a breathing tube can be inserted.
     - Newer cricothyrotomy kits employ a Seldinger catheter wire and dilator technique.
     - A catheter attached to syringe is inserted through the cricothyroid membrane, while pulling back, when air is aspirated, the syringe is removed and a guidewire is passed through the catheter into the trachea, a dilator is then passed over the guidewire removed and finally the tube/introducer is inserted over the guidewire into the trachea.
     - Contraindications include:

a. Airway trauma rendering access across the cricothyroid membrane futile
b. Age less than 10 as their smaller airways increases the risk of laryngeal trauma

- Alternatives and Adjuncts
  ○ Supraglottic airway devices:
  1. Serve as an intermediate between face mask ventilation and endotracheal intubation
  2. Can be used as conduits for endobronchial intubation and are often used for both spontaneously and mechanically ventilated patients during general anesthesia.
  3. Supraglottic devices can all be attached to a respiratory circuit or breathing bag.
  4. They all have a sealing device that redirects air to the glottis and occlude the esophagus in varying degrees.
  5. They do not offer the same protection against aspiration of stomach content as cuffed endotracheal tubes do.
  6. Options include:
     - Laryngeal mask airway
     - Esophageal–tracheal combitube
     - King laryngeal tube

- Laryngeal Mask Airway (LMA)
  ○ Often used for elective cases in fasting patients
  ○ It can be a rescue device as described in the difficult airway algorithm.
  ○ It can be used as a planned intubating conduit in difficult airways.
  ○ It can also be used in CPR situations if the patient is unresponsive with no gag.
  ○ There are various LMA designs on the market:
  1. The I-Gel uses a heat activated "gel occlude" that molds to the individual's hypopharyngeal anatomy once placed.
  2. The ProSEAL allows for passage of a gastric tube and the Fastrach intubating LMA is designed for use as an intubating conduit.
  ○ Contraindicated:
  1. Morbidly obese
  2. Patients where peak inspiratory pressures during ventilation will exceed 20 cm H_2O (e.g., restrictive airway disease)
  3. Individuals at higher risk of aspiration such as gestation more than 14 weeks, hiatal hernias, gastroparesis, and others
  4. A relative contraindication is pharyngeal pathology.
  ○ Advantages over a face mask include:
  1. Better seal in heavily bearded patients

2. A lower incidence of facial nerve and eye trauma
3. An allowance for hands-free operation.
   ○ Advantages over endotracheal tubes include:
   1. Less laryngo- and bronchospasm (especially in setting of upper respiratory tract infection)
   2. Less laryngo- and bronchospasm (especially in setting of upper respiratory tract infection)
   ○ Disadvantages include:
   1. Increased risk of airway trauma
   2. Need for deeper anesthetic depth
   3. Note that obstruction after insertion is commonly because of a pushed down epiglottis or laryngospasm.
   4. A sore throat is a common complaint in the PACU following LMA use.
   5. Hypoglossal, recurrent laryngeal and lingual nerve injuries are possible.
- Esophageal–Tracheal Combitube
  ○ Consists of two fused tubes.
  ○ The blue tube is longer and has an occluded distal tip, with a series of side perforations.
  ○ The short tube is clear with no side perforations and an open distal tip.
  ○ It is inserted blindly and advanced until two black rings are at the teeth.
  ○ Once the Combitube is placed, both its proximal (100 mL) and the distal (15 mL) cuffs are inflated.
  ○ The idea is that if the distal lumen is in the esophagus (more than 9/10 times), gas will flow from the side perforations and into the larynx.
  ○ The clear tube (shorter tube) can be used for gastric decompression.
- King Laryngeal Tube (LT)
  ○ A popular supraglottic airway device among emergency medical response teams
  ○ It consists of a single tube with a small esophageal balloon and a large hypopharyngeal balloon.
  ○ It only has one inflation line, compared with the two of the Combitube.
  ○ Ventilation of the lungs is achieved through air that exits between the two balloons.
  ○ It has a suction port distal to the esophageal balloon.
  ○ It is inserted blindly, and both the cuffs inflate at the same time.
  ○ A common reason for difficult ventilation is a tube placed too deeply.
- Endobronchial Intubation
  ○ There are four absolute indications for one lung ventilation:
    1. Protective isolation, confining bleeding or infection to one lung

2. Control of ventilation distribution in settings like bronchopleural fistula, giant cyst or bullae at risk of rupture and trauma/lung transplant with major bronchial disruption
3. Unilateral lung lavage
4. Video-assisted thoracoscopic surgery (VATS)
   ○ Three techniques can be used:
   1. Placement of a double-lumen tube
   2. Use of a single-lumen tube in conjunction with a bronchial blocker
   3. Inserting a single-lumen tube into a mainstem bronchus.
   4. It is important to know the advantages and disadvantages of one technique over the other.
   ○ Double-Lumen Tube (DTL):
   1. DLTs all share the following trademarks: Longer bronchial lumen that fits in the left or right bronchus, a tracheal and bronchial cuff, and a preformed curve.
   2. DLT is sized by height.
   3. The most commonly used sizes are 35, 37, 39, and 41 Fr.
   4. Bronchial anatomy dictates the differences between a right and left-sided DLT.
   5. Left-sided bronchial tube is used for most surgical situations since the left upper lobe orifice is 5 cm from the carina. This anatomy allows plenty of room to position the blocker optimally.
   6. The right-sided DLT has a proximal portal allowing for ventilation through the very proximal right upper lobe orifice (usually just 1–2.5 cm from the carina).
   7. Although more difficult to place, right-sided DLTs should be considered for:
      - Left-sided lung transplantation or pneumonectomy
      - When left main bronchus anatomy is distorted by tumor or compression from outside by a mass or thoracic aortic aneurysm.
   8. Malpositioning errors during and after intubation are common.
      - Tracheal intubation is usually accomplished under direct visualization with a Macintosh 3 blade.
      - Upon passage of the bronchial end through the vocal cords, the tube is rotated 90 degrees counterclockwise (left-sided tube) or clockwise (right-sided tube).
      - However, this technique does not ensure proper bronchial entry.
      - If the tube is inserted too deep, the carina could obstruct the tracheal orifice, causing obstruction and poor ventilation if the tracheal side is ventilating.
      - *Underinsertion* can also occur, and you will hear no breath sounds and see no end-tidal

CO_2 ($etCO_2$) when the tracheal lumen is used as the endobronchial cuff is in the trachea.

9. A flexible fiberoptic scope is invaluable in troubleshooting situations of malpositioning.
   - A useful landmark is the right upper lobe, which is unique in that it has three take-off branches.
10. Advantages:
    - Excellent lung isolation with the ability to quickly ventilate either or both lungs
    - Rapid lung deflation
    - Ability to suction either lung
11. Disadvantages:
    - Tube's size and stiffness: difficulty with intubation and tracheal/bronchial trauma.
    - Often must be switched out with single-lumen tubes for the ICU if the patient is to remain intubated.
- Bronchial blockers:
  1. Passed through a single-lumen endotracheal tube and can be used to selectively block off one bronchial orifice at time.
  2. It has a high-volume, low-pressure spherical-shaped cuff, and an inner lumen diameter of 1.4 mm.
  3. The distance markings are placed unilateral to the natural bend in the distal tip.
  4. Once the patient is intubated, bilateral breath sounds heard and the endotracheal tube secured, the bronchial blocker is initially placed blindly.
  5. However, the blocker MUST be positioned, advanced, and inflated under direct visualization.
  6. Advantages over a DLT:
     - Ease of placement
     - Lower incidence of trauma
     - No need to reintubate at the conclusion of the case
  7. Disadvantages:
     - Blocker does not block the lung as reliably as a double lumen tube.
     - More subject to displacing into the trachea during surgical manipulation
     - This leads to inability to ventilate or poor lung isolation.
     - The smaller lumen also makes suctioning of secretions difficult.
- Intubation and Tube Change Adjuncts
  - Bougies (Eschmann tracheal tube introducer):
    1. 24 inches (60 cm) in length, typically 15 Fr (5 mm diameter) with a curved tip
    2. There is a 10 Fr pediatric version for tubes as small as 4–6 mm.
    3. Some have a central lumen with a port for ventilation and is good option for endotracheal tube

exchange. It is made of braided polyester with a resin coating. This allows it to be both flexible and stiff at body temperature.

4. The bougie is useful in a situation where laryngeal visualization is poor but an approximate location can be ascertained (as in incomplete lifting of the epiglottis).
5. The bougie is passed through the glottis and functions as a guide for the endotracheal tube loaded over it.
6. The bougie is stiff enough to cause serious damage or even perforate the trachea; attempt to place a bougie under direct vision with a laryngoscope rather than blindly.
7. A rare, but real complication is that the bougie damages the trachea at the carina, causing bilateral tension pneumothorax. This may be hard to diagnose as the breath sounds, though poor, can be equal and classical tracheal shift does not happen.
8. It is *not* recommended for routine use in exchanging endotracheal tubes.
9. For endotracheal tube exchange, a standard tube exchanger should be used. They tend to be softer and more flexible.
- Soft and rigid tube change catheter:
  1. Most soft and rigid tube change devices have lumens that are hollow and will allow insufflation or jetting of oxygen if necessary.
  2. The same caution exists for advancing a tube whose cuff is above the cords.
  3. Examples include the *Cook Airway Exchange Catheter* and the *Aintree Intubation Catheter*.
  4. As the name suggests, it is used for replacement/ exchange of a DLT, or an endotracheal tube/ tracheostomy tube, when one is already in place.
  5. Tube change catheters are long, flexible, with length markings and round tips.
  6. They have a hollow central lumen with holes at each end and a connector that can attach to an Ambubag.
  7. *Cook Airway Exchange Catheter* comes in 5, 10, 15 Fr with varying length.
  8. Use the biggest size feasible. Smaller sizes are prone to kinking, slipping out into the esophagus or have so much give that the tip of the "railroaded" ETT gets stuck against the arytenoid cartilage-if this happens rotate the ETT tube, its bevel should allow it to slide over the arytenoid cartilage.
  9. Make sure the exchange catheter is lubricated before it is passed through the existing tube into the airway. Oxygen insufflation can be performed until the new ETT is placed.
  10. The old ETT is removed, and the new tube is railroaded over the catheter as a guide.
  11. It is highly suggested that a laryngoscope or video-laryngoscope be used to optimize the view of the larynx or ensure that the exchange catheter is not

dislodged. It also displaces soft tissues that might resist passage of the new tube.

- Endotracheal Tube Types
  - Endotracheal tubes maintain airway patency, permits oxygenation and ventilation, allows for suctioning of secretions, lower the risk of aspiration of gastric contents/oropharyngeal secretions, and facilitate the use of inhalation anesthetics.
  - Endotracheal tubes are made of PVC (polyvinylchloride) and are single-use. They have a number of characteristic features with variation of design.
  - Endotracheal tubes have a left-facing bevel at the tip and a Murphy eye.
  - The Murphy eye provides an alternate gas passage if the bevel tip becomes occlusive.
  - The PVC does not absorb X-rays, and for this reason most PVC tubes contain a **radio-opaque line**, which makes them visible on chest radiographs.
  - The bevel is left-facing rather than right-facing to allow the endotracheal tube tip an easier pass through the vocal cords.
  - Endotracheal tubes are placed with the right hand in a right-to-left direction toward the larynx.
  - Most endotracheal tubes used today have **low pressure–high volume** type cuffs. This design has comparatively large volume and allows for large contact area between cuff and trachea at lower pressures.
    1. The problem is that this balloon like cuff can make folds when inflated, creating little tracks through which gastric/oropharyngeal fluid can flow into the trachea. Thus, they have a higher risk of aspiration.
  - In contrast, **high pressure–low volume** cuffs are thought to provide better protection against aspiration. Because of their much smaller cuff–trachea contact area and higher inflation pressures used, cuff folds are less likely to develop, at the expense of more likely tracheal mucosal ischemia.
  - "Laser tube":
    1. Has a cuff design that is high pressure–low volume.
    2. Laser tubes are made of PVC, which is highly flammable in presence of the laser light and oxygen.
    3. The thoracic surgeon may employ a laser to ablate granulation tissue or webs that causes airway narrowing in the lung.
    4. The laser tube's PVC core is wrapped in an inner metallic foil and an outer nonreflective core.
    5. The cuff is most vulnerable as it is not protected.
    6. The pilot balloon is filled with blue dye granules, which dissolve when filled with water.
    7. This blue dye will leak into the trachea and the hope is that it will be noticed in the airways during bronchoscopy.

  - Nasal and oral endotracheal tubes:
    1. Also known as RAE tubes after Ring, Adair, and Elwyn, its inventors.
    2. The RAE facilitate oral and some facial, ophthalmologic surgery by moving the outer part of the endobronchial tube out of the way.
    3. It has a preformed bend, and the point of greatest angle is indicated by a little black bar.
    4. RAE endotracheal tubes are the same in all other aspects as standard endotracheal tubes.
    5. The "south-facing" tube's connector is facing the patient's feet and the "north facing" tube (or nasal RAE) has a connector facing toward the head of the patient.
    6. Disadvantages:
       - Preformed shape limits insertion depth, the bend naturally sits best at the lower lip or nostril.
       - An alternative would be to use an armored tube that can be bent out of the surgeon's way without kinking.
  - Armored tubes:
    1. Look just like standard ET tubes, but as the name suggests it is armored or reinforced tubes with an embedded metal wire coil in its wall
    2. It still has a typical left-facing bevel tip and Murphy eye.
    3. It does not have a radio-opaque line, as the tubes contain metal.
    4. The armored tubes lack a fixed bend, and a stylet will be necessary to ensure successful intubation.
    5. Disadvantages:
       - Metal coil has memory; it will not expand once a patient bites into it.
       - It is important to use a bite block to prevent this complication.
       - Armored endotracheal tubes are classified as MR-conditional (considered generally safe in MRI environment, with no real heating in the magnetic field).
       - It is interesting to note that NO endotracheal tube is designated as MRI-safe, because of the metal spring in the pilot balloon.
  - Microlaryngoscopy tube (commonly called MLT, for massive, long tube):
    1. Adult length endotracheal tubes with pediatric-sized diameter, long but thin
    2. The microlaryngoscopy tube is also designed with an "adult" size cuff.
    3. They come in three sizes: 4, 5, and 6 mm.
    4. They are used for laryngeal surgery.
    5. The smaller diameter optimizes the surgical view.
    6. The smaller diameter of these tubes means higher resistance to gas flows, which translates to higher airway pressures for a given tidal volume.
    7. Lower I:E ratios may be needed to allow for complete expiration.

- Extubation
  - More of an art than a science
  - Historically two paths: (1) Awake extubation, where patient is responding to commands. (2) Deep extubation, where patient fully anesthetized but spontaneously breathing.
  - Following one of the two paths was deemed necessary to avoid the pitfalls of phase 2 (laryngospasm, aspiration, hyperactivity). In the United States, option 1 was favored as it was deemed safer.
  - More recent clinical experience with modern anesthetics, multimodal pain management, and antiemetic medication has raised doubts as to the existence of true phase 2 emergence in modern practice.
  - The risk to healthcare personnel of airborne infection as demonstrated by the COVID-19 pandemic has placed a greater premium on avoiding excessive patient coughing and hyperactivity requiring physical restraint.
  - Adjuvants such as dexmedetomidine, tramadol, lidocaine, ketamine, propofol, and opioids have all been used to smooth out extubation in deep, moderately sedated, or awake patients.
  - When available, sugammadex and quantitative neuromuscular monitoring have been efficacious facilitators
  - Regardless of technique, the most dangerous time point is immediately after extubation, where laryngospasm, breath-holding, and airway obstruction are most likely to occur. Heightened vigilance is crucial during this time.

- Standards for Basic Anesthetic Monitoring
  - Divided into two standards:

Standard I

- The "showing up" mandate-trained anesthesia personnel must be present at all times throughout the delivery of a general, regional, or MAC anesthetic.

Standard II

Continuous evaluation of **oxygenation, ventilation, circulation**, and **temperature** throughout the case.

Oxygenation
- Inhaled gas oxygen analyzer (when anesthesia machine used)
- Pulse oximetry (All anesthetics)

Ventilation
- Qualitative end-tidal CO_2 (GA)
- Quantitative end-tidal CO_2 (ET tube/LMA)
- Disconnect alarm (when anesthesia machine used)

Circulation
- Electrocardiography
- Blood pressure
- Pulse oximetry

Temperature
- Temperature probe when clinically significant changes in temperature are expected.

Further Reading

Aintree Intubation Catheter. Available at: http://vam.anest.ufl.edu/airwaydevice/aintree/index.html

American Society of Anesthesiologists Committee of Quality Management and Departmental Administration. Continuum of Depth of Sedation: Definition of General Anesthesia and Levels of Sedation/Analgesia. Last amended by the ASA House of Delegates on October 15, 2014.

American Society of Anesthesiologists Committee of Standards and Practice Parameters. Standards for Basic Anesthetic Monitors. Last amended by the ASA House of Delegates on October 28, 2015.

American Society of Anesthesiologists Task Force on Management of the Difficult Airway. Practice guidelines for management of the difficult airway: an updated report by the American Society of Anesthesiologists Task Force on

Management of the Difficult Airway. *Anesthesiology.* 2013;**118**;2:1–20.

Barash PG, Cullen BF, Stoelting RK, et al., editors. *Clinical Anesthesia*, 7th ed. Lippincott Williams & Wilkins, 2013.

Barash PG, Cullen BF, Stoelting RK, et al., editors. *Clinical Anesthesia*, 7th ed. Lippincott Williams & Wilkins, 2013; pp 774–776.

Butterworth JF IV, Mackey DC, Wasnick JD. *Morgan & Mikhail's Clinical Anesthesiology*, 5th ed. McGraw-Hill, 2013.

Dority J, Hassan ZU, Chau D. Anesthetic implications of obesity in the surgical patient. *Clin Colon Rectal Surg.* 2011;**24** (4):222–228.

Forman S, Yang R. Administration of general anesthesia. In Dunn PF, Alston TA, Baker KH, et al., editors. *Clinical Anesthesia Procedures of the Massachusetts General Hospital*, 7th ed. Lippincott Williams & Wilkins, 2007; pp 228–232.

Gavel G, Walker R. Laryngospasm in anesthesia. *Continuing Education in Anaesthesia Critical Care & Pain* 2014;**14** (2):47–51.

Gelb K, Leslie K, Stanski D, Shafer S. Monitoring the depth of anesthesia. In Miller RD, Eriksson LI, Fleisher LA, et al., editors. *Miller's Anesthesia*, 7th ed. Elsevier Saunders, 2010; pp 1229–1265.

Guidelines for fiberoptic guided tracheal intubation through supraglottic airway device using Aintree Intubation Catheter. Difficult Airway Society, National Health Services, United Kingdom.

Henderson J. Airway management in the adult. In Miller RD, Eriksson LI, Fleisher LA, et al., editors. *Miller's Anesthesia*, 7th ed. Elsevier Churchill Livingstone, 2010; pp 1573–1610.

Kim HJ, Asai T. High flow nasal oxygenation for anesthesia management. *Korean J Anesthesiol* 2019;**72**(6):527–547.

Miller RD, Eriksson LI, Fleisher LA, et al., editors. *Miller's Anesthesia*, 8th ed. Elsevier Saunders, 2014; pp. 2209–2210.

Nolan JP, Wilson ME. Endotracheal intubation in patients with potential cervical spine injuries: an indication for the gum elastic-bougie. *Anes* 1993;**49**:630–633.

Pommerenke C, Lipp M, Collo J. [The micro laryngeal tube – a new tube for direct laryngoscopy in the ENT field]. In German. *Anaesthesia Progress*. 1989 Mar;38(3):144–146.

Reed A. The difficult airway. In Reed AP, Yudkowitz FS, editors. *Clinical Cases in Anesthesia*. Elsevier Churchill Livingstone, 2005; pp 247–260.

Ring WH, Adair JC, Elwyn RA. A new pediatric endotracheal tube. *Anesthesia Analgesia* 1975;**54**(2):273–274.

Savarese J. Upcoming improvements in relaxation & reversal. In Morgan GE, Mikhail MS, Murray MJ, editors. *Clinical Anesthesiology*, 4th ed. McGraw-Hill, 2006; p 217.

Silbert K, Long J, Haddy S. Extubation and the risks of coughing and laryngospasms in the era of coronavirus disease-19 (COVID-19). *Cureus* 2020;**12**(5):e8196.

Turk M, Gravenstein D. Aintree Intubation Catheter technique in unanticipated difficult intubation. Retrieved January, 28, 2015, from University of Florida Department of Anesthesiology, Centre for Simulation, Advanced Learning and Technology, Virtual Anesthesia Machine website: http://vam.anest.ufl.edu/airwaydevice/aintree/index.html

Welcome to MRIsafety.com! Available at: www.mrisafety.com

Monitored Anesthesia Care and Sedation

Ethan O. Bryson

Levels of Sedation

Monitored anesthesia care (MAC) is defined as "a specific anesthesia service in which an anesthesiologist has been requested to participate in the care of a patient undergoing a diagnostic or therapeutic procedure."[1] MAC can be as simple as the placement and observance of standard American Society of Anesthesiologists (ASA) monitors during a procedure without sedation or intervention, the administration of anxiolytics, or the administration of anesthetics that bring the patient to a deeper level of sedation. Sedation is defined as a continuum of states, and often during the course of an anesthetic the depth of sedation will fluctuate, depending on the level of stimulation or anesthetic concentration.

Levels of sedation are defined by the patient's physical state and degree of responsiveness, not on the dose or type of medication administered:[2]

- Minimal sedation:
  1. Responds appropriately to verbal stimulus
  2. Spontaneous respirations
  3. No airway or cardiovascular compromise
- Moderate sedation:
  1. Responds appropriately to either verbal or tactile stimulation
  2. Adequate respirations
  3. No airway or cardiovascular interventions required
- Deep sedation:
  1. No response to verbal or tactile stimulation, responds only to painful stimulus
  2. Respirations may be inadequate
  3. Airway interventions may be required (jaw-thrust, chin-lift, oral airway)
  4. Cardiovascular interventions not required
- General anesthesia:
  1. No response, even to painful stimulus
  2. Respirations may be inadequate
  3. Airway interventions may be required (laryngeal mask airway [LMA] or endotracheal tube [ETT] insertion)
  4. Cardiovascular function may be impaired

Techniques

There are many different techniques that are used to produce anxiolysis, analgesia and anesthesia. Any one of these alone may bring a patient to more than one depth of anesthesia depending upon the characteristics of the patient and the dose of the medication used. In general, the intended level of sedation can be reached by the following:[3,4]

- Minimal sedation:
  - Administration of a single intravenous (IV) anxiolytic (e.g., midazolam)
  - Peripheral nerve blocks without sedation
  - Local or topical anesthesia
  - Administration of less than 50% nitrous oxide (N_2O) in oxygen with no other sedative or analgesic medications by any route
  - A single, oral sedative or analgesic medication administered in doses appropriate for the unsupervised treatment of insomnia, anxiety, or pain.
- Moderate sedation:
  - Administration of more than one IV agent (e.g., midazolam and fentanyl) at doses appropriate to maintain response to verbal or tactile stimulation
  - Administration of IV agents via infusion (e.g., propofol or dexmedetomidine) at doses appropriate to maintain response to verbal or tactile stimulation
- Deep sedation:
  - Administration of multiple IV agents (e.g., midazolam, fentanyl, ketamine, propofol, "Ketofol," dexmedetomidine) or a single agent at doses appropriate to blunt the response to painful stimulus while maintaining spontaneous respirations, with or without intervention.

Risks and Complications

Because the depth of sedation fluctuates during the procedure depending on the level and intensity of stimulation as balanced by the concentration of medications provided, anyone who administers these medications must be properly trained to "rescue" the patient from an unanticipated, deeper level of sedation including agitation, loss of spontaneous respirations and hemodynamic instability.[5,6]

- Unanticipated response to sedation
  - Some patients may become agitated, require more anesthesia than anticipated, or quickly pass from a state of light sedation into a much deeper plane depending on a number of factors including:
    - Comorbid conditions that alter the physiologic response to anesthesia (e.g., extremes of age, chronic obstructive pulmonary disease [COPD], morbid obesity)
    - Medications that increase or decrease tolerance to anesthetics (e.g., chronic benzodiazepine use, antidepressants)
    - Airway anatomy leading to obstruction with resulting hypoxia or hypercarbia
- Loss of patent airway or loss of respiratory drive
  - With sedation, the muscles of the pharynx are relaxed and lead to either partial or full airway obstruction, which can result in hypoxia or hypercarbia despite respiratory effort. Rescue maneuvers may include:
    - Head-tilt
    - Chin-lift
    - Jaw-thrust
    - Insertion of an airway device (e.g., oral airway, nasal trumpet, LMA, ETT)
  - When respiratory drive itself is blunted or compromised, rescue maneuvers may include the administration of reversal agents (e.g., naloxone, flumazenil)
- Cardiovascular compromise
  - Relaxation of the vasculature often accompanies deeper levels of sedation and may require cardiovascular support. Rescue interventions may include:
    - Administration of fluids
    - Administration of vasopressors (e.g., phenylephrine, ephedrine)
    - Basic or advanced cardiovascular life support techniques (Basic Life Support [BLS], Advanced Cardiovascular Life Support [ACLS])

ASA Guidelines for Sedation and Sedation Guidelines for Non-Anesthesiologists

ASA Guidelines for Sedation refer to medication provided for procedures performed in a variety of settings, including hospitals, freestanding clinics, physician, dental, and other offices.[2]

- The medical history of every patient should be reviewed with a focus on items that could possibly alter the response to anesthetic agents including:
  - Cardiovascular, pulmonary, or neurological abnormalities
  - Prior adverse events with anesthesia
  - Current medications
  - Allergies to medications or anesthetic agents
  - Time of last oral intake
  - History of tobacco, alcohol, or substance use or misuse
- A focused physical examination should be performed.
  - Pre-procedure vital signs should be determined
  - Auscultation of the heart and lungs should be performed
  - An airway evaluation to determine the potential for obstruction under anesthesia is essential
- In patients with certain underlying medical conditions (e.g., end-stage renal disease requiring hemodialysis, COPD requiring oxygen therapy), pre-procedure laboratory testing should be performed if there is an increased likelihood that the results of such tests will affect patient management or alter the choice of anesthetic.

ASA Guidelines for sedation when anesthesia is administered by practitioners who are not specialists in anesthesiology:

- These guidelines do not apply to patients receiving general anesthesia or major conduction anesthesia (e.g., spinal or epidural/caudal block)
- When anesthesia is administered, the operating practitioner or another licensed physician should have specific training in sedation, anesthesia, and rescue techniques appropriate to the type of sedation or anesthesia being provided.

References

1. American Society of Anesthesiologists Committee of Origin: Quality Management and Departmental Administration. Continuum of depth of sedation: definition of general anesthesia and levels of sedation/analgesia. (Approved by the ASA House of Delegates on October 13, 1999, and last amended on October 15, 2014).

2. American Society of Anesthesiologists Task Force on Sedation and Analgesia by Non-Anesthesiologists.

Practice Guidelines for Sedation and Analgesia by Non-Anesthesiologists: an updated report. *Anesthesiology* 2002; **96**:1004–1017.

3. American Dental Association. Guidelines for the use of general anesthesia and sedation by dentists. Adopted by the ADA house of delegates October 2016.

4. Das S, Ghosh S. Monitored anesthesia care: an overview. *J Anaesthesiol Clin Pharmacol* 2015;**31**(1):27–29.

5. Bhananker SM, Posner KL, Cheney FW, et al. Injury and liability associated with monitored anesthesia care: a closed claims analysis. *Anesthesiology* 2006;**104**(2):228–234.

6. Agostoni M, Fanti L, Gemma M, et al. Adverse events during monitored anesthesia care for GI endoscopy: an 8-year experience. *Gastrointest Endosc* 2011;**74**(2):266–275.

Intravenous Fluid Therapy in the Perioperative Period

Stefan A. Ianchulev and Charles P. Plant

Water, Electrolytes, Glucose Requirement, Disposition

- History
  - In the early 1800s, Robert Lewins introduced the treatment of cholera victims with intravenous (IV) administration of alkalinized salt solution in substitution of the "quantity of serum lost."
  - Later, Sidney Ringer developed a physiological salt solution for rehydration of children with gastroenteritis, which was then modified by Alexis Hartmann.[1]
  - The first mass use of albumin, developed from the fractionation of human blood, was for treatment of burn victims after the attack on Pearl Harbor in 1941.[1]
- Current research
  - Grocott et al. in 2012 published a systematic review on the definition of goals and outcomes of resuscitation following surgery where they describe the quality of available studies as mediocre at best.[2]

- Total body water and plasma

Total body water	Plasma volume	Plasma content		
60–70% body weight	~ 3L	Inorganic ions	Albumin	Small molecules

- Endothelial function: Selective permeability
  - Starling's equation underscores the important forces (hydrostatic and oncotic) affecting fluid distribution between capillary and interstitial space (see Figure 19.1):

$$J_v = K_f[(P_c-P_i) - \sigma \ (\pi_c-\pi_i)]$$

J_v – net filtration or net fluid movement
K_f – filtration coefficient
P_c and P_i – the hydrostatic pressures in the capillaries and interstitial space, respectively
σ – reflection coefficient
π_c and π_i – capillary and interstitial oncotic pressure, respectively

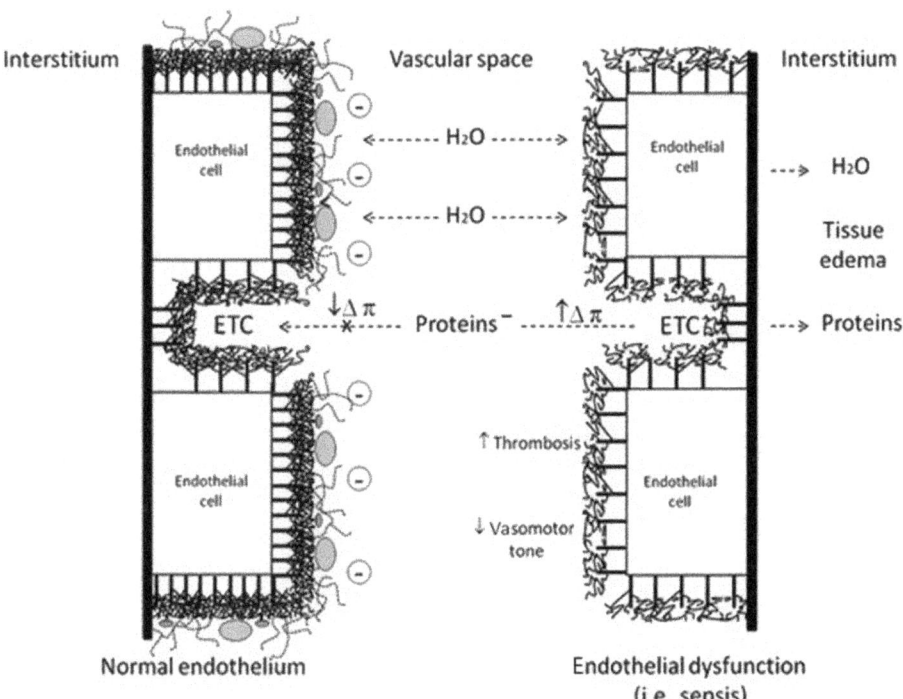

Figure 19.1 Glycocalyx characteristics in normal endothelium (left) and during endothelial dysfunction (right). ETC: endothelial cleft. Source: Chelazzi C, Villa G, Mancinelli P, et al. *Crit Care* 2015;19:26. doi:10.1186/s13054-015-0741-z.

- Na$^+$, K$^+$, Cl$^-$ ions: ATP-dependent process maintains a gradient across the membrane.
- Albumin and other larger molecules remain intravascularly due to endothelial properties.
- Natural driving force and thus fluid movement is from capillary to interstitial space, where the excess fluid is cleared by the lymphatics.
- Endothelial function disruption possibly due to surgery, inflammatory process, and direct injury leads to:
  - Changes in the interstitial fluid composition
  - Reduction of the oncotic pressure difference leading to further extravasation of fluid and resulting in tissue edema,
  - Compromise of local perfusion and accumulation of toxic byproducts, causing a vicious cycle of worsening edema.
- Perioperative fluid therapy goals:
  - Maintain the intravascular compartment volume to assure adequate delivery of oxygen and nutrients to the organs while maintaining good clearance of metabolic byproducts.
  - Ideal resuscitation fluid:
    - Should produce predictable and sustainable increase in the intravascular volume
    - Resemble closely the composition of extracellular fluid
    - Be easily metabolized and freely excreted
    - Be devoid of metabolic or systemic effects
    - Be inexpensive[1]

Resuscitation Fluids

- Crystalloids
  - History: Hartog Hamburger Studies 1882 – red blood cells best preserved in 0.9% saline[1]
  - Balanced solutions – ionic solution and osmolality close to plasma
  - Approximately 20% remain in the intravascular compartment.
  - Crystalloid buffers: Sodium bicarbonate, lactate, acetate, gluconate, and malate.
    - Sodium bicarbonate is not suited for long-term storage.
    - Excess administration of buffer containing solutions causes alkalemia, hyperlactatemia, and hypotonicity.[1]
  - Resuscitation with normal saline (NS) can cause hyperchloremic acidosis.
  - Use of chloride-restrictive fluid strategy with calcium-free balanced fluids has yielded a lower incidence of creatinine rise and renal replacement therapy.[3]
  - Hypertonic saline in traumatic brain-injured patients did not show any short- or long-term improvement of survival.[1]
  - Some reports on crystalloids inducing hypercoagulable states.

- Plasma volume expansion rule:
  Plasma volume expansion = Volume infused/Volume of distribution
- Colloids: Dissolved large molecular weight substances.
  - Naturally occurring colloids: Albumin
    - Produced from fractionation of blood, which is then heat-treated to prevent transmission of infections and then suspended in saline
    - Exists as 4–5% and 20%
    - The SAFE and FEAST studies, in pediatric populations, did not show any significant differences between albumin and saline groups in resuscitation end points compared with saline.[4,5]
  - Semisynthetic Colloids:
    - Gelatins – bovine collagen derivatives. Some preparations can contain Ca^{2+} or other inorganic ions.
    - Dextrans – biosynthesized sucrose derivatives, best described by their molecular weight (Dextran 40–40,000 Da, Dextran 70–70,000 Da)
    - Hetastarches – derivatives of amylopectine. They are divided into high molecular weight, medium molecular weight, and low molecular weight and are dissolved in NS or balanced solutions.
    - Effects of semisynthetic colloids:
      - Improved viscosity due to hemodilutional effect
      - Red blood cell aggregation increased by large molecular colloids but decreased by medium and low molecular colloids
      - All colloids affect renal function.
      - Gelatins have higher incidence of allergic reactions.
      - No mortality benefit shown in CHEST study with HES 6%[6]

Fluid Requirements and Fluid-Deficit Calculations

- **Maintenance Rule:**
  - 4–2–1 rule:
    - 4 mL/kg first 10 kg,
    - 2 mL/kg second 10 kg,
    - 1 mL/kg – remainder of the weight.
- **Fasting Fluid Deficit:**
  - Number of hours Maintenance fluid requirement = Fluid deficit
    - Replacement administered over the first 3 hours.
  - Current enhanced recovery after surgery (ERAS) protocols recommend carbohydrate drinks up until 2 hours before surgery.
    - These patients may not have such significant deficit compared to those who fasted 6 hours or more.

- **Insensible Losses:**
  - Losses due to dehumidification of breathing air, large exposed intracavitary areas.
  - In the past, those losses were estimated to be as large as 12 mL/kg/hr in major abdominal or thoracic surgeries.
  - Today it is thought that the insensible losses do not exceed 2 mL/kg/hr.
- **Blood Loss:**
  - Best substitute for lost blood is whole blood.
    - Difficult to come by and associated with infectious and immunologic problems.
  - Replacement of minor blood losses with crystalloids or colloids is acceptable substitute.
  - Hematocrit decreases to 21% can be well tolerated by some patients.
  - Lower Hct can be associated with good outcome if O_2 demand is decreased.
  - Recommendations:
    - Substitute individual components – red blood cells (PRBC), plasma (FFP, Cryo), platelets, recombinant clotting factors.
    - Major trauma: 1:1:1 ratio of PRBC:FFP:Plt.
- **Perioperative Fluid Management:**
  - Goal-directed therapy (GDT): Protocolized fluid administration based on continuous assessment of fluid deficit.
    - Need for invasive or noninvasive continuous assessment devices.
    - Shoemaker: Oxygen delivery optimization therapy. Important to measure biological markers associated with hypo-perfusion.
    - Arterial line contour assessment – calibrated and non-calibrated devices. Dependent on tidal volumes of 8 mL/kg IBW.
    - Swan–Ganz catheters for continuous cardiac output – currently out of favor due to complications, invasiveness, and user familiarity.
    - Tissue perfusion model – gastric tonometry, laser Doppler flowmetry, micro-dialysis catheters, transcutaneous oxygen saturation measurements, and tissue pH monitors.
  - Effects of GDT:
    - Improved nausea and vomiting[7]
    - Reduced pain scores[7]
    - Better outcomes in abdominal surgery with restrictive fluid administration[8]
    - Shorter length of stay[9]
  - Pitfalls in perioperative fluid management algorithms:
    - Indices generally accepted in the past like urine output (UO) can be reduced due to anesthetic agents and surgical stress (volume kinetic analysis of the distribution of 0.9% saline in conscious vs. isoflurane-anesthetized sheep; isoflurane but not

mechanical ventilation promotes extravascular fluid accumulation during crystalloid volume loading), blood pressure (BP), heart rate (HR), central venous pressure (CVP), pulmonary artery occlusion pressure (PAOP) have been deemed as inadequate markers for optimization of cardiac output (CO) and mixed venous saturation S_vO_2 in recent years.[6]
- CVP does not correlate with preload responsiveness. Swan–Ganz catheter has fallen out of favor. [10,11]
- Static (BP, CO, PAOP, HR, LVDEP) vs. dynamic (CO, SV, SVV) parameters, and upstream (DO$_2$, CVP, PAP) vs. downstream (SvO$_2$, SV, stroke volume variation, pulse contour analysis, near-infrared spectroscopy-based tissue oxygenation, lactate) indices.
- Shoemaker observed that supra-normal oxygen delivery of greater than 600 mL/m^2/min can lead to improved outcomes in high-risk patients.[12]
- Velmahos et al. concluded that in the severely injured patients, those who could achieve supra-maximal values of oxygen delivery, fared better.[13]
  - Noninvasive Technologies:
    - POCUS – point-of-care ultrasound assessment of the heart, vessels, abdomen and chest to institute the best therapy based on contractility, volume status and responsiveness. Some limitations in the intraoperative period due to access, as well as ability to establish good scanning windows. Recent artificial intelligence modes added to handheld devices.
    - Pleth variability index
    - Pulse wave transit time and pulse wave contour index
    - Thoracic bioimpedance and bioreactance devices

Normal Saline (NS) vs. Lactated Ringer's vs. Plasma-Lyte

- Type of crystalloid best for resuscitation has not been established (Table 19.1).
- Most commonly utilized crystalloids are 0.9% NS, lactated Ringer's solution, Plasma-Lyte, and dextrose 5% in water.
- Each solution differs in its ionic composition, strong ion difference to plasma, and fluid pH (Table 19.1).
- NS has been associated with decreased renal artery flow and reduced renal cortical tissue perfusion in subjects who received 2 L of NS over 1 hour as compared with Plasma-Lyte 148.[14]
- Impaired gastrointestinal and hematological pathways, thrombin generation and platelet activation due to NS.[15]
- Increased incidence of renal insufficiency but not mortality or length of stay with NS;[16] however, a recent study, SPLIT, did not show difference on AKI, renal replacement therapy, mortality, or LOS.[17]

Table 19.1 Characteristics of common crystalloid solutions compared to human plasma[20]

	Plasma	0.9% saline	Compound sodium lactate (lactate buffered solution)	Ringer's lactate (lactate buffered solution)	Ionosteril® (acetate buffered solution)	Sterofundin ISO® (acetate & malate buffered solution)	Plasma-Lyte 148® (acetate & gluconate buffered solution)
Sodium (mmol/L)	136–145	154	129	130	137	145	140
Potassium (mmol/L)	3.5–5.0		5	4	4	4	5
Magnesium (mmol/L)	0.8–1.0				1.25	1	1.5
Calcium (mmol/L)	2.2–2.6		2.5	3	1.65	2.5	
Chloride (mmol/L)	98–106	154	109	109	110	127	98
Acetate (mmol/L)					36.8	24	27
Gluconate (mmol/L)							23
Lactate (mmol/L)			29	28			
Malate (mmol/L)						5	
eSID (mEq/L)	42		27	28	36.8	25.5	50
Theoretical osmolarity (mosmol/L)	291	308	278	273	291	309	295
Actual or measured aosmolality (mosmol/kg H_2O)	287	286	256	256	270	Not stated	271
pH	7.35–7.45	4.5–7	5–7	5.0–7	6.9–7.9	5.1–5.9	4–8

All values are in mEq/L, except calculated osmolarity, which is in mOsm/L. Plasma-Lyte A is "Multiple Electrolyte Injection, Type 1, USP," from Baxter Healthcare Corporation; Normosol-R is "Multiple Electrolyte Injection, Type 1, USP," from Hospira, Inc.; Isolyte S is from B. Braun Medical Inc.; Ringer's acetate is "Sterofundin ISO, Isotonic Electrolyte Solution," from B. Braun; lactated Ringer's is "lactated Ringer's Injection, USP," from Baxter Healthcare Corporation; Hartmann's solution is "Compound Sodium Lactate" from Baxter Healthcare Corporation; and 0.9% saline is "Sodium Chloride Injection, USP," from Baxter Healthcare Corporation.

Strategies for Fluid Management

- Ambulatory surgery: Minimal fluid loss and less preoperative volume depletion due to ERAS protocols, thus it is not much of an issue.
- Moderately invasive surgical procedures: Usually not significant blood loss. Patients with preexisting cardiac disease (CAD, CHF, etc.) restrictive fluid management is recommended, and the use of noninvasive monitoring devices can be beneficial for fluid therapy management in patients who have cardiac disease.
- Major surgery: The fluid losses should be replaced and a zero-balance fluid therapy should be the goal.[18] Avoid replacement of "third space losses," as this may lead to fluid overload and current evidence is not supporting it.[19]
- Regional anesthesia: Avoid preload with fluids.

References

1. Myburgh JA, Mythen MG. Resuscitation fluids. *N Engl J Med* 2013;**369**(13):1243–1251.

2. Grocott MP, Dushianthan A, Hamilton MA, et al. Perioperative increase in global blood flow to explicit defined goals and outcomes following surgery. *Cochrane Database Syst Rev* 2012;**11**:CD004082.

3. Reddy S, Weinberg L, Young P. Crystalloid fluid therapy. *Crit Care* 2016;**20**:59.

4. Finfer S, Bellomo R, Boyce N, et al. A comparison of albumin and saline for fluid resuscitation in the intensive care unit. *N Engl J Med* 2004;**350**(22): 2247–2256.

5. Maitland K, Kiguli S, Opoka RO, et al. Mortality after fluid bolus in African children with severe infection. *N Engl J Med* 2011;**364** (26):2483–2495.

6. Grocott MP, Mythen MG, Gan TJ. Perioperative fluid management and clinical outcomes in adults. *Anesth Analg* 2005;**100** (4):1093–1106.

7. Chappell D, Jacob M, Hofmann-Kiefer K, Conzen P, Rehm M. A rational approach to perioperative fluid management. *Anesthesiology* 2008;**109**(4):723–740.

8. Nisanevich V, Felsenstein I, Almogy G, et al. Effect of intraoperative fluid management on outcome after intraabdominal surgery. *Anesthesiology* 2005;**103**(1):25–32.

9. Thacker JK, Mountford WK, Ernst FR, Krukas MR, Mythen MM. Perioperative fluid utilization variability and association with outcomes: considerations for enhanced recovery efforts in sample US surgical populations. *Ann Surg* 2016;**263**(3):502–510.

10. Tseng GS, Wall MH. Endpoints of resuscitation: what are they anyway? *Semin Cardiothorac Vasc Anesth* 2014;**18**(4):352–362.

11. Marik PE. Obituary: pulmonary artery catheter 1970 to 2013. *Ann Intensive Care* 2013;**3**(1):38.

12. Shoemaker WC, Appel PL, Kram HB, Waxman K, Lee TS. Prospective trial of supranormal values of survivors as therapeutic goals in high-risk surgical patients. *Chest* 1988;**94** (6):1176–1186.

13. Velmahos GC, Demetriades D, Shoemaker WC, et al. Endpoints of resuscitation of critically injured patients: normal or supranormal? A prospective randomized trial. *Ann Surg* 2000;**232**(3):409–418.

14. Chowdhury AH, Cox EF, Francis ST, Lobo DN. A randomized, controlled, double-blind crossover study on the effects of 2-L infusions of 0.9% saline and Plasma-Lyte® 148 on renal blood flow velocity and renal cortical tissue perfusion in healthy volunteers. *Ann Surg* 2012;**256**(1):18–24.

15. Brummel-Ziedins K, Whelihan MF, Ziedins EG, Mann KG. The resuscitative fluid you choose may potentiate bleeding. *J Trauma* 2006;**61** (6):1350–1358.

16. Yunos NM, Bellomo R, Glassford N, et al. Chloride-liberal vs. chloride-restrictive intravenous fluid administration and acute kidney injury: an extended analysis. *Intensive Care Med* 2015;**41**(2):257–264.

17. Young P, Bailey M, Beasley R, et al. Effect of a buffered crystalloid solution vs saline on acute kidney injury among patients in the intensive care unit: the SPLIT randomized clinical trial. *JAMA* 2015;**314**(16):1701–1710.

18. Brandstrup B. Fluid therapy for the surgical patient. *Best Pract Res Clin Anaesthesiol* 2006;**20**(2):265–283.

19. Brandstrup B, Svensen C, Engquist A. Hemorrhage and operation cause a contraction of the extracellular space needing replacement–evidence and implications? A systematic review. *Surgery* 2006 Mar;**139**(3):419–432. doi: 10.1016/j.surg.2005.07.035. PMID: 16546507

20. Semler MW, Kellum JA. Balanced crystalloid solutions. *Am J Respir Crit Care Med* 2019;**199**(8):952–960.

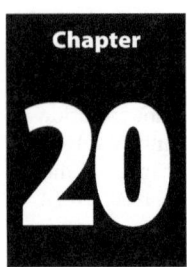

Complications of Anesthesia: Etiology, Prevention, and Treatment

Andrew Glasgow Perez, MD

- Common causes of anesthesia-related *brain damage/death*
  1. **Cardiovascular**: Multifactorial (arrhythmia, hypotension, etc.), pulmonary embolism, hypovolemia, stroke, hemorrhage, myocardial infarction
  2. **Respiratory**: Difficult intubation, inadequate ventilation/oxygenation, esophageal intubation, premature extubation, aspiration, airway obstruction
  3. **Medication related**: Wrong drug/dose, allergic or adverse reaction, malignant hyperthermia
  4. **Equipment related**: Equipment *misuse* more common than *malfunction*. Gas delivery problems most often associated with death
  5. **Block related**: High spinal/epidural, intravascular injection, absorption
- Common complication during MAC: *Respiratory event*, due to *oversedation*[1]
- Common cause of anesthesia litigation→ *dental injury*
- As claims related to surgery *decrease*, claims related to acute/chronic pain have *increased*, an association with the opioid epidemic

Airway-Related Injury

Upper Airway: Facial nerve and mental nerve paresis
  ○ Risk: Pressure from mask rim, jaw thrusts

Nasal: Epistaxis; nasal septum necrosis; retropharyngeal abscess, sinusitis
  ○ Risk: Nasal foreign body (tube/temp probe), mask
  ○ Avoid nasal passage in patient with *basilar skull fractures* or severe facial trauma → potential for cranial intubation

Laryngeal: Vocal cord paresis; arytenoid disarticulation; granuloma formation
  ○ Risk: Routine and emergent intubations

Tracheal: *Early complications* – tracheal lacerations; hemorrhage; recurrent laryngeal nerve injury; discomfort from tracheostomy. *Late complications* – tracheal stenosis; tracheo-esophageal fistulas; trachea-innominate fistula; tracheomalacia
  ○ Risk: emergent tracheostomy, ETT movement, stylette, LTAs, ETT cuff > 25 mmHg

Pharyngeal/Esophageal Tears: Abscess; esophageal perforation, mediastinitis
  ○ Risk: Age > 60, female, difficult intubation, esophageal intubation, NGT, TEE
  ○ Mortality rate up to 50%, monitor esophageal intubations closely

Temporomandibular Joint (TMJ) Injuries: TMJ disarticulation; pain
  ○ Risk: Female, age < 60 years old, American Society of Anesthesiologists Physical Status Classification ASA1/2

Dental Injuries: Fracture; tooth avulsion
  ○ Risk: Laryngoscopy/intubation, airway manipulation, poor dentition, 5th–7th decade, and characteristics associated with difficult laryngoscopy Occurrence rate: 0.04–0.05%

Airway Injuries:
  ○ Prevention: Identify risk factors and potential causes of trauma; utilize teeth guards, oral airway, videolaryngoscope or fiberoptic bronchoscope, small endotracheal tube (ETT), ETT cuff < 25 mmHg; request additional support if known or suspected difficult intubation; nasogastric tube (NGT) and transesophageal echocardiography (TEE) experience
  ○ Treatment: Early identification and referral – ENT, GI, oral and maxillofacial surgery (OMFS), or dental

Respiratory Events

COVID-19

Surgery in patients with recent or active COVID-19 is associated with an increased morbidity and mortality.

- Prevention: Elective surgery should ideally not be undertaken within 2 weeks of a new diagnosis of COVID-19, or longer if symptoms persist.
- Treatment: Antiviral medications, pulmonary support, specialist consult

Pediatric Respiratory Events

Increased risk due to smaller airways, heightened airway reactivity, and higher oxygen consumption.

- Risk factors: History of reactive airway disease (RAD) (+/– exposure to wildfire smoke, tobacco, fine particulate matter), prematurity, younger age, obesity, obstructive sleep apnea (OSA), upper respiratory infection (URI)

- Prevention: Ensure adequate depth of anesthesia, pretreatment with ß-2 agonist, and postponing elective procedures in high-risk patients
- Treatment: Positive pressure, deepening anesthetic, ß-2 agonist

Bronchospasm/Laryngospasm

- Etiology: ETT, pungent airway irritants, desflurane, secretions, cold air exposure
- Risk factors: Reactive airway disease, recent URI (e.g., COVID-19), gastroesophageal reflux disease (GERD), pediatric patients
- Prevention: Vigilance, adequate anesthetic depth, pretreat with ß-2 agonist
- Treatment: Inhaled ß-2 agonist, deepen anesthetic, +/− steroids, +/− epinephrine, (specific for laryngospasm, positive pressure, muscle relaxant)

    Negative Pressure Pulmonary Edema (NPPE): Inspiration against closed airway. Occurs in 4% of cases of laryngospasm, 0.05–0.1% of general anesthetics
- Risk factors: Male, young, OSA, acromegaly, difficult intubation, ENT surgery[2]
- Signs and symptoms: Acute respiratory distress in an otherwise healthy patient, pink frothy pulmonary secretions, chest radiography (CXR) with bilateral interstitial alveolar infiltrates
- Prevention: Bite block/spacer
- Treatment: Positive end-expiratory pressure (PEEP) via mechanical ventilation or continuous positive airway pressure (CPAP). Potential role with ß-2 agonists, low tidal volume ventilation strategies, and diuresis; however, further study is indicated.
- Resolution: Usually occurs in 3–12 hours; however, complete resolution may take 12–48 hours. Intubation > 48 hours associated with increased morbidity and mortality.

Aspiration

Aspiration of Gastric Contents

- Risk factors: Emergency surgery, difficult intubation, pain, diabetes, obesity, pregnancy, smoking, alcohol, drug abuse, opioids, gastrointestinal pathology (GERD, hiatal hernia, bowel obstruction), light anesthesia, and unexpected motor response

Aspiration Management: Laryngeal Mask Airways (LMA)

If regurgitation occurs with LMA:
1. Place in Trendelenburg position and give 100% O_2.
2. Determine risk and benefits of keeping LMA in place vs. placing an ETT tube.
3. Consider evaluating regurgitation with fiberoptic visualization of trachea and bronchi

Other LMA complications: LMA overinflation or N_2O-related distention and use of lidocaine gel → hypoglossal, lingual, and recurrent laryngeal nerve damage (usually temporary)

Aspiration Pneumonitis
- If no symptoms after 2 hours, aspiration unlikely to become serious.
- Particulate aspiration may require bronchopulmonary lavage.
- Avoid (1) neutralizing solutions, (2) prophylactic steroids, (3) prophylactic antibiotics → may increase risk of pneumonia.

Ocular Injuries

See Table 20.1.

Vascular Complications

These include arterial/venous thrombosis, guidewire or catheter embolism, cardiac tamponade, pneumothorax, hemothorax, pulmonary artery rupture, carotid artery puncture, central line-associated bloodstream infection (CLABSI), ectopy, hematoma.

Table 20.1 Ocular injuries, symptoms, and rates

	Corneal abrasion	Acute angle closure glaucoma	Anterior ischemic optic neuropathy	Posterior ischemic optic neuropathy
Pain	YES	YES	NO	NO
Vision	Photophobia	Blurred	Blindness	Blindness
Patient risk factors	Exophthalmos, proptosis, dry eyes	Female, elderly, glaucoma, HTN	HTN, DM, CAD, PVD, smoker, degenerative eye, CVA	HTN, DM, CAD, PVD, smoker, degenerative eye, CVA, male, obesity
Surgical and anesthesia risks	Prone, lateral	Bucking, coughing, anti-muscarinic, pressors, high blood pressure	Cardiopulmonary bypass	Prone spine surgery (prolonged, fusion, hypovolemia, hypotension)
Rate	0.034–0.17%	Rare	0.06%	0.013–0.2%

CAD: coronary artery disease; DM: diabetes mellitus; CVA: cerebrovascular accident; HTN: hypertension; PVD: peripheral vascular disease.

Central retinal artery occlusion: Common cause of postoperative visual loss, seen most often after prone spine surgeries, caused by extrinsic compression on eye.[3,4]

Central Lines

Acute Complications

- Serious: Most common acute complications are *hematoma* or *arterial injury* followed by *cardiac tamponade*.
- Less serious: Most common non-serious complication is *ventricular ectopy*.

Late Complications

- Infection: CLABSI occurs in 0.8/1,000 central line days
- Thrombosis: PICC> CVC>port; jugular>subclavian

Safety Steps

- Where possible, use single lumen, heparin-bonded catheters (less risk of infection and thrombus), with bactericidal impregnated patches (less risk of infection) and remove ASAP.
- Confirm proper placement: Visualization of wire under ultrasound, manometry, pressure waveform monitoring, blood gas measurement, observing color and nonpulsatile flow

Left-Sided Versus Right-Sided Central Line

- Cupola of the pleura is higher on the left (↑ risk of pneumothorax)
- Thoracic duct may be injured on the left
- Left internal jugular (LIJ) is usually smaller and there is greater degree of overlap with adjacent carotid artery compared to right internal jugular (RIJ)
- Left-sided central lines enter the superior vena cava (SVC) at a more *oblique angle* → greater risk of vascular perforation and cardiac tamponade

Pulmonary Arterial Catheter (PAC):

Minor complications common 50%; major complications 0.1–0.5%

- **Complications with placement:** Arrhythmias (pretreatment with lidocaine does not prevent arrhythmia), ventricular fibrillation, right bundle branch block (RBBB), complete heart block, hematoma, scar, pain
- **Complications with residence:** Knots, thromboembolism, pulmonary infarction, infection/endocarditis, endocardial damage, cardiac valve injury, pulmonary artery rupture, pulmonary artery pseudo-aneurysm, misinterpretation of data
- **Misuse of equipment:** Causes 3× more adverse events than equipment malfunction

Arterial Line Complications:

Vascular insufficiency/thrombosis, vasospasm

- Risk factors: vasospastic arterial disease, previous injury, thrombocytosis, protracted shock, high-dose vasopressor administration, prolonged cannulation, and infection
- Complications with femoral artery > radial artery

- Brachial lines are associated with potential damage to the median nerve
- Bloodstream infections with arterial lines are 1:1,000 catheter days

Intra-osseous (IO) Line Complications

- Extravasation of fluid and meds → compartment syndrome or muscle necrosis, due to improper placement/supervision
- Hematoma, pain, fracture, growth plate injury, fat micro-emboli
- Infection: osteomyelitis and cellulitis (limit use to < 72 hours)
- Tibial IO lines have *higher flow* rates, while humeral IO lines *reach central circulation faster*

Avoid growth plate in pediatric patients; avoid placement in fractured bone. IO lines are relatively contraindicated in patients with osteogenesis imperfecta/osteoporosis.

Position-Related Peripheral Nerve Complications

Peripheral Neurological Complications
Caused by compression, stretch, ischemia, trauma, and intrinsic patient risk factors – diabetes mellitus (DM), multiple sclerosis (MS), chemotherapy, prolonged immobility, smoking, body habitus, patient position.

- Not every nerve injury is due to improper positioning, some are related to events occurring out of the OR.

Ulnar Injury: Most common, occurring in 1:2,700 patients.
  - Risk factors: Male, both thin and obese patients, prolonged hospital stay
  - More common under general anesthesia (GA), although 15% of ulnar injuries occur under monitored anesthesia care (MAC) or lower extremity regional technique; supinate arm

Brachial Plexus
- Risk factors: Stretching or direct compression at axilla (lateral decubitus position)

Peroneal Injury
- Risk factors: Lithotomy (> 2 hours), pressure on lateral aspect of upper fibula (candy cane stirrups), extreme angle, hypotension, thin body habitus, older age, vascular disease, DM, cigarette smoking

Management of Postoperative Neuropathy: For mild symptoms that persist > 24 hours, consult a neurologist or physiatrist, as physiological testing can determine whether the condition is acute or chronic. If severe, more urgent neurological consultation warranted.

Thermodysregulation

Types of Heat Loss
- Radiation: Heat loss to structures not in contact with body

- Convection: Heat loss to cooler air surrounding body
- Conduction: Heat loss to structures in contact with body
- Evaporation: Heat loss through loss of moisture, respiration, disinfecting prep, surgical hair clipping

Redistribution

- Movement of heat from the core to periphery is the principal mechanism of heat loss during the first hour/stage of anesthesia

Hypothermia

- Risk Factors: Regional and GA impairs thermoregulation; low ambient temperature of the operating room; pediatric patients; low BMI
- **Prevention**/Treatment: Forced air warming done 30 minutes prior, prevents phase I cooling. Once in the OR, consider warming the operating room, warming IV fluids, heated humidification of inhaled gases, and forced air warming (most cost effective)

Special precaution with **sickle cell disease, Raynaud's, hyperkalemic familial periodic paralysis, MS**

Complications of Hypothermia

- Cardiac arrhythmias and ischemia
- Increase in systemic vascular resistance (SVR), stress response, and postoperative protein catabolism
- Left shift of Hgb-O_2 saturation curve
- Platelet dysfunction
- Altered mental status, delayed emergence
- Impaired renal function, wound healing
- Delayed drug metabolism

Postop shivering can increase oxygen consumption as much as 5×, → decrease oxygen saturation, which can increase the risk of myocardial infarction (MI).

Active Cooling of Febrile Patient

- May fail to reduce core temperature
- Induces autonomic nervous system activation
- Leads to shivering and potentially patient discomfort

Nonmalignant Hyperthermia/Passive Hyperthermia

- Most common in pediatric patients due to improper monitoring, avoid in multiple sclerosis
- Treatment is to stop active warming and remove insulating layers

Malignant Hyperthermia (MH)[5]

- 1:15,000 pediatric patients, 1:40,000–50,000 adult patients
- Mortality rate 5% with early detection
- **Risk Factors:**
  Central-core disease, multi-minicore myopathy, King–Denborough syndrome
- Mostly autosomal dominant, involving ch19q3.1 ryanodine receptor type 1 (RYR1)
- Muscular males have increased potential reaction for MH

- Mechanism: Uncontrolled release of intracellular calcium from sarcoplasmic reticulum of skeletal muscle; calcium removes inhibition of troponin → sustained muscle contraction
- Increase ATPase activity → increase aerobic and anaerobic metabolism

Signs of Malignant Hypothermia

- Increase CO_2 production → respiratory acidosis
- Increase O_2 consumption → decreased O_2 supply and delivery → lactic acidosis
- Skin mottling (cyanosis), tachycardia, hypertension, arrhythmias, rigidity, and hyperthermia (*late sign*)
- Treatment: Call for help and stop volatile agent/succinylcholine
- Terminate surgery if possible or continue with nontriggering agent
- Give 100% FiO_2 at 10 L flows & hyperventilate
- Dantrolene 1–2.5 mg/kg → up to 10 mg/kg
- Call *MHAUS Hotline*
- Check VBG/ABG and core temp
- Manage hyperkalemia, acidosis, and hyperthermia
- Monitor urine output and consider arterial line/central line, +/– diuresis
- Avoid calcium channel blockers

Allergic Reactions

Hypersensitivity – Most common cause of perioperative hypersensitivity is cefazolin

Anaphylaxis – IgE mediated (Type I): Diagnosed with elevated tryptase level (> 11.5 ng/mL) (Figure 20.1)

Principal culprits: Muscle relaxants (1:3,500–1:20,000 anesthetics), rocuronium, succinylcholine

Latex Allergies:

- Decreasing overall as ORs are reducing latex
- Patient risk factors: *spina bifida, spinal cord injury, congenital genitourinary (GU) abnormality, rubber factory and health care worker*

Sugammadex:

- Increasing in frequency, dose-dependent

Antibiotics:

- In PCN allergic patients, less than 1% develop reaction to cephalosporins

Nonimmune-Mediated Anaphylaxis: Mast cell activation directly or via complement (not IgE) → inflammatory response; more common than "true" anaphylaxis

Chronic Environmental Exposure, Fertility, Carcinogenicity, Teratogenicity, Scavenging

- N_2O exposure has deleterious reproductive and teratogenic effects in animals (Table 20.2).

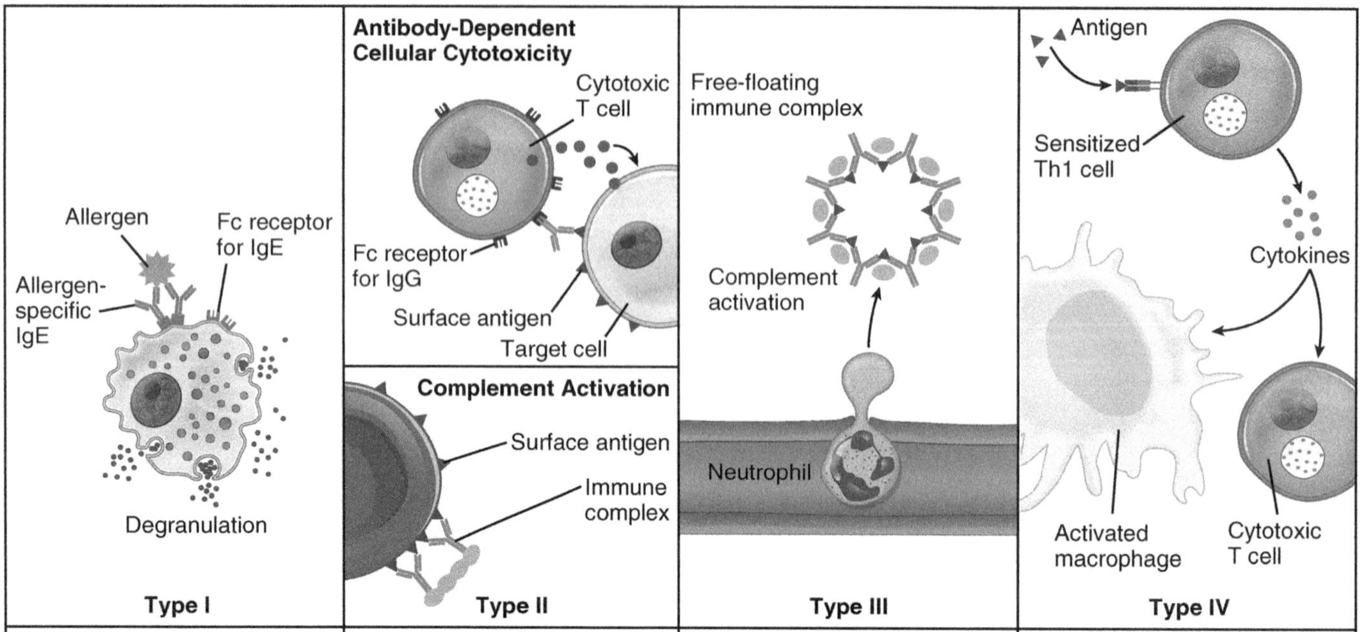

IgE-Mediated Hypersensitivity	IgG-Mediated Cytotoxic Hypersensitivity	Immune Complex-Mediated Hypersensitivity	Cell-Mediated Hypersensitivity
IgE is bound to mast cells via its Fc portion. When an allergen binds to these antibodies, crosslinking of IgE induces degranulation.	Cells are destroyed by bound antibody, either by activation of complement or by a cytotoxic T cell with an Fc receptor for the antibody (ADCC).	Antigen–antibody complexes are deposited in tissues, causing activation of complement, which attracts neutrophils to the site.	Th1 cells secrete cytokines, which activate macrophages and cytotoxic T cells and can cause macrophage accumulation at the site.
Causes localized and systemic anaphylaxis, seasonal allergies including hay fever, food allergies such as those to shellfish and peanuts, hives, and eczema.	Red blood cells destroyed by complement and antibody during a transfusion of mismatched blood type or during erythroblastosis fetalis.	Most common forms of immune complex disease are seen in glomerulonephritis, rheumatoid arthritis, and systemic lupus erythematosus.	Most common forms are contact dermatitis, tuberculin reaction, autoimmune diseases such as diabetes mellitus type I, multiple sclerosis, and rheumatoid arthritis.

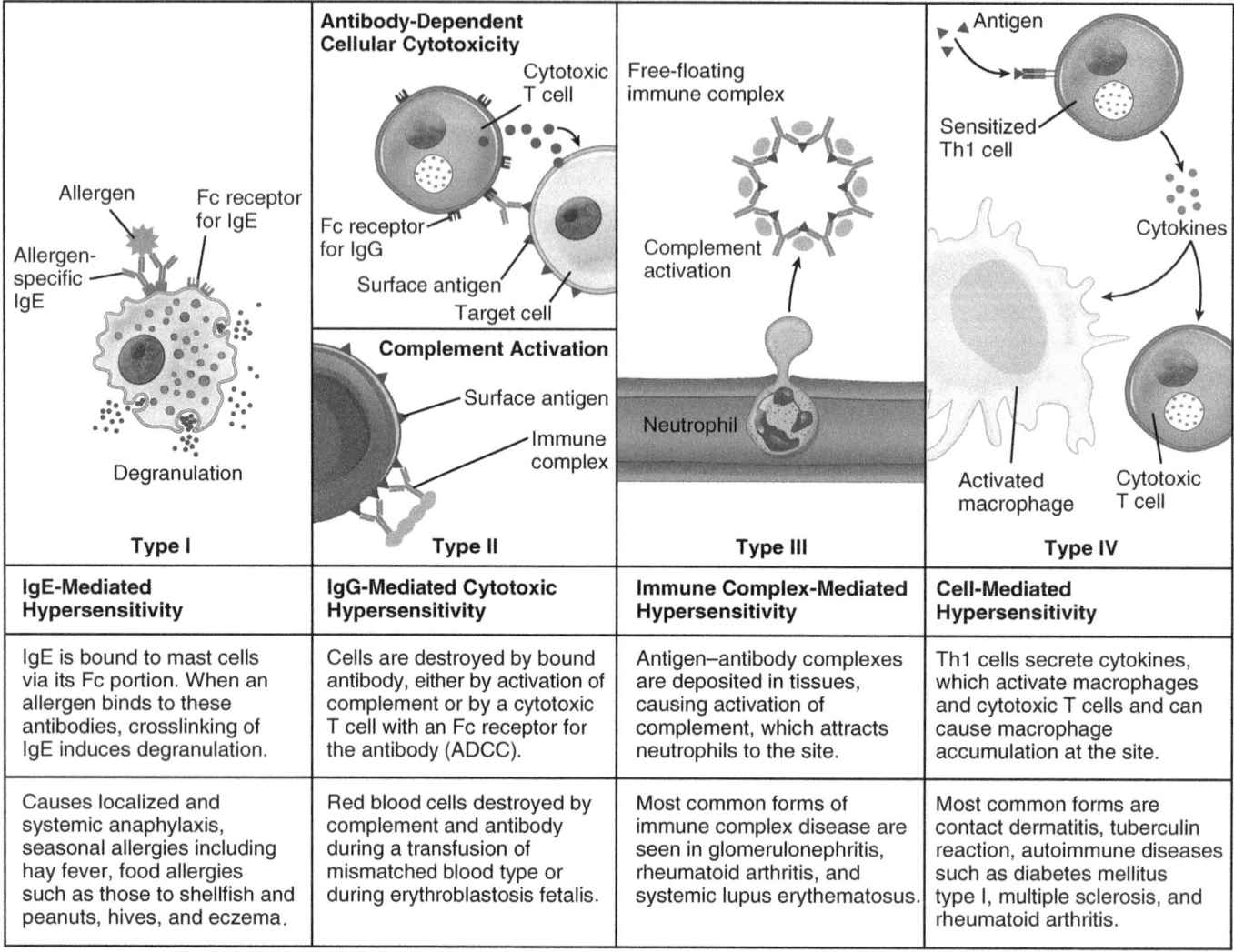

Figure 20.1 Hypersensitivity reaction types.[6]

Table 20.2 OSHA: anesthetic gases: guidelines for workplace exposure

	OSHA N_2O max	OSHA volatile max
N_2O alone	25 ppm	–
Volatile alone	–	2 ppm
N_2O & volatile	25 ppm	0.5 ppm
Level attainable without scavenging	3,000 ppm	50 ppm

- Healthcare providers (HCP) have increased risk of miscarriage, infertility; however, may be unrelated to operating room.
- Trace concentrations of anesthetic vapors do not present a health hazard.
- Efforts should be made to keep anesthetic vapors to a minimum.

Table 20.3 OSHA maximum limit of radiation for occupational exposure*

Prospective annual limit	5 rems/year
Retrospective annual limit	10–15 rems/year
Pregnant women	0.5 rems/gestation

* Average exposure in the United States is 0.080–0.2 rem/year.

Sources of Contamination: Inhalation induction, uncuffed ETT, LMAs, circuit disconnects, inadequate scavenging
Postanesthesia Care Unit (PACU) → unsafe levels of anesthetic gas if air not circulated properly[7]

Radiation Exposure

Ionizing radiation (i.e., X-ray, fluoroscopy, mammogram, CT scan) is associated with cardiovascular disease, thyroid cancer, leukemia, cataracts, glaucoma, dermatitis, and potential effects on fertility (Table 20.3).[8,9]

Table 20.4 Risk of transmission and postexposure prophylaxis (PEP) after needlestick, HBV, HCV, HIV[*]

	HBV	HCV	HIV
Risk	≈ 22–30% HBeAg positive source ≈ 1–6% HBeAg negative source	1.8% (negligible for mucous membrane)	0.3% (0.09% for mucous membrane)
PEP/ Test	If HBsAg (+) source or unknown: **Unvaccinated**: HBIg and HBV vaccinated w/in 24 hr **Vaccinated**: ✔ anti-HBsAb level If > 10 mIU/mL→ done If < 10 mIU/mL→ give HBIg and HBV vaccine boost If HBsAg (–) source **Unvaccinated**: Give HBV vaccine **Vaccinated**: No treatment	Pre-exposure prophylaxis not recommended Provider should have HCV status checked w/in 24 hours & then again > 3 weeks	4-week course of two anti-retroviral medications; three if deemed high risk Provider should have HIV status checked at time of needlestick & at follow-up

[*] Abbreviated table: See CDC MMWR Recommendations and Reports[10] for details.

- 6 feet of air = 9 inches of concrete = 2.5 mm of lead.
- Dosage of radiation $\approx 1/(\text{Distance})^2$

HCP should utilize lead glass partitions, lead aprons with thyroid shields, and protective eyewear and carry radiation detection badges.

Infectious Diseases

Herpetic Whitlow

- Risk: Direct contact with HSV-1, 2 sores
- Prevention: Avoid visible sores, wear gloves
- Treatment: topical 5% acyclovir ointment

HPV Recurrent Respiratory Papillomatosis (RRP) or Laryngeal Papillomatosis

- Risk: Laser surgery of patient with HPV (low risk)
- Prevention: N-95 masks and local exhaust ventilation, ventilated OR
- Treatment: Surgery

Needlestick Injury[10]

- *Seroconversion rate* depends on infectivity of organism, degree of viremia, size of inoculum, and the immune status of health care provider (Table 20.4).

References

1. Metzner J, Posner KL, Lam MS, Domino KB. Closed claims' analysis. *Best Pract Res Clin Anaesthesiol* 2011;**25**(2):263–276.

2. Ware LB, Matthay MA. Acute pulmonary edema. *N Engl J Med* 2005;**353**:2788–2796.

3. Nuttall GA, Garrity JA, Dearani JA, et al. Risk factors for ischemic optic neuropathy after cardiopulmonary bypass: a matched case/control Study. *Anesth Analg* 2001;**93**(6):1410–1416.

4. Buono LM, Foroozan R. Perioperative posterior ischemic optic neuropathy: review of the literature *Surv Ophthalm* 2005;**50**(1):15–26.

5. Malignant Hyperthermia Association of the United States. Managing an MH Crisis. 2017. Available at: www.mhaus.org/healthcare-professionals/managing-a-crisis (accessed February 7, 2017).

6. *Anatomy & Physiology*. Connexions 2013. © 1999–2024, Rice University. Available at: http://cnx.org/content/col11496/1.6/. OpenStax CC BY 3.0 (accessed December 10, 2022).

7. US Department of Labor: Occupational Safety and Health Administration. Anesthetic gases: guidelines for workplace exposures. 2017. Available at: www.osha.gov/dts/osta/anestheticgases/ (accessed February 7, 2017).

8. Hamada N, Fujimichi Y. Classification of radiation effects for dose limitation purposes: history, current situation and future prospects. *J Radiat Res* 2014;**55**(4):629–640.

9. US Department of Labor: Occupational Safety and Health Administration. Maximum Permissible Dose Equivalent for Occupational Exposure. Available at: www.osha.gov/SLTC/radiationionizing/introtoionizing/ionizingattachmentsix.html (Accessed February 7, 2017).

10. Centers for Disease Control. Updated US Public Health Service Guidelines for the Management of Occupational Exposures to HBV, HCV, and HiV and Recommendations for Postexposure Prophylaxis. *MMWR* June 29, 2001;**50**(RR11):1–42. Available at: www.cdc.gov/mmwr/PDF/RR/RR5011.pdf (Accessed February 7, 2017).

Postanesthesia Recovery Period: Analgesics

Deborah C. Mokuolu and Rebecca E. Lee

- **Postoperative Analgesic Routes**
  - **Intravenous**
    - Fastest, most common route of medication delivery
    - Medication doses can quickly be titrated to effect
    - Administration by healthcare providers as IV push or infusion, or by the patient through patient-controlled analgesia
      - **Patient-controlled analgesia (PCA)**
        - Device programmed with specific medication, rate of constant (background) infusion, bolus (demand) dose, and lockout interval
        - Commonly used drugs: fentanyl, morphine, hydromorphone
        - Improved *patient satisfaction* due to control over delivery of pain medications and improve pain scores
        - May increase *total opioid consumption*
  - **Oral**
    - Second most common route of medication delivery postoperatively
    - Useful in ambulatory setting and for patients without IV access
    - Bioavailability of oral medications varies widely
    - Generally longer duration of action than IV, but limited utility for managing severe pain due to delayed onset and peak effect
    - Not feasible in NPO patients or those with significant postoperative nausea and vomiting (PONV)
  - **Subcutaneous**
    - Drug injected into subcutaneous fat and absorbed into systemic circulation
    - Generally, less painful than IM injection
    - Option for patients without IV access and unable to tolerate PO
    - Variable drug absorption
    - Larger doses required to reach desired effect
  - **Transcutaneous**
    - Drug absorbed across skin into systemic circulation
    - Option for patients without IV access
    - Transcutaneous patches can slowly release drug into circulation over prolonged periods, providing *long-acting pain relief*
    - *Slow and* often *unpredictable absorption* – drug must be lipophilic for adequate absorption to occur (e.g., fentanyl patch)
  - **Transmucosal**
    - Drug absorbed across mucus membranes into systemic circulation
      - For example, rectal, sublingual, buccal
    - Useful for patients without IV access
    - Generally faster than transcutaneous but unpredictable absorption
  - **Intramuscular**
    - Drug injected directly into muscle
    - Patients without IV access or unable to tolerate PO
    - Pain at injection site affects tolerability
  - **Epidural**
    - Excellent modality of analgesia for a wide range of procedures
    - Ability to use local anesthetics and opioids separately or in combination
    - Epidural opioids diffuse into CSF acting on mu receptors in the spinal cord located in the substantia gelatinosa of the posterior horn (Rexed lamina II)
      - Some systemic absorption also occurs
    - Can be placed at many levels of the spinal cord (caudal to cervical), depending on the procedure and desired application:
      - **Caudal** – groin, pelvic, lower extremity surgery (commonly used in pediatrics)
      - **Lumbar** – abdominal, pelvic, lower extremity surgery
      - **Thoracic** – thoracic, upper and lower abdominal, rib fractures
      - **Cervical** – steroid injection by pain management physicians
    - Placement of epidural is dependent on patient willingness, anatomy, recent anticoagulation, or infection
  - **Spinal**
    - Intrathecal injection – benefit of rapid onset when using local anesthetics or opioids
      - Both act directly on target receptors in the CNS without systemic effects

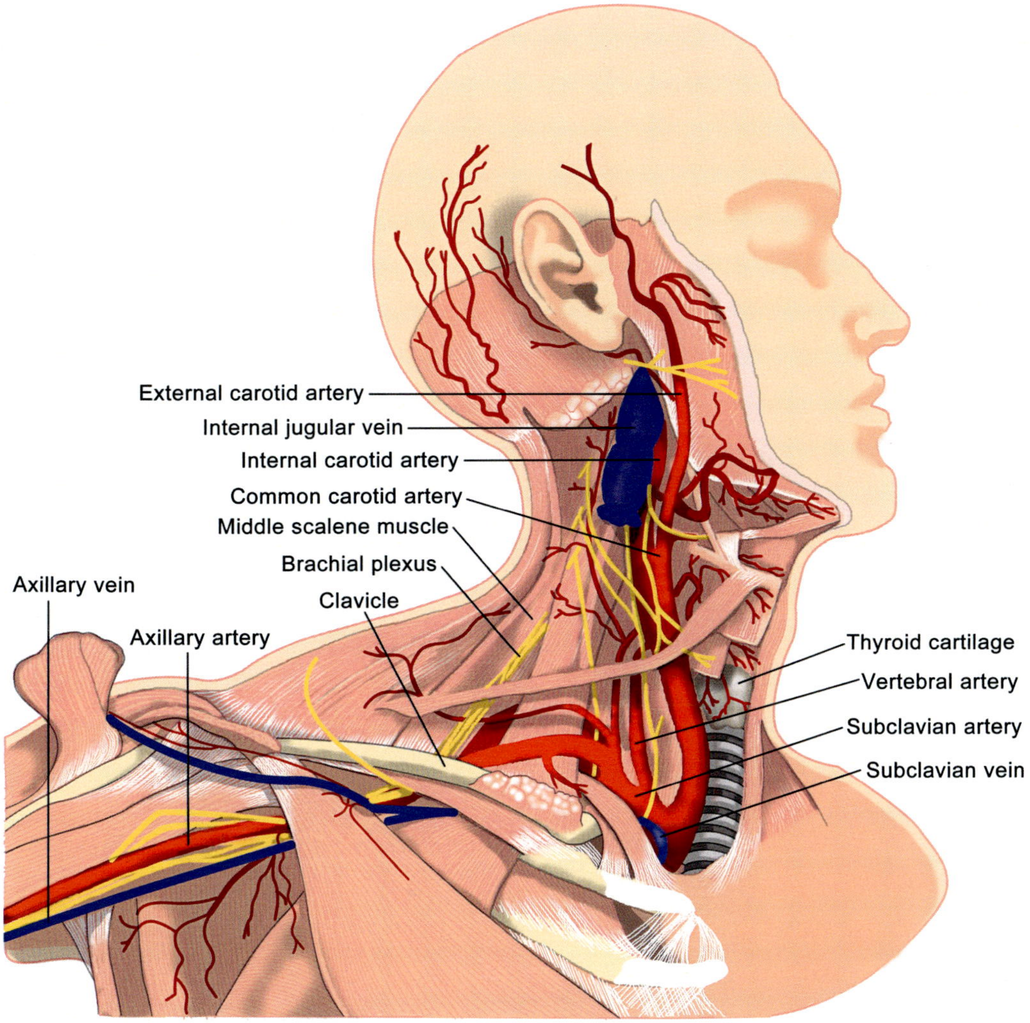

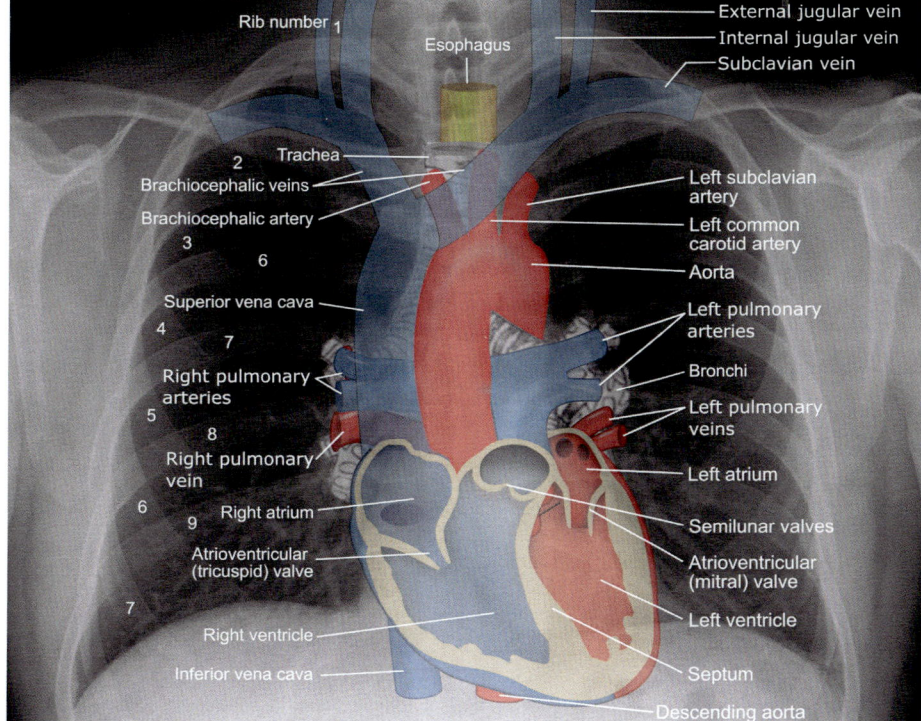

Figure 1.1 Normal anatomical relationships of the major vessels, nerves, bones, and muscles of the neck and axilla.

External carotid artery
Internal jugular vein
Internal carotid artery
Common carotid artery
Middle scalene muscle
Brachial plexus
Clavicle
Axillary vein
Axillary artery

Thyroid cartilage
Vertebral artery
Subclavian artery
Subclavian vein

Figure 1.3 Normal radiograph of the chest. Superimposed on this image are outlines of some of the major topographical landmarks of the chest.

Rib number 1
Esophagus
External jugular vein
Internal jugular vein
Subclavian vein
2 Trachea
Brachiocephalic veins
Brachiocephalic artery
3   6
Superior vena cava
4   7
Right pulmonary arteries
5   8
Right pulmonary vein
6   9   Right atrium
Atrioventricular (tricuspid) valve
7
Right ventricle
Inferior vena cava

Left subclavian artery
Left common carotid artery
Aorta
Left pulmonary arteries
Bronchi
Left pulmonary veins
Left atrium
Semilunar valves
Atrioventricular (mitral) valve
Left ventricle
Septum
Descending aorta

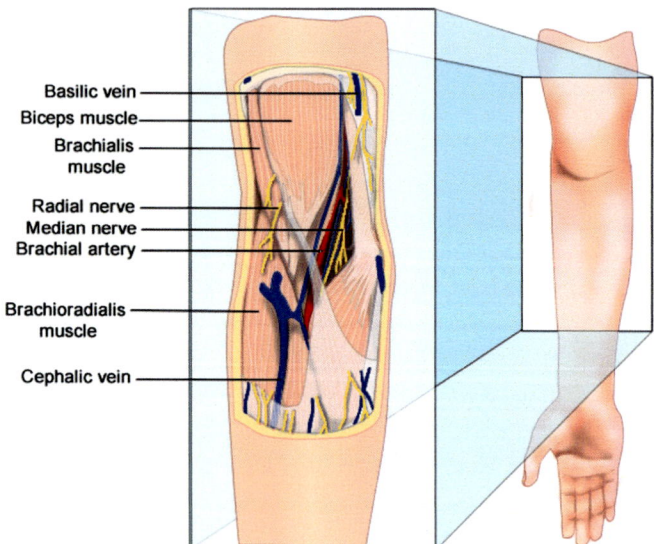

Figure 1.4 Normal anatomical relationships of the major vessels and nerves, bones, and muscles of the antecubital fossa.

Basilic vein
Biceps muscle
Brachialis muscle
Radial nerve
Median nerve
Brachial artery
Brachioradialis muscle
Cephalic vein

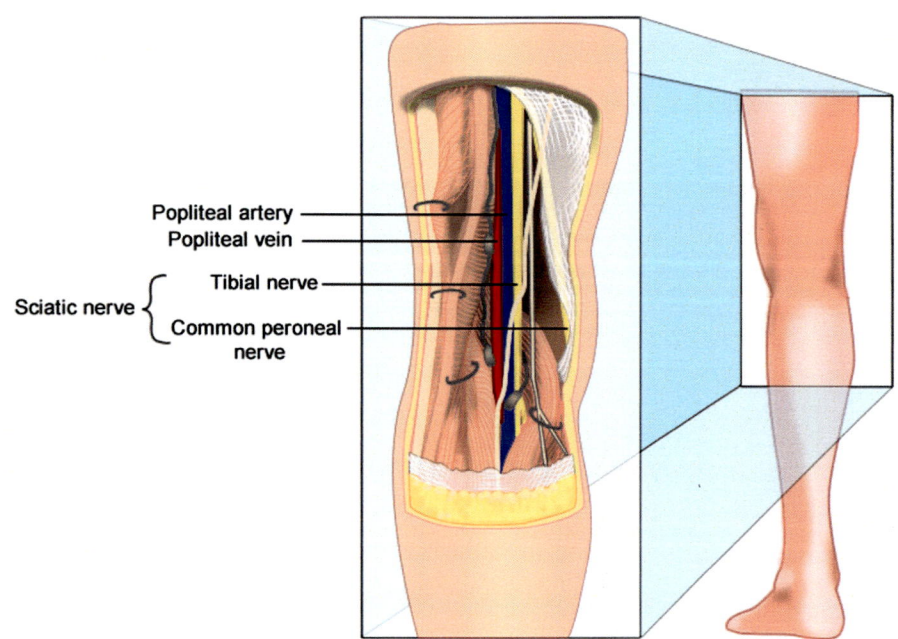

Figure 1.5 Normal anatomical relationships of the major vessels, nerves, bones, and muscles of the popliteal fossa (medial to lateral).

Popliteal artery
Popliteal vein
Sciatic nerve { Tibial nerve
Common peroneal nerve

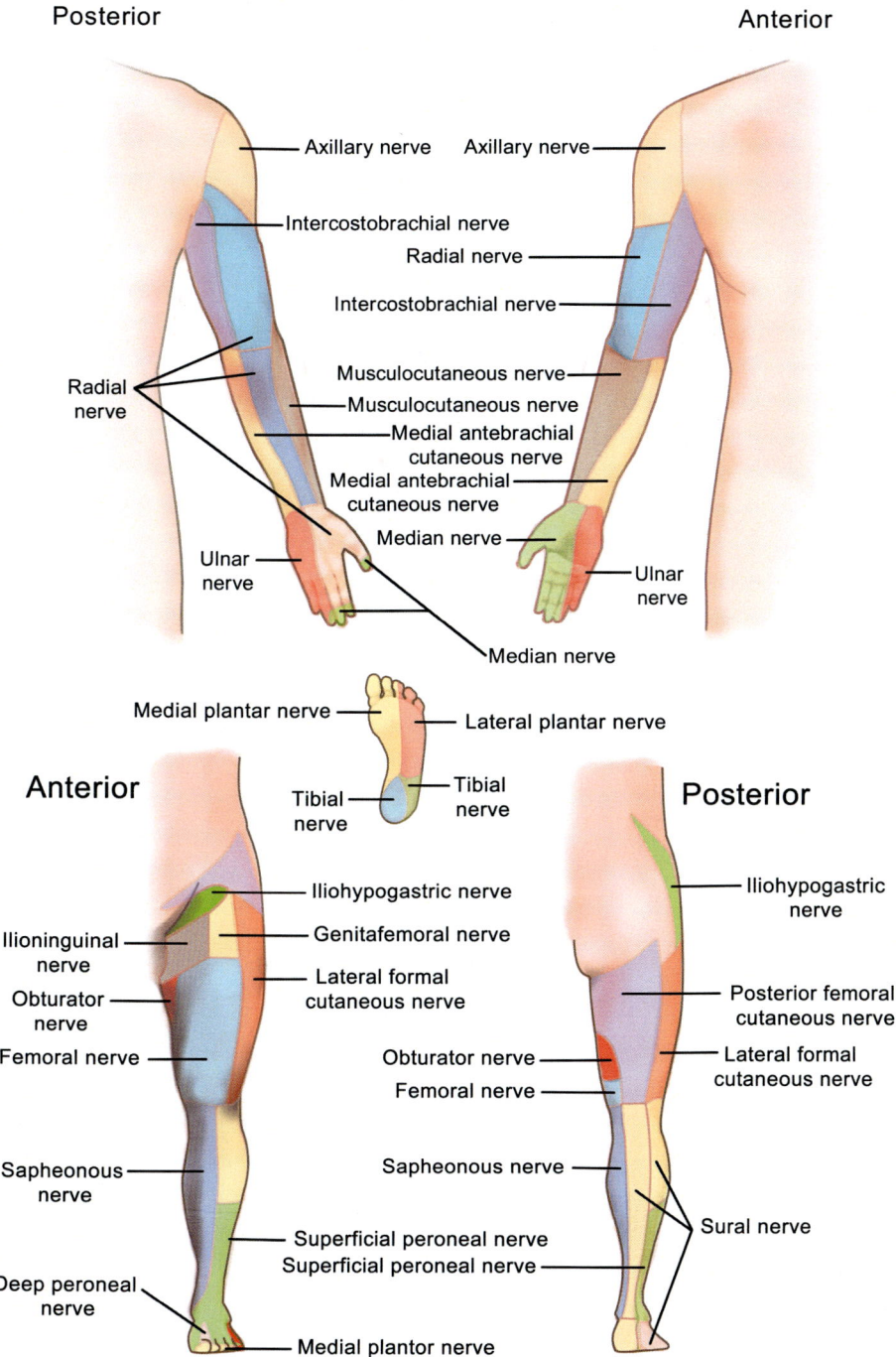

Posterior

Anterior

Axillary nerve

Axillary nerve

Intercostobrachial nerve

Radial nerve

Intercostobrachial nerve

Musculocutaneous nerve

Musculocutaneous nerve

Radial nerve

Medial antebrachial cutaneous nerve

Medial antebrachial cutaneous nerve

Median nerve

Ulnar nerve

Ulnar nerve

Median nerve

Medial plantar nerve

Lateral plantar nerve

Tibial nerve

Tibial nerve

Anterior

Posterior

Iliohypogastric nerve

Iliohypogastric nerve

Ilioninguinal nerve

Genitafemoral nerve

Obturator nerve

Lateral formal cutaneous nerve

Posterior femoral cutaneous nerve

Femoral nerve

Obturator nerve

Lateral formal cutaneous nerve

Femoral nerve

Sapheonous nerve

Sapheonous nerve

Sural nerve

Superficial peroneal nerve

Superficial peroneal nerve

Deep peroneal nerve

Medial plantor nerve

Figure 1.6 Distribution of the major cutaneous nerve branches of the upper and lower extremities.

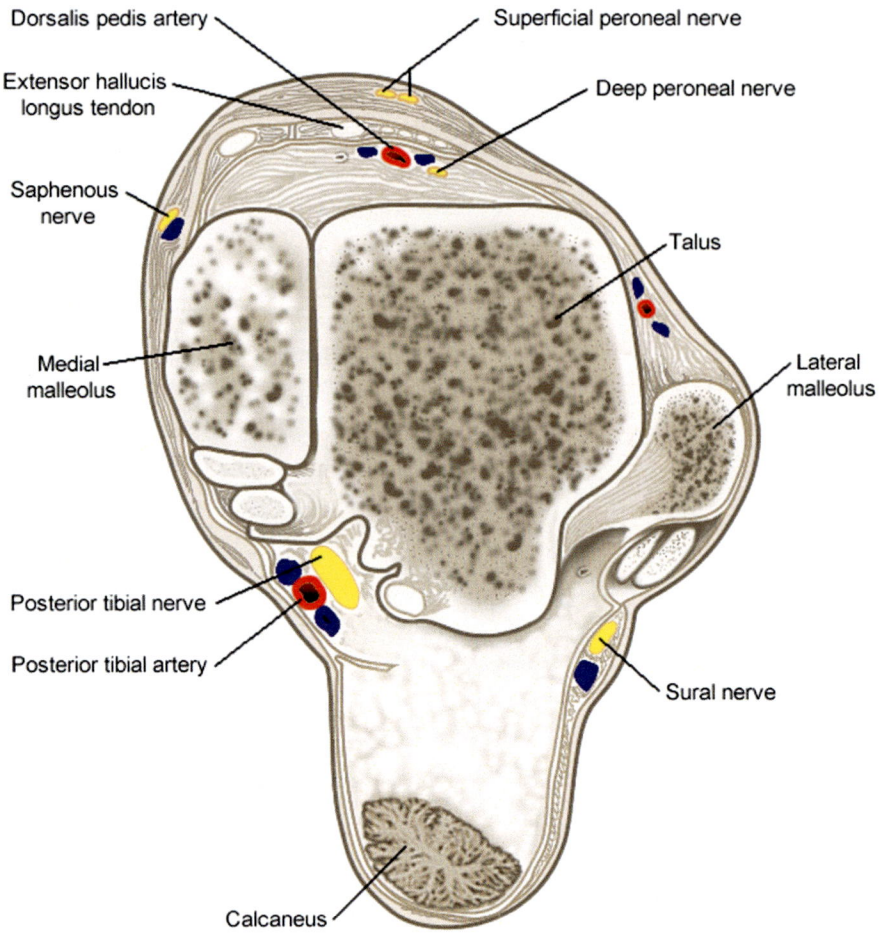

Figure 1.7 Normal anatomical relationship of the major vessels, nerves, bones, and the ankle.

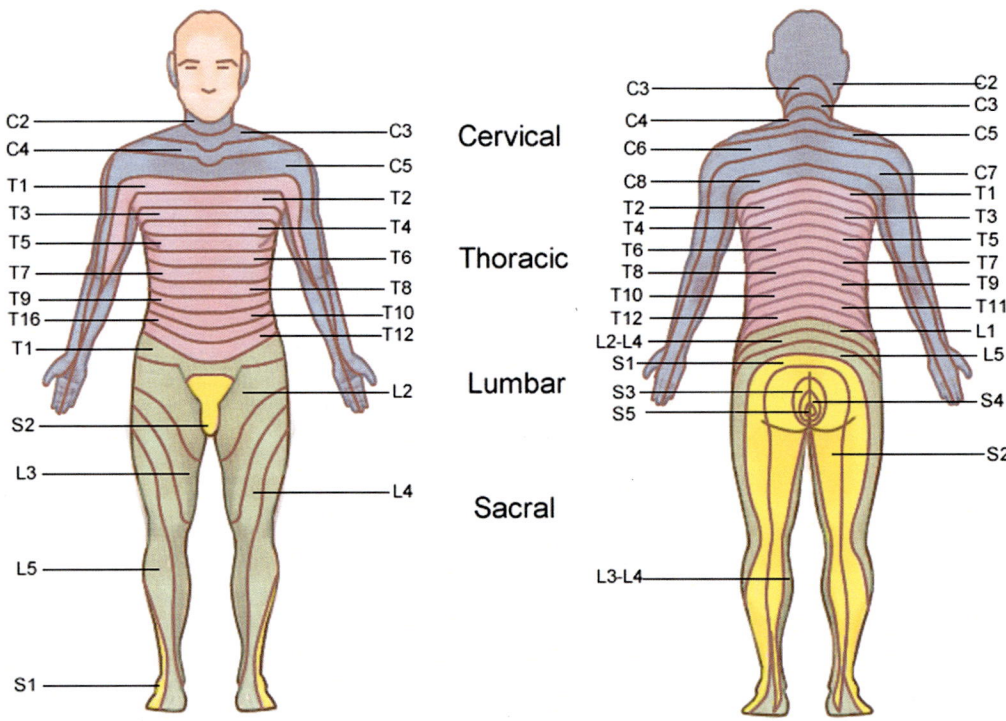

Figure 1.11 Dermatome map.

Cervical (C1–C7)
Cricoid Cartilage
Vertebra Prominens
Angle of Louis
Thoracic (T1–T12)
Inferior Angle of Scapula
Lumbar (L1–L5)
Iliac Crest
Sacral (S1–S5)

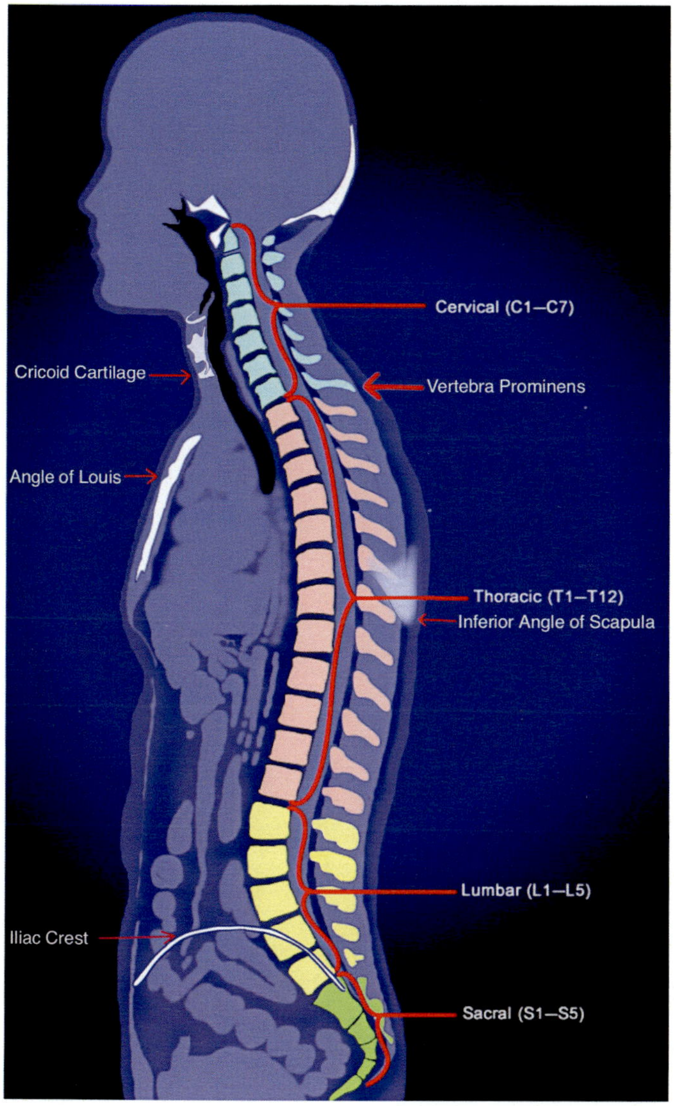

Figure 1.12 Spinal anatomy and relevant surface anatomy.

NITROUS OXIDE
OXYGEN
MEDICAL AIR

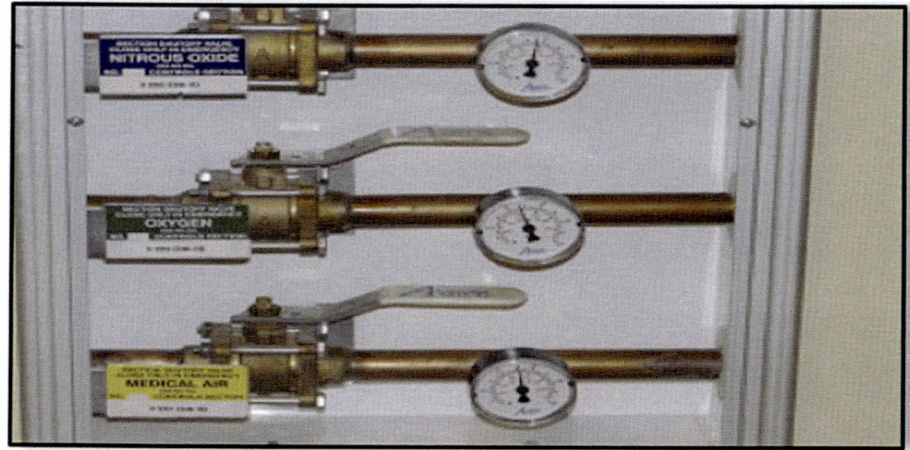

Figure 4.7 Gas-specific shutoff valves, required to be located outside of each operating room to enable control of pipeline supply in the event of emergencies such as fires.

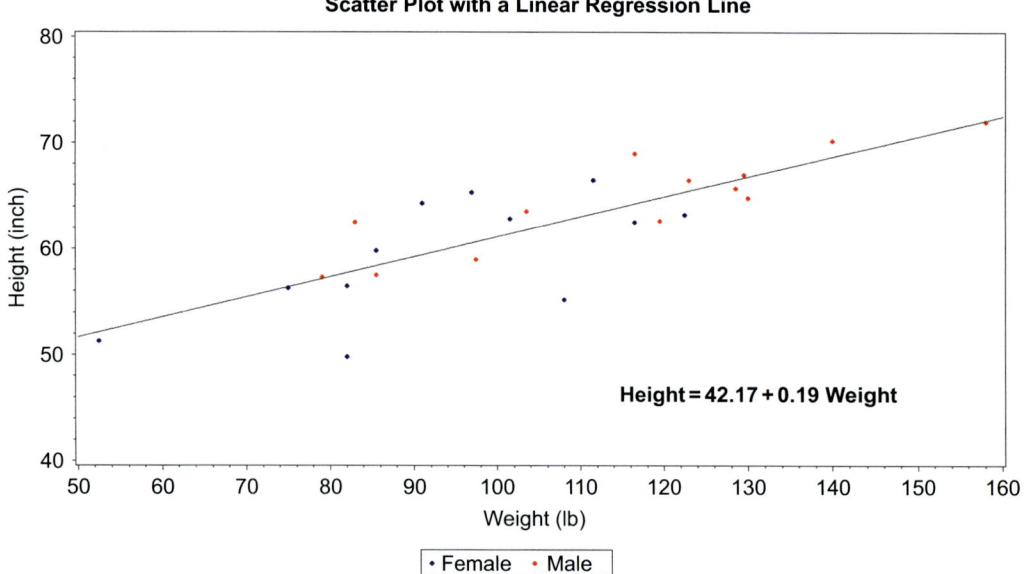

Scatter Plot with a Linear Regression Line

Height = 42.17 + 0.19 Weight

· Female   · Male

Figure 7.1 Example of a linear equation used to model the relationship between height (in.) and weight (lb) in children aged 11–17.

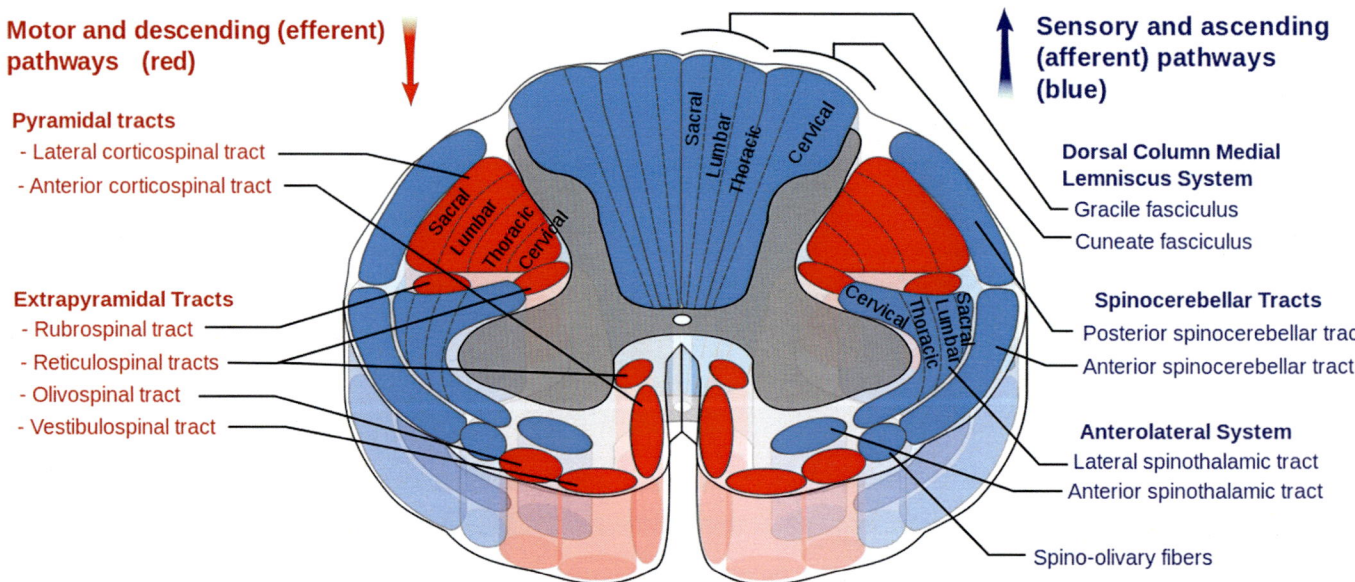

Motor and descending (efferent) pathways (red)

Pyramidal tracts
- Lateral corticospinal tract
- Anterior corticospinal tract

Extrapyramidal Tracts
- Rubrospinal tract
- Reticulospinal tracts
- Olivospinal tract
- Vestibulospinal tract

Sensory and ascending (afferent) pathways (blue)

Dorsal Column Medial Lemniscus System
- Gracile fasciculus
- Cuneate fasciculus

Spinocerebellar Tracts
- Posterior spinocerebellar tract
- Anterior spinocerebellar tract

Anterolateral System
- Lateral spinothalamic tract
- Anterior spinothalamic tract

- Spino-olivary fibers

Figure 23.3 Spinal cord and spinal cord tracts.

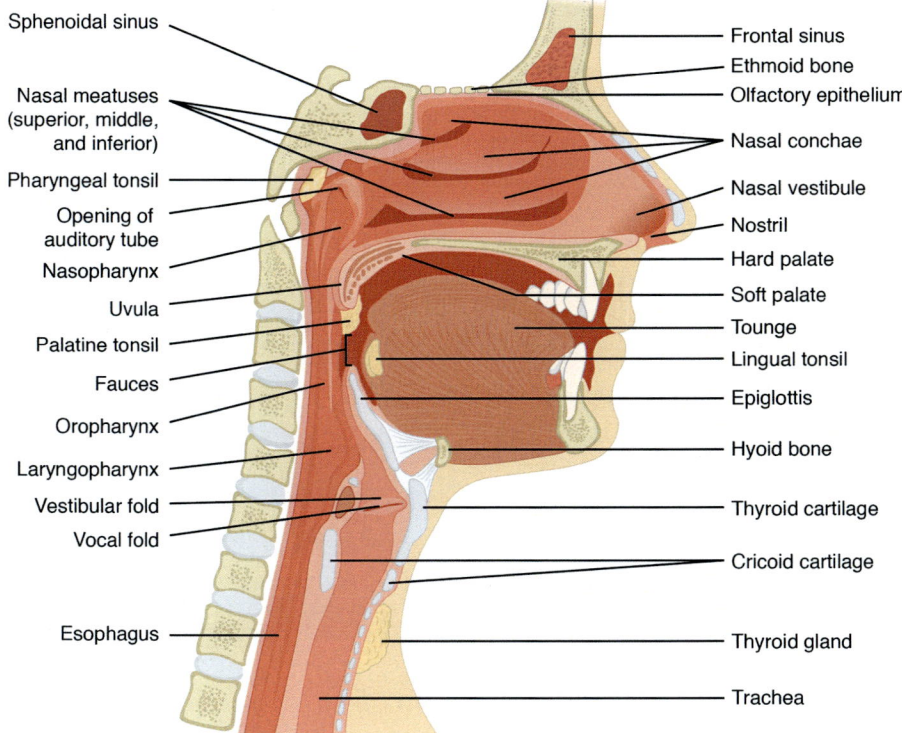

Figure 28.1 Pharynx.

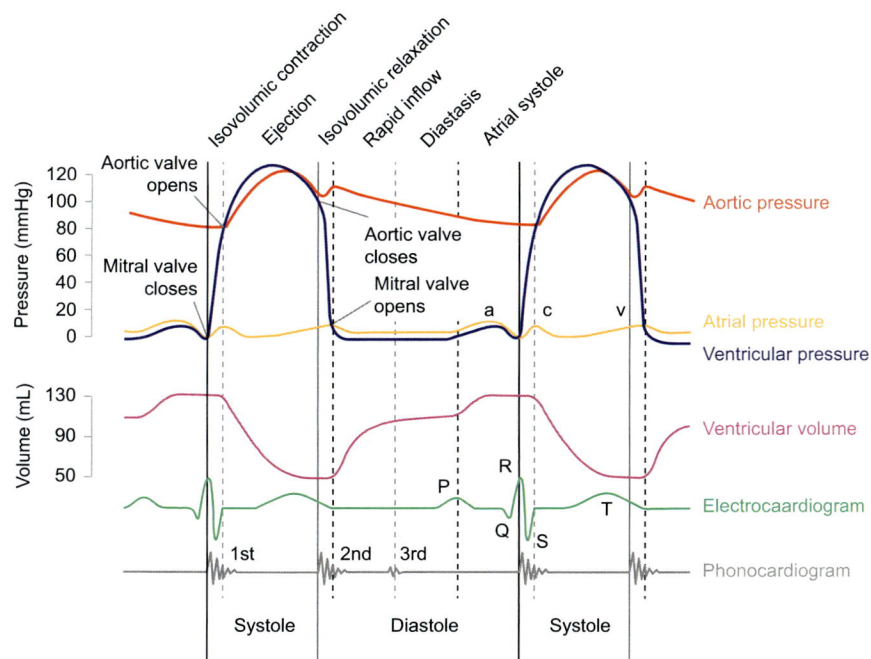

Figure 30.1 Wiggers diagram. Cardiac cycle demonstrating electrical, mechanical, valve, pressure, and heart sound synchronicity during systolic and diastolic events.
From https://en.wikipedia.org/wiki/Wiggers_diagram

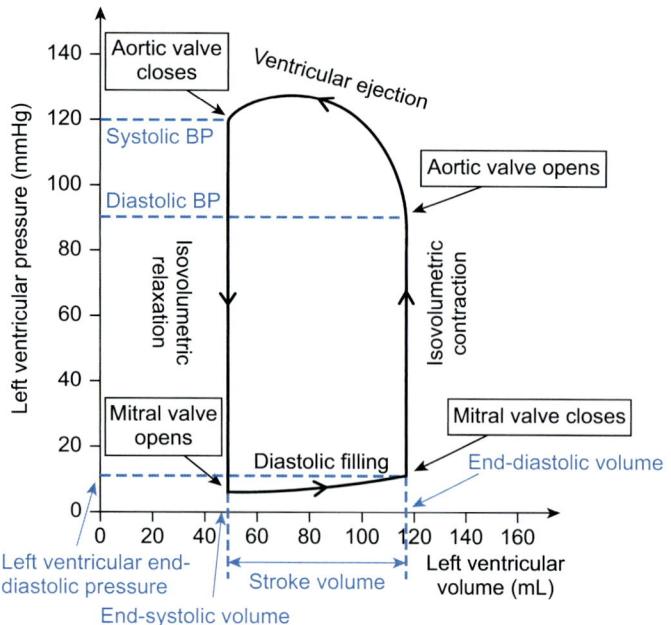

Figure 30.2 Stylized LV pressure–volume loop demonstrating a normal ventricle through four phases: isovolumetric contraction (no change in volume, increase in pressure), ventricular ejection, isovolumetric relaxation (no change in volume, decrease in pressure), ventricular diastole.
From Chambers D, Huang C, Matthews G. Cardiac pressure–volume loops. In *Basic Physiology for Anaesthetists*. Cambridge University Press, 2019; pp 136–140. doi:10.1017/9781108565011.034.

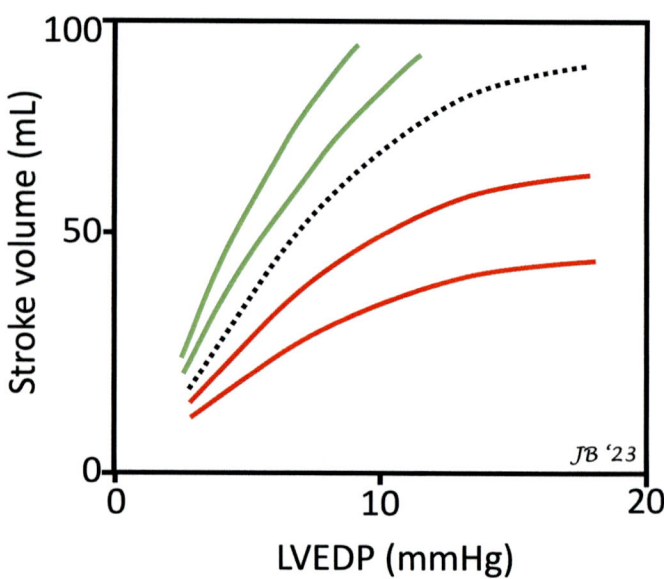

Figure 30.4 Frank–Starling curve. Relationship between LV filling, pressure, and stroke volume illustrated by family of curves. Black dotted curve represents "normal" curve where increased stroke volume is proportional to increasing LVEDP. Green curves depict hearts with reduced afterload and/or increased inotropy. Red curves depict hearts with increased afterload and/or reduced inotropy. Created by J. Brodt.

In-Hospital Cardiac Arrest Sequence

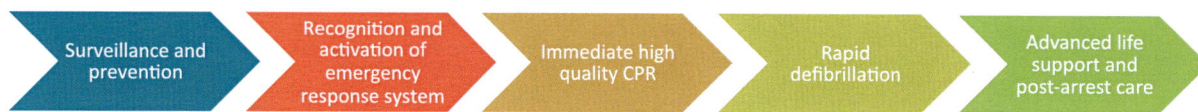

Out-of-Hospital Cardiac Arrest Sequence

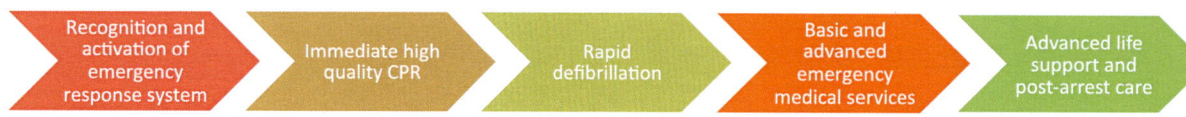

Figure 31.1 Difference between in-hospital and out-of-hospital cardiac arrest algorithm. Adapted from the ACLS *2020 Handbook of Emergency Cardiovascular Care for Healthcare Providers*.

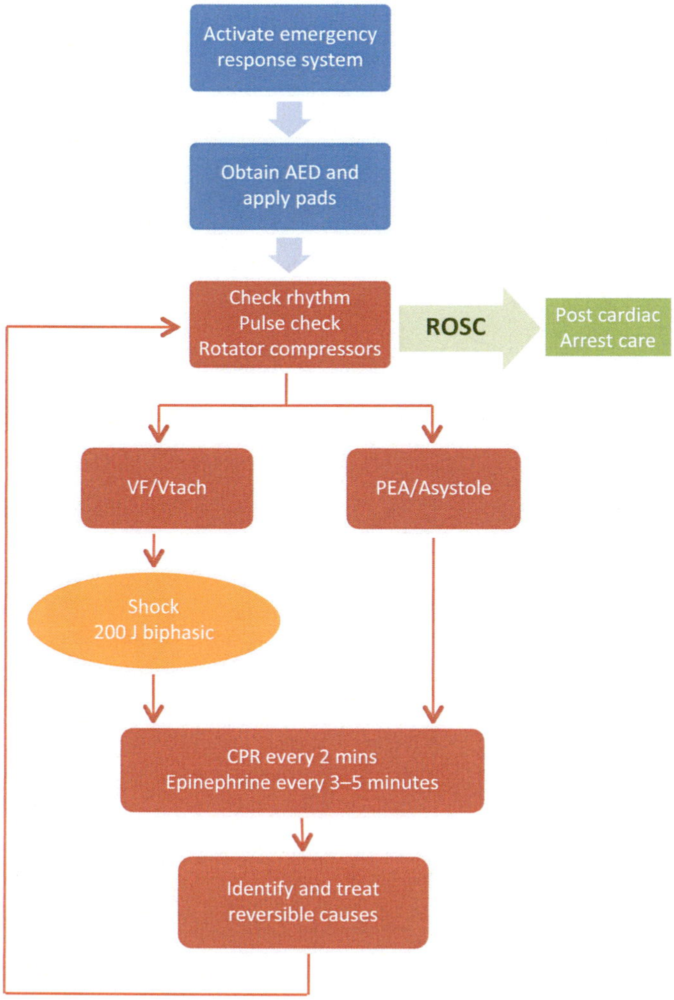

Figure 31.2 Cardiac arrest algorithm. Adapted from the *2020 Handbook of Emergency Cardiovascular Care for Healthcare Providers.*

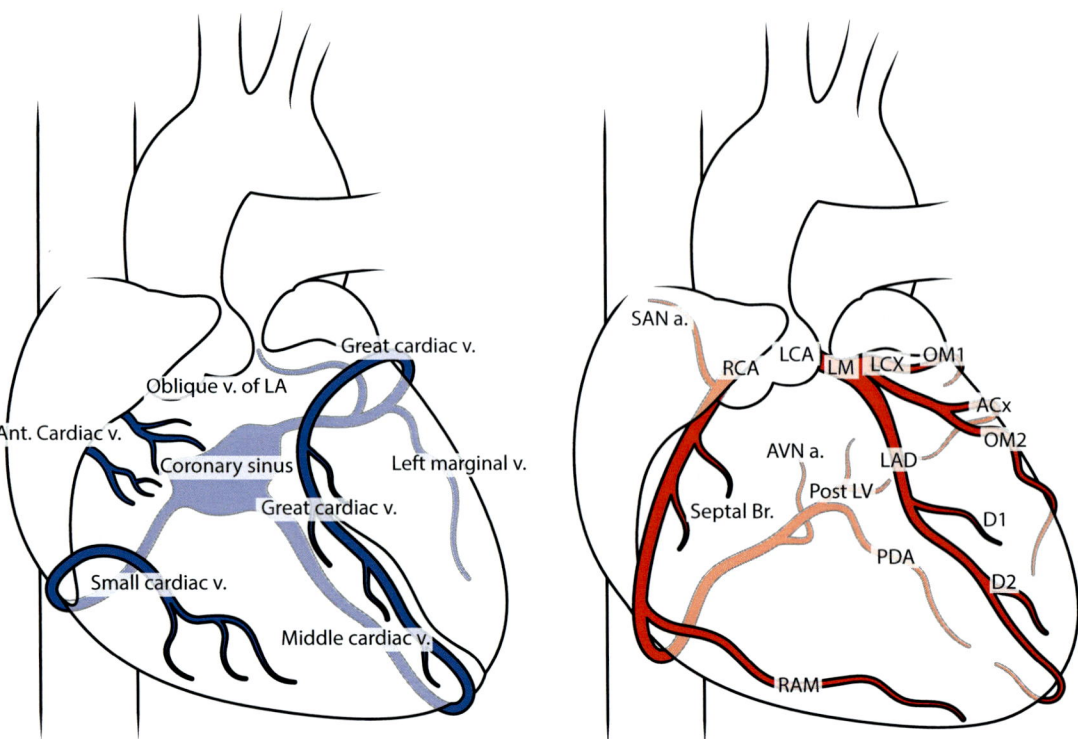

Figure 32.1 Cardiac arterial and venous circulation – anterior view. ACx: atrial circumflex artery; AVN a.: atrioventricular nodal artery; DM1: first diagonal; D2: second diagonal; LAD: left anterior descending artery; LCA: left coronary artery; LCX: left circumflex; LM: left main coronary artery; OM1: first obtuse marginal; OM2: second obtuse marginal; PDA: posterior descending artery; Post.LV: posterior left ventricular artery; RAM: right anterior marginal; RCA: right coronary artery; SAN a.: sino-atrial nodal artery.

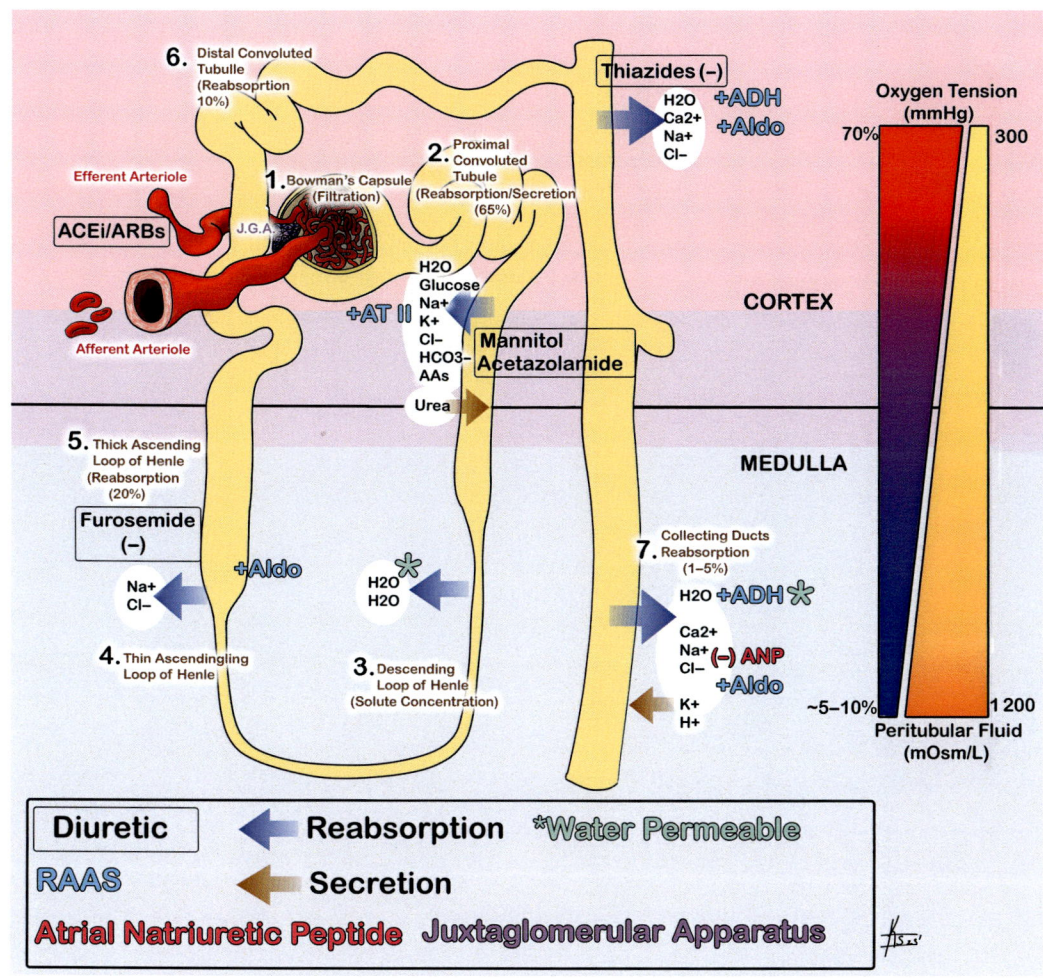

Figure 35.1 Nephron system.

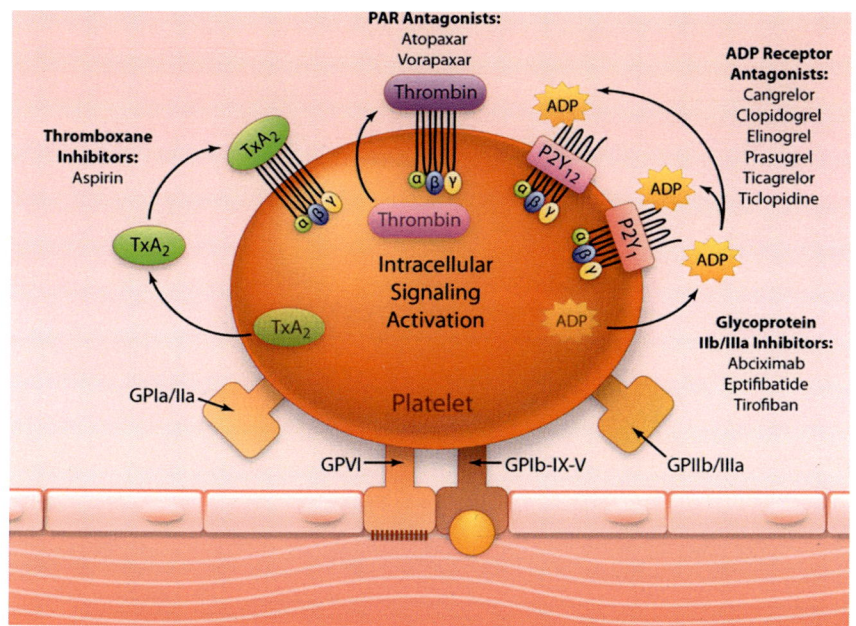

Figure 37.1 Formation of a platelet plug.

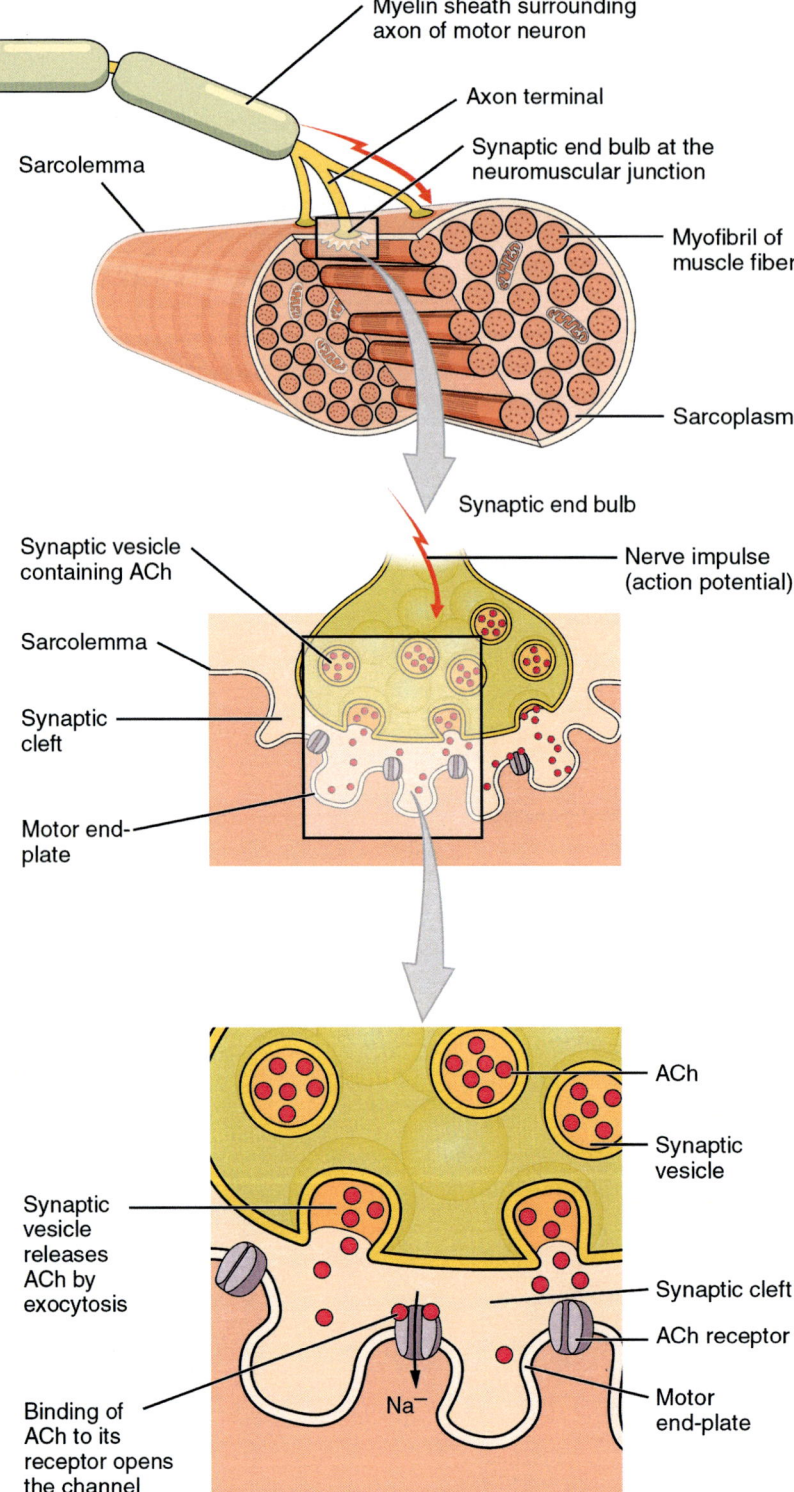

Myelin sheath surrounding
axon of motor neuron

Axon terminal

Synaptic end bulb at the
neuromuscular junction

Sarcolemma

Myofibril of
muscle fiber

Sarcoplasm

Synaptic end bulb

Synaptic vesicle
containing ACh

Nerve impulse
(action potential)

Sarcolemma

Synaptic
cleft

Motor end-
plate

ACh

Synaptic
vesicle

Synaptic
vesicle
releases
ACh by
exocytosis

Synaptic cleft

ACh receptor

Motor
end-plate

Binding of
ACh to its
receptor opens
the channel

Na⁻

Figure 41.1 Neuromuscular junction, motor end plate, and innervation. Source: OpenStax College. "Anatomy and Physiology." OpenStax CNX, OpenStax College, June 19, 2013, cnx.org/content/col11496/1.6/

- Intrathecal opioids can provide prolonged analgesia from a single injection, particularly if hydrophilic (e.g., preservative-free morphine)
  - Delayed respiratory depression up to 24 hours possible due to eventual rostral spread of cerebrospinal fluid
  - Duration and level of block from local anesthetics depends on specific drug properties, total dose, level of injection, patient positioning, and baricity
- **Intrapleural**
  - Local anesthetics and/or analgesics injected in the intrapleural space
  - Produces a multilevel intercostal block for thoracotomies and other thoracic procedure
  - Less reliable technique as the effects vary and depend on patient positioning and volume of injected drug
  - High rate of systemic absorption
- **Opioids**
  - **Mechanism of Action**
    - Binds to four major opioid receptors located within the central nervous system: mu, kappa, delta, sigma
      - $\mu 1$ = supraspinal analgesia
      - $\mu 2$ = respiratory depression & decreased GI motility
      - kappa = spinal analgesia, shivering, ↓ADH
      - delta = antidepressant
    - Binding activates G proteins → membrane hyperpolarization
    - Inhibits nociceptive neuronal pathways by preventing release and response to acetylcholine and substance P
  - Can ↑ the apneic threshold and ↓ hypoxic respiratory drive, a significant concern postoperatively
  - Tables 21.1 and 21.2 describe commonly used postoperative opioid agonists and agonist-antagonists
- **Local Anesthetics (LA)** – bind to intracellular voltage-dependent sodium channels
  - **Lidocaine** – short-acting amide
    - Common uses: Intravenous, topical, infiltration, epidural, peripheral nerve block, and transdermal
      - Intravenous infusions – USEFUL as part of multimodal pain management strategy. Data supports use during and after major abdominal surgery – reducing postoperative pain and opioid requirements. Postoperative infusion doses range from 1 to 2 mg/kg/hr
      - Transdermal patch – 5% lidocaine patch applied directly to skin overlying painful area. When applied for the recommended maximum duration of 12 hours/day, systemic absorption is minimal
      - IV regional anesthesia (Bier Block) – Lidocaine is the drug of choice when performing IV regional anesthesia for the management of intra- and postoperative pain

- **Chloroprocaine** – short-acting ester
  - Common uses: Infiltration, epidural, peripheral nerve block
  - Fastest-acting LA
  - Low systemic toxicity permits use of high concentrations
  - Development of tachyphylaxis with repeated use
- **Mepivacaine** – medium-acting amide LA
  - Common uses include: infiltration, epidural, peripheral nerve block
- **Bupivacaine, ropivacaine** – long-acting amide LA
  - Common uses: infiltration (bupivacaine), peripheral nerve or plexus block, epidural, intrathecal
  - Contraindicated in IV regional anesthesia due to risk of systemic toxicity
  - Ropivacaine – less lipophilic → less motor block, decreased potential of cardiotoxicity and CNS toxicity
- **Liposomal bupivacaine** (Exparel)
  - Lipid-based delivery system to extend duration of bupivacaine analgesia up to 72 hours; ~ 100 × cost of regular bupivacaine
  - Hussain et al.'s 2021 meta-analysis – statistically significant but clinically unimportant improvement in postoperative pain scores (insignificant once vendor-sponsored studies were excluded). No additional benefits found
  - Avoid simultaneous infiltration of non-bupivacaine local anesthetic + liposomal bupivacaine as it can produce immediate release of bupivacaine by disrupting liposomal drug delivery vehicle
- **Alpha-2 Agonists**
  - **Clonidine** – specific, central-acting alpha-2 agonist with hypnotic, sedative, anxiolytic, sympatholytic, analgesic properties
    - Intra- and postoperative use associated with improved pain control and decreased opioid requirements
    - Most efficacious when administered via neuraxial route (epidural, intrathecal) either alone or in combination with local anesthetics
    - Side effects include sedation and hypotension
  - **Dexmedetomidine** – specific, central-acting alpha-2 agonist with similar effects as clonidine but with higher specificity for alpha-2 receptors
    - Intraoperative use as part of multimodal pain management strategy decreases intra- and postoperative opioid requirements
    - Postoperatively can be used as a low dose intravenous infusion (0.2–0.7 mcg/kg/hr) or added to neuraxial or peripheral local anesthetics to potentiate their effect

Table 21.1 Commonly used postoperative opioid agonists

Drug	Route	Dose (adult)	Onset	Duration of action	Comments
Morphine	IV IM Oral (immediate release) Oral (extended release) Epidural (bolus) Epidural (continuous) Intrathecal	2–15 mg 5–20 mg 10–30 mg 15–60 mg (or greater) 1–5 mg 0.1–1 mg/hr 0.1–0.3 mg	5–10 min 10–30 min 30 min Variable 30–60 min 30–60 min 30–60 min	4–5 hr 4–5 hr 3–5 hr 8–12 hr 12–24 hr Continuous 18–24 hr	– Risk of respiratory depression and excess sedation in renal failure (from morphine-6-glucoronide metabolite)
Fentanyl	IV IM Transdermal Transmucosal Epidural (bolus) Epidural (continuous) Intrathecal	25–100 µg 25–100 µg 12.5–100 µg /hr 100–200 µg 50–100 µg 25–100 µg/hr 5–25 µg	Immediate 7–8 min 6 hr 5–15 min 5–10 min 5–10 min Immediate	30–60 min 1–2 hr 72–96 hr Variable 60 min Continuous 60 min	– Can rarely cause chest wall rigidity (especially in children)
Meperidine	IV IM SubQ Oral	50–75 mg 50–75 mg 50–75 mg 50–150 mg	5 min 10–15 min 10–15 min 10–15 min	2–3 hr 2–4 hr 2–4 hr 2–4 hr	– Smaller doses used for postop shivering (12.5–25 mg IV) – Metabolite normeperidine lowers seizure threshold – Mild anticholinergic effect
Hydromorphone	IV SubQ Oral Epidural (bolus) Epidural (continuous) Intrathecal	0.2–1 mg 0.8–1 mg 2–4 mg 0.5–1 mg 0.1–0.2 mg/hr 0.04-.1 mg	5–10 min 5–10 min 15–60 min 15 min 15 min 5 min	3–4 hr 3–4 hr 3–4 hr 8–12 hr Continuous 10–20 hr	– Safer in renal failure vs. morphine (no renally excreted active metabolites)
Methadone	IV Oral	2.5–10 mg 5–10 mg	10–20 min 30–60 min	6–8 hr Variable	– Watch for QTc prolongation – Exhibits NMDA antagonism, MAOI activity
Codeine	Oral	15–60 mg	30–60 min	4–6 hr	– Metabolized by CYP2D6 to morphine – "Slow" metabolizers show increased drug sensitivity – "Fast" metabolizers show drug resistance – Avoid in pediatric tonsillectomy patients
Oxycodone	Oral (immediate release) Oral (extended release)	5–15 mg 10–80 mg	10–30 min 60 min	3–6 hr 12 hr	– Commonly combined with acetaminophen
Hydrocodone	Oral	5–10 mg	10–30 min	4–6 hr	– Commonly combined with acetaminophen
Tramadol	Oral	50–100 mg	30–60 min	4–6 hr	– Also exhibits SNRI activity – Generally not recommended in children < 17 years old

Route and dosing information taken from Apfel 2014; Hindle 2008; Nicholau 2014. See Further Reading.

- **Nonsteroidal Anti-Inflammatory Drugs (NSAIDs)**
  - Analgesic, anti-inflammatory, anti-pyretic compounds
  - Mechanism: Inhibition of cyclooxygenase leads to decreased synthesis of prostaglandins
  - When given alone – provide analgesia for mild and moderate pain
  - When given as adjuncts and part of a multimodal analgesic regimen, can provide significant pain relief and decrease opioid consumption
  - Common side effects: GI upset/ulceration, platelet dysfunction, renal dysfunction
  - Selective COX-2 inhibitors theoretically have fewer GI and platelet effects but show increased risk of stroke and myocardial infarction.

Table 21.2 Opioid agonist–antagonists

Drug	Route	Dose (adult)	Onset	Duration of action
Buprenorphine (partial μ agonist, κ antagonist)	IV IM	0.3–0.6 mg 0.3–0.6 mg	5–15 min 15–30 min	6–13 hr 6–13 hr
Butorphanol (κ agonist, partial μ antagonist)	IV IM	0.5–2 mg q3-4 hr 2 mg q3-4 hr	30–60 min	8–24 hr (dose-dependent)
Nalbuphine (κ agonist, partial μ antagonist)	IV IM Subq	10 mg/70 kg q3-6 hr	2–3 min 5–15 min 5–15 min	3–6 hr 3–6 hr 3–6 hr
Pentazocine (κ agonist, partial μ antagonist)	IV IM Subq	5–30 mg q3-4 hr	15 min	1 hr 2 hr 2 hr

Route and dosing information taken from Nicholau 2014; Hindle 2008; Apfel 2014.

Table 21.3 Common postoperative nonsteroidal anti-inflammatory drugs (NSAIDs)

Drug	Route	Dose (adult)	Onset	Duration of action
Ibuprofen (COX-1 & COX-2)	Oral IV	200–400 mg q4-6 hr 400–800 mg q6 hr	30–60 min	4–8 hr 4–8 hr
Naproxen (COX-1 & COX-2)	Oral	250–500 mg q6-8 hr	30–60 min	6–10 hr
Ketorolac (COX-1 & COX-2)	IV or IM	15–30 mg q6 hr	30–60 min	3–6 hr
Celecoxib (COX-2)	Oral	400 mg once or 200 mg q12 hr	30–60 min	8–12 hr
Diclofenac	Oral Topical	50 mg 2–3 × daily Apply twice daily	30–60 min Variable	8–12 hr Variable
Meloxicam	Oral	7.5–15 mg daily	30–60 min	Up to 24 hr
Indomethacin	Oral	20–40 mg q12 hr	30–60 min	4–6 hr
Acetaminophen (COX-2 & COX-3} (Analgesic, antipyretic only)	Oral Rectal IV	325–1 000 mg q4–6 hr 325–600 mg q4–6 hr 650–1 000 mg q6 hr	30–60 min	4–6 hr

Route and dosing information taken from Apfel 2014; Hindle 2008; Nicholau 2014. See Further Reading.

- ○ Table 21.3 describes commonly used postoperative NSAIDs.
- **N-Methyl-Aspartate (NMDA) Receptor Blockers**
  - ○ **Ketamine**
    - Sedative-hypnotic NMDA receptor antagonist with activity at opioid, cholinergic, monoaminergic receptors
    - Also acts as Na+ channel blocker
    - Results in dissociative state producing anesthesia and analgesia
    - Side effects – salivation, hallucinations (attenuated by benzodiazepine administration), bronchodilation, sympathomimetic activity
  - ○ **Magnesium**
    - In the CNS acts as a non-competitive NMDA receptor antagonist
    - When infused as adjunct intraoperatively in doses of 8 mg/kg/hr, some studies demonstrate decreased perioperative pain
    - Potentiates the effects of neuraxial narcotics when given intrathecally
    - Side effects include hypotonia
  - ○ **Amantadine**
    - Noncompetitive NMDA antagonist
    - Most often used for chronic neuropathic, musculoskeletal, postoperative pain
- **Tricyclic Antidepressants (TCAs)**
  - ○ Examples – amitriptyline, nortriptyline, imipramine, clomipramine
  - ○ Primarily act in the CNS as serotonin-norepinephrine reuptake inhibitors
  - ○ Demonstrate efficacy in treating neuropathic pain and fibromyalgia, but also as adjuncts in the postop period
  - ○ Mechanism of analgesia likely related to neuromodulation of descending pain pathways
- **Selective Serotonin/Norepinephrine Inhibitors (SNRIs)**
  - ○ Examples – venlafaxine, duloxetine
  - ○ Mechanism thought to be similar to TCAs

- **Gabapentinoids**
  - Examples – gabapentin, pregabalin
  - Inhibit α-2-σ voltage-gated calcium channels in the CNS → modulate nociceptive pathways
  - Effective in treating neuropathic, chronic, and postoperative pain
  - Synergistic effects when given in conjunction with NSAIDs and narcotics
  - Can be given preoperatively for multimodal postoperative pain control
- **Other Regional Techniques**
  - **Peripheral nerve and plexus blocks**
    - Provide excellent intra- and postoperative analgesia for surgery involving the upper and lower extremities
    - Local anesthetics are injected and/or infused around a peripheral nerve or plexus, resulting in anesthesia in those nerve distributions.
  - **Transverse abdominal plain (TAP) blocks**
    - Controls incisional pain after large abdominal surgeries
    - Local anesthetic delivered in fascial plane between transversus abdominis and internal oblique, blocking somatic afferents from T8–L1
    - No effect on visceral pain
  - **Rectus sheath block**
    - Useful for postop analgesia for midline abdominal surgeries, especially umbilical hernia repairs
    - Local anesthetic is injected between rectus abdominis and posterior rectus sheath
      - Acts on T9–T11 dermatomes
  - **Paravertebral blocks**
    - Used to manage pain from thoracic, breast, upper abdominal surgery, rib fractures
    - Local anesthetic is injected into paravertebral space along the spinal column, targeting the spinal nerves as they exit the intervertebral foramina
    - Results in ipsilateral somatic and sympathetic block in a dermatomal distribution
    - Complications – pneumothorax, intravascular injection, epidural, or intrathecal injection
- **Postoperative Analgesia – Other Techniques**
  - **Transcutaneous electrical nerve stimulation (TENS)**
    - Involves placement of transcutaneous electrodes to deliver current resulting in nerve excitation
    - Continuous stimulation of nerve pathways results in downregulation of nociceptive impulse transmission (gate-theory)
    - Useful as adjunct in postoperative period
    - Associated with reduced postoperative analgesic use, however efficacy varies by study and many patients cannot tolerate the sensation of electrical stimulation

  - **Cryotherapy (Cryoanalgesia)**
    - Temporary but prolonged neurolysis (weeks to months) by freezing and thawing peripheral nerves using cold cryo probe
    - Mostly used for post-thoracotomy pain
    - Analgesia may not reach full effect for 48 hours
  - **Acupuncture**
    - Involves insertion of needles into discrete, anatomically defined points (meridians)
    - Needles may be twisted or have electrical current applied
    - Mechanism of action has been debated, but possibly related to release of endogenous opioids.
    - Naloxone administration can reverse effects of acupuncture.
    - In some studies, acupuncture appears to reduce postoperative pain, decrease opioid-requirements, and decrease opioid-related side effects.
    - Relatively safe, devoid of systemic effects
  - **Hypnosis**
    - Relaxation technique meant to alter arousal and decrease sympathetic tone associated with pain
    - Pain perception altered by having patient focus on other sensations, localize pain to another site, and dissociate from a painful experience
    - Benefit greatest for patients with pre-existing musculoskeletal disorders

Postoperative Management of Medication-Assisted Treatment (MAT) for Opioid Use Disorder (OUD)

- **Methadone**: Full mu agonist
  - Continue full dose perioperatively
  - Can aid in analgesia
  - Half-life of 12–72 hours, analgesic duration of 6–8 hours, consider split dosing to BID or TID
- **Buprenorphine**: Partial mu agonist, kappa antagonist
  - Continue perioperatively, can consider decreasing dose
    - Less than 8–12 mg total sublingual dose: continue regimen
    - More than 8–12 mg total sublingual dose: decrease to 8–12 mg daily dose in divided doses
  - Ceiling effect, very high-affinity binding for mu receptor, difficult to displace with perioperative opioid. Choose opioids with high binding affinity such as sufentanil or hydromorphone
  - Half-life of 20–37 hours, analgesic duration of 6–13 hours, highly variable based on route of administration
- **Oral naltrexone**: Pure mu antagonist
  - Discontinue 3–5 days prior to elective procedures
  - Half-life of 4 hours, active metabolite 9 hours
  - Used for alcohol or opioid dependence

- **Depot naltrexone:** Pure mu antagonist
  - Stop 1 month prior to elective procedures
  - Monthly high-dose subcutaneous injection
  - Maximal mu antagonism effect peaks mid-month and wanes by the end of 4 weeks

Further Reading

Apfel C. Postoperative nausea and vomiting. In Miller RD, Eriksson LI, Fleisher LA, et al., editors. *Miller's Anesthesia*, 8th ed. Elsevier Saunders, 2014, chapter 97, pp 2947–2973.

Butterworth JF IV, Mackey DC, Wasnick JD. *Morgan and Mikhail's Clinical Anesthesiology*, 7th ed. McGraw-Hill / Medical, 2022.

Chou G, Gordon DB, de Leon-Casasola OA, et al. Management of postoperative pain: a clinical practice guideline from the American Pain Society, the American Society of Regional Anesthesia and Pain Medicine, and the American Society of Anesthesiologists' Committee on Regional Anesthesia, Executive Committee, and Administrative Council. *J Pain* 2016;**17** (2):131–157.

Hindle A. Intrathecal opioids in the management of acute postoperative pain. *Contin Educ Anaesth Crit Care Pain* 2008;**8** (3):81–85.

Hussain N, Brull R, Sheehy B, et al. Perineural liposomal bupivacaine is not superior to nonliposomal bupivacaine for peripheral nerve block analgesia. *Anesthesiology* 2021;**134**(2):147–164.

Malhotra A, Malhotra V, Rawal N. Perioperative pain management. In Yao F-S F, Fontes ML, Malhotra V, editors. *Yao & Artusio's Anesthesiology: Problem-Oriented Patient Management*, 8th ed. Lippincott Williams & Wilkins, 2016; chapter 51.

McNicol E, Ferguson M, Hudcova J. Patient controlled opioid analgesia versus non-patient controlled opioid analgesia for postoperative pain. *Cochrane Database Syst Rev* 2015;**2015**(6):CD003348. doi:10.1002/14651858.CD003348.pub3

Nicholau TK. The postanesthesia care unit. In Miller RD, Eriksson LI, Fleisher LA, et al., editors. *Miller's Anesthesia*, 8th ed. Elsevier Saunders, 2014; chapter 96, pp 2924–2946.

Sinatra RS, Jahr JS, Watkins-Pitchford JM, editors. *The Essence of Analgesia and Analgesics*. Cambridge Medicine. Cambridge University Press, 2010.

Weibel S, Jokinen J, Pace NL, et al. Efficacy and safety of intravenous lidocaine for postoperative analgesia and recovery after surgery: a systematic review with trial sequential analysis. *Br J Anaesth* 2016;**116** (6):770–783.

Postoperative Period: Consequences of Anesthesia and of Surgical Incisions

Deborah C. Mokuolu, Renee L. Davis, and Rebecca E. Lee

Respiratory Consequences of Anesthesia and Surgery

- **Loss of Pharyngeal Tone**
  - Most common cause of postoperative/post-anesthesia airway obstruction → loss of tone → soft tissue/airway collapse → airway obstruction
  - Cumulative effects of anesthetics, neuromuscular blockade, opioids
  - Treatment:
    - Jaw-thrust, continuous positive airway pressure (CPAP), oral/nasal airway, laryngeal mask airway, intubation
    - Reverse pharmacological agents with naloxone, flumazenil, neostigmine/sugammadex

- **Residual Neuromuscular Blockade**
  - Affects diaphragm, pharyngeal muscles, accessory muscles of respiration → risk of respiratory failure
  - Treatment: Reverse with neostigmine + glycopyrrolate or sugammadex, support airway

- **Atelectasis**
  - Dependent lung fields in anesthetized patients
    - Multifactorial – prolonged patient immobility, changes in respiratory physiology, decreased lung volumes, impaired gas exchange, obesity, postoperative pain
  - Treatment intraoperatively – positive end-expiratory pressure (PEEP), recruitment maneuvers
  - Treatment postoperatively – CPAP, incentive spirometry, pain control, upright repositioning

- **Laryngospasm**
  - Sudden vocal cord spasm → partial or complete occlusion of larynx
  - Most susceptible at emergence and immediately post-extubation (children > adults)
  - Increased risk with volatile anesthetics ≫ propofol
  - Treatment: Laryngospasm notch pressure (Larson's maneuver), CPAP, propofol + succinylcholine 20–40 mg

- **Bronchospasm**
  - Increased in patients with preexisting reactive airway disease
  - Triggers: Pharyngeal or tracheal stimulation, suctioning, light anesthesia, or aspiration

  - Treatment: Inhaled beta agonists, IV/inhaled anticholinergics, IV epinephrine, deepen anesthesia with iso-/sevoflurane (bronchodilation)

- **Airway Edema**
  - Oropharyngeal swelling
  - More likely to occur in:
    - Prolonged prone or Trendelenburg position
    - Large-volume fluid administration or head/neck/airway surgery
  - Facial swelling may be absent – this does not predict lack of oropharyngeal or laryngeal edema

- **Airway Hematoma**
  - Devastating complication of head/neck/airway procedures by direct airway compression
  - Treatment: Urgent hematoma evacuation, then endotracheal intubation, emergent tracheostomy

- **Obstructive Sleep Apnea (OSA)**
  - Redundant oropharyngeal tissue or anatomic abnormalities → airway obstruction when asleep or anesthetized
  - Underdiagnosed and majority are NOT obese
  - CPAP and judicious use of sedatives

- **CO_2 Narcosis**
  - Volatile anesthetics/opioids decrease the brain's sensitivity to hypercarbia
  - Depressed respiratory drive → decreased minute ventilation
  - Signs: patient confused or obtunded, coma
  - Treatment: Naloxone 0.04 mg every 5 minutes as needed

- **Diffusion Hypoxia**
  - Nitrous oxide (N_2O): Rapid diffusion of N_2O into alveoli upon discontinuation
  - Dilutes alveolar oxygen → decreasing PAO_2 → arterial hypoxemia
  - Administer supplemental oxygen after discontinuing nitrous oxide
  - May persist up to 10 minutes

- **Postobstructive (Negative Pressure) Pulmonary Edema**
  - Inspiration against closed glottis → transudative edema from exaggerated negative intrathoracic pressure
    - Obstructed endotracheal tube or laryngospasm
  - Chest radiography: Bilateral fluffy pulmonary infiltrates
  - Supportive treatment: Supplemental oxygen, diuresis, possible positive pressure ventilation

- **Transfusion-Related Acute Lung Injury (TRALI)**
  - Non-cardiogenic pulmonary edema occurring within 6 hours of blood transfusion, especially plasma-derived components
  - Mechanism may be secondary to leukocyte antibodies in the transfused product causing inflammation, vascular leakage, edema
- **Pulmonary Embolism**
  - Consider if sudden onset hypoxemia, dyspnea, tachycardia, hypotension, possible chest pain
  - May be a result of embolization from deep vein thrombosis, fat (long bone trauma/surgery), or amniotic fluid (following delivery)
- **Pneumonia**
  - Occurs in up to 9% of high-risk surgery patients
  - General anesthesia itself can predispose to pneumonia due to alterations in:
    - Mucociliary clearance, forced vital capacity, alveolar macrophage activity
  - Increased risk in patients requiring extended postoperative ventilatory support
- **Pneumothorax**
  - Entrainment of air into pleural cavity leads to lung collapse
  - Common causes:
    - Surgical trauma
    - Rupture of surface blebs
    - Central line placement
    - Aggressive positive pressure ventilation
    - Bronchoscopy
  - Signs: Hypoxia, tachycardia, decreased breath sounds, hypotension
    - Circulatory collapse possible with tension pneumothorax
  - Management:
    - 100% FiO_2, needle decompression, chest tube placement

Cardiovascular Consequences of General and Regional Anesthesia

- **Postoperative Hypertension**
  - Preexisting hypertension at greatest risk
    - Carotid endarterectomies and intracranial surgeries are most commonly associated with postoperative hypertension
  - Other causes of hypertension:
    - Pain leading ↑ sympathetic tone
      - Treatment: Pain medication, regional anesthetic/analgesic techniques
    - Hypercarbia
      - Treatment: Ventilatory support

- Urinary retention/bladder distention
  - Treatment: Bladder catheterization
- Intubated patients with inadequate sedation
  - Treatment: Sedation, pain control
- Nausea and vomiting
  - See postoperative nausea and vomiting (PONV) in the Nausea and Vomiting section
- **Postoperative Hypotension**
  - Etiologies:
    - Hypovolemic
      - Insufficient fluid resuscitation, surgical bleeding, third-space translocation
      - Treatment: IV crystalloid, colloid, blood products, vasopressors, cardiac inotropes
    - Cardiogenic
      - Pump failure from myocardial ischemia or infarction, cardiac tamponade, dysrhythmias, cardiomyopathy
      - Diagnosis – ECG monitoring, echocardiography, central venous pressure monitoring, consider pulmonary artery catheter monitoring
      - Treatment depends on etiology: vasopressors, inotropes, volume resuscitation, anti-arrhythmics, cardioversion, or defibrillation
    - Distributive
      - Sympathectomy: Due to neuraxial/regional anesthetic techniques or surgical complication. Treatment may include volume resuscitation and vasopressors
      - Allergic reactions: Anaphylactic and anaphylactoid reactions. Most common triggers: neuromuscular blockers > antibiotics > latex
      - Systemic inflammatory response syndrome/sepsis: → decreased systemic vascular resistance and hypotension.
  - Management: Cardiovascular support and treatment of inciting cause or infectious agent
- **Arrhythmias**
  - **Sinus Bradycardia**
    - Medication-related:
      - Anticholinesterases, opioids, beta-blockers
    - Procedure-related:
      - Increased intracranial pressure or intraocular pressure, bowel distention, high spinal anesthesia
  - **Sinus Tachycardia**
    - Common causes: Pain, hypovolemia, agitation, fever/hyperthermia, sepsis, medications (anticholinergics)
  - **Atrial Dysrhythmias**
    - Atrial fibrillation (AFib), atrial flutter, premature atrial complexes (PACs)
    - New-onset atrial dysrhythmias may occur in up to 10% of patients postoperatively, higher rates after cardiothoracic procedures

- For acute-onset Afib, treat by controlling the ventricular response rate with beta blockers and calcium channel blockers
- **Ventricular Dysrhythmias**
  - Immediately postop – premature ventricular contractions (PVCs) and ventricular bigeminy are most commonly encountered
    - Can be secondary to underlying cardiac pathology, electrolyte abnormalities, hypercapnia, and increased sympathetic tone
    - PVCs – frequently benign and usually managed by treating the above causes
  - Ventricular tachydysrhythmias (e.g., ventricular tachycardia, ventricular fibrillation) are rare but can occur, especially in patients with underlying cardiac pathology

Nausea and Vomiting

- Postoperative nausea and vomiting (PONV) – up to 30% of patients; second most common postoperative complaint after pain
- **Physiology**
  - Nausea – subjective feeling of the need to vomit
  - Vomiting (emesis) – actual oral expulsion of gastrointestinal contents
  - Input from the cerebral cortex, GI tract vagal afferents, the vestibular system, and the central chemoreceptor trigger zone (CRTZ) act on the area postrema in the medulla oblongata
  - Efferent signals are sent to visceral and somatic nuclei → physical act of emesis with the accompanying sympathetic and vagal symptoms (e.g., sweating, tachycardia, salivation)
  - Neurotransmitters implicated in nausea and vomiting pathways:
    - Serotonin (5-HT), acetylcholine (Ach), substance P, dopamine (DA), and histamine
- **Etiology**[1]
  - **Gastrointestinal Toxins**
    - Examples: hypertonic saline, copper sulfate, ipecac syrup
    - Releases 5-HT from enterochromaffin cells, stimulating vagal afferents to the brainstem and activation of area postrema
  - **Circulating Toxins and Drugs**
    - Direct stimulation of the CRTZ
    - The CRTZ uniquely lacks a blood–brain barrier, allowing detection of emetogenic substances in the bloodstream
    - Intravenous and volatile anesthetics, opioids, and a myriad of other substances can trigger nausea and vomiting in this manner

- Activation of the Vestibular System
  - Classically implicated in motion sickness, Meniere's disease, procedures involving the inner ear
  - Opioids *may* also increase sensitivity of the vestibular system
- **Risk Factors**
  - **Patient-Related Factors**
    - Female sex (strongest predictor)
    - Non-smokers
    - History of PONV or motion sickness
    - Older age, anxiety, history of migraines have been implicated, but data are less convincing
  - **Anesthesia-Related Factors**
    - Perioperative opioids
    - All volatile anesthetics and nitrous oxide – additive risk with simultaneous nitrous oxide and volatile administration
    - ↑ duration →↑ risk
  - **Surgical-Related Factors**
    - Strabismus surgery in children (but not adults) – most well-established independent surgical risk factor
      - Most commonly implicated procedures:
    - Middle- and inner-ear surgeries, adenoidectomy/ tonsillectomy, gynecological and laparoscopic abdominal surgery
- **Risk Assessment**
  - In **adults**, an additive scoring system can be used to predict the risk of PONV:
    - 1 point for each of the following: female gender, nonsmoking status, history of PONV or motion sickness, postoperative opioid use
    - Table 22.1 describes the relationship between number of risk factors and risk of PONV in adults.
  - The pediatric population utilizes a similar additive scoring system:
    - 1 point is given for each of the following: surgical duration ≥ 30 min, age ≥ 3, strabismus surgery, history of PONV in patient or immediate relative
    - Table 22.2 describes the relationship between number of risk factors and incidence of POV in children.
- **Preventive Strategies**
  - Limit exposure to opioids, volatile anesthetics, nitrous oxide when feasible
  - Administering propofol for induction and maintenance can decrease early PONV (defined as initial 6 hours postop)
  - Opt for regional over general anesthesia
  - Multimodal pain management strategy to reduce need for perioperative opioids

Table 22.1 Simplified risk score for postoperative nausea and vomiting (PONV) in adults

Number of risk factors	Risk of PONV
0	10%
1	20%
2	40%
3	60%
4	80%

Source: Modified from Apfel C, Laara E, Koivuranta M, et al. A simplified risk score for predicting postoperative nausea and vomiting: conclusions from cross-validations between two centers. *Anesthesiology* 1999;91:693–700.

Table 22.2 Simplified risk score for postoperative vomiting (POV) in children

Number of risk factors	Incidence of POV
0	9%
1	10%
2	30%
3	55%
4	70%

Source: Modified from Eberhart LH, Geldner G, Kranke P, et al. The development and validation of a risk score to predict the probability of postoperative vomiting in pediatric patients. *Anesth Analg* 2004;99:1630–1637.

○ Administer PONV prophylactic medications
  ▪ Low-risk patients (0 risk factors) (see above) – no prophylaxis is warranted
  ▪ 1 risk factor – single prophylactic agent (ondansetron) should be used, with the option of adding a second agent (dexamethasone)
  ▪ Higher risk patients: > two risk factors – at least two agents should be used
○ Perioperative hydration with crystalloid
  ▪ Some studies show liberal crystalloid supplementation as an effective antiemetic
  ▪ Mechanism – possibly decreases release of arginine vasopressin (known to have emetic properties) during episodes of hypovolemia
- **Failed or Absent Prophylaxis**
  ○ If pharmacological prophylaxis fails, an antiemetic should be administered from a class of drug different from those given for prevention
    ▪ Minimal benefit from re-dosing the same agent
  ○ Propofol 20 mg IV can be a rescue antiemetic; however, the effects are generally short lived
  ○ Ondansetron dose as a rescue agent (1 mg) is less than the prophylaxis dose (4 mg)

- **Antiemetic Agents**
  ○ Table 22.3 includes commonly used agents for PONV prophylaxis and treatment
- **Multimodal Therapy**
  ○ Greatest quantifiable decrease in PONV observed when adding a single prophylactic agent
  ○ Utilization of more agents will further reduce risk, however the benefits become less pronounced
    ▪ Especially true once two agents are given
  ○ Combining multiple pharmacological agents with other preventive strategies (e.g., hydration, oxygen, total intravenous anesthetic) significantly decrease overall PONV incidence
- **Acupressure and Acupuncture**
  ○ Stimulation of the P6 meridian pressure point of the wrist reduces risk of nausea and vomiting to a similar degree as traditional antiemetics
- **Antacids, Histamine-2 (H_2) Blockers, and Proton Pump Inhibitors (PPIs)**
  ○ Effective for pre- and postop neutralization of gastric acids
  ○ Examples:
    ▪ Antacids – calcium carbonate tablets, citric acid/sodium citrate
    ▪ H_2 blockers – cimetidine, famotidine, ranitidine
    ▪ PPIs – omeprazole, esomeprazole, lansoprazole, pantoprazole
  ○ No direct antiemetic effects
  ○ Possibly useful as adjuncts for preventing and treating GERD, indigestion, and dyspepsia, which may contribute to PONV

Neuromuscular Consequences of Anesthesia
- **Residual Paralysis**
  ○ Due to incomplete antagonism of non-depolarizing neuromuscular blocking drugs
  ○ Associated with:
    ▪ Generalized muscle weakness
    ▪ Difficulty in phonation – laryngeal muscle weakness
    ▪ Diplopia – extraocular muscle weakness
    ▪ Difficulty swallowing, ↑ aspiration risk – impaired coordination of pharyngeal constriction and relaxation of upper esophageal sphincter
    ▪ Upper airway obstruction – pharyngeal muscle weakness
    ▪ Atelectasis
  ○ Ultimate consequence may be hypoxia, hypercarbia, respiratory failure, prolonged ventilator time, and other complications
- **Muscle Soreness**
  ○ Succinylcholine-associated myalgias
  ○ Reported rates as high as 89%

Table 22.3 Commonly used agents for PONV

Drug	Mechanism	Dose (adult)	Comments
Ondansetron	5-HT_3 (serotonin) antagonist	4 mg IV (ppx) 1 mg IV (rescue)	– More effective when given near end of surgery – QTc prolonging – Caution in patients taking other serotonergic agents due to risk of serotonin syndrome
Dolasetron	5-HT_3 antagonist	12.5–50 mg IV	
Granisetron	5-HT_3 antagonist	1 mg IV	
Metoclopramide	D_2 (dopamine) antagonist Minor 5-HT_3 antagonist	10–50 mg IV	– Minimal antiemetic benefit from 10 mg dose, greater efficacy at 25 or 50 mg – Promotes gastric motility – QTc prolonging
Droperidol	D_2 antagonist	1 mg IV 0.5 mg IM	– FDA black box warning for QTc prolongation has made its use more controversial, although at doses used for PONV the risk is likely minimal
Haloperidol	$D_{2,3,4}$ antagonist 5-HT_2 antagonist	0.5–1 mg IV 0.5 mg IM	– QTc prolonging – IV use is off-label
Prochlorperazine	D_2 antagonist	6.25–12.5 mg IV/IM 3–6 mg buccal	
Diphenhydramine	H_1 (histamine) antagonist	12.5–50 mg IV	– Anticholinergic side effects – Caution in elderly and other at risk of delirium
Promethazine	H_1 antagonist	12.5–25 IV/IM	
Aprepitant	NK1 (neurokinin) antagonist	40 mg PO	– Blocks substance P binding to NK receptor – Better at preventing vomiting than nausea – Expensive – Must be administered hours before surgery
Dexamethasone	Unknown	4–8 mg	– Effective only as prophylaxis – Administer shortly after induction – Similar PONV benefit with either 4 or 8 mg
Scopolamine	Muscarinic acetylcholine antagonist	1.5 mg transdermal patch × 24 hr	– Can be applied night before surgery or immediately preop because takes 4 hours to take effect

Drug information, route, and dosing taken from Apfel 2014 and Prashant et al. 2016. See Further Reading.

- Less common in children and patients over age 50
- Possibly less common in those with greater muscle fitness
- Mechanism not entirely understood, but possibly from uncoordinated muscle contractions leading to muscle fiber rupture/damage
- Prevention
  - NSAIDs, lidocaine, and small doses of nondepolarizing muscle relaxants may lessen the risk of myalgias
- **Recovery of Airway Reflexes**
  - Examples of airway reflexes include
    - Pharyngeal (gag) reflex – prevents unintended objects from entering the pharynx
      - Mechanism: CN IX glossopharyngeal afferents → CN X vagal efferents
    - Cough reflex – enhances clearance of secretions/airway particulates and protects from aspiration of foreign objects
      - Mechanism: Internal branch of superior laryngeal nerve (sensory) →recurrent laryngeal nerve (motor)

- Anesthesia and neuromuscular blockade blunt protective airway reflexes

Neurological Consequences of Anesthesia

- **Confusion**
  - Depressed level of consciousness from anesthesia → impairs memory, attention, reaction time
  - May last for hours postoperatively, despite outward appearance of wakefulness and alertness
  - Commonly manifests as unawareness of surroundings, repetitive questioning, emotional lability
- **Delirium**
  - Acute, fluctuating disturbance in cognition, awareness, and/or level of consciousness unexplained by preexisting neurocognitive disorder(s)
  - Incidence: 10% in patients ≥ 50 years old undergoing elective surgery
    - Highest in surgical repair of hip fractures and bilateral knee replacements
  - **Patient Risk Factors**
    - Advanced age (≥ 70 years old)
    - Preoperative cognitive impairment
    - Decreased functional status

- Alcohol abuse
- Severe illness
- Vision impairment
- History of delirium
  - **Intra- and Postoperative Risk Factors**
    - Bleeding (Hct < 30%)
    - Blood transfusions
    - Use of anticholinergics, antihistamines, narcotics, and sedative-hypnotics
  - **Management**
    - Exclude and treat iatrogenic causes – electrolyte abnormalities, hypoxia, dehydration, endocrine dysfunction, pain, infection, anemia, and others
    - Repeatedly reorient to surroundings
    - Promote sleep hygiene, remove excessive stimulation
    - Remove restraints and tethers if possible such as monitors, catheters, and physical restraints
    - Judiciously utilize typical and atypical antipsychotics
- **Postoperative Cognitive Dysfunction (POCD)**
  - Deterioration in cognitive function lasting days, weeks, months, or longer after undergoing anesthesia
  - **Risk Factors**
    - Cardiac surgery but has been well-described after non-cardiac surgery
      - Incidence as high as 70% at 1 week, up to 40% at 1 year

- Lengthy surgery and/or time under general anesthesia
- Intraoperative organ ischemia and damages
- Age > 60
- Preexisting cerebral, cardiac, or vascular disease
- History of alcohol abuse
  - **Mechanism**
    - Unclear, but likely a complex interplay of genetics, drug toxicity, inflammatory mediators, hormones, tissue hypoxia
- **Delayed Emergence from Anesthesia**
  - **Pharmacological**
    - Residual effects of administered anesthetics
    - Excessive sedation
    - Inadequate neuromuscular blockade reversal
    - Central anticholinergic syndrome
      - Treatment: physostigmine – crosses blood brain barrier
    - Illicit substances intoxication
  - **Metabolic**
    - Electrolyte, glucose, or acid/base abnormalities, hypo/hyperthermia
    - Other systemic disorders – e.g., hepatic or uremic encephalopathy
      - **Neurological:** Ischemic or embolic stroke, TIA, intracerebral hemorrhage, seizures, increased intracranial pressure

Further Reading

Apfel C, Laara E, Koivurant M, et al. A simplified risk score for predicting postoperative nausea and vomiting: conclusions from cross-validations between two centers. *Anesthesiology* 1999; **91**:693–700.

Apfel C. Postoperative nausea and vomiting. In Miller RD, Eriksson LI, Fleisher LA, et al., editors. *Miller's Anesthesia*, 8th ed. Elsevier Saunders, 2014, chapter 97, pp 2947–2973.

Butterworth JF IV, Mackey DC, Wasnick JD. *Morgan and Mikhail's Clinical Anesthesiology*, 5th ed. McGraw-Hill, 2013.

Eberhart LH, Geldner G, Kranke P, et al. The development and validation of a risk score to predict the probability of

postoperative vomiting in pediatric patients. *Anesth Analg* 2004;**99**:1630–1637.

Gan TJ, Diemunsch P, Habib AS, et al. Consensus guidelines for the management of postoperative nausea and vomiting. *Anesth Analg* 2014;**118**(1):85–113.

Miller MO. Evaluation and management of delirium in hospitalized older patients. *Am Fam Physician* 2008 Dec 1;**78**(11):1265–1270.

Nicholau TK. The postanesthesia care unit. In Miller RD, Eriksson LI, Fleisher LA, et al., editors. *Miller's Anesthesia*, 8th ed. Elsevier Saunders, 2014; chapter 96, pp 2924–2946.

Prashant S, Yoon SS, Kuo B. Nausea: a review of pathophysiology and

therapeutics. *Therap Adv Gastroenterol* 2016;**9**(1):98–112.

Rasmussen LS, Stygall JS, Newman SP. Cognitive dysfunction and other long-term complications of surgery and anesthesia. In Miller RD, Eriksson LI, Fleisher LA, et al., editors. *Miller's Anesthesia*, 8th ed. Elsevier Saunders, 2014; chapter 99, pp 2999–3010.

Sinatra RS, Jahr JS, Watkins-Pitchford JM, editors. *The Essence of Analgesia and Analgesics*. Cambridge Medicine. Cambridge University Press, 2010.

Wong SF, Chung F. Succinylcholine-associated postoperative myalgia. *Anaesthesia* 2000;**55**(2):144–152.

Central and Peripheral Nervous System

Connie Yue and Jung Kim

Brain

Cerebral Blood Supply

- Anterior cerebral circulation: Provided by anterior cerebral arteries (ACA) and middle cerebral artery (MCA) from internal branch of carotid artery.

    ACA stroke: Contralateral lower limb motor and sensory defect.

    MCA stroke: Contralateral facial and upper limb motor and sensory defect.

- Posterior cerebral circulation: Provided by vertebral arteries.
- Circle of Willis provides collateral circulation (Figure 23.1).
- Cerebral cortex and subcortical structures (Figure 23.2).
- Reference table (Table 23.1).

Table 23.1 Reference table

Cerebral perfusion pressure (CPP)	80–100 mmHg
Intracranial pressure (ICP)	5–12 mmHg
Cerebral blood flow (CBF)	50 mL/100 g/min
Cerebral metabolic rate of oxygen (CMRO₂)	3 mL/100 g/min 50 mL/min
Cerebrospinal fluid (CSF) pressure	8–15 mmHg
CSF volume	150 mL

Cerebral Blood Flow and Cerebral Metabolism

- CPP = MAP – ICP or CVP whichever is higher.
- CBF receives about 15% of cardiac output.

Physiological Factors That Affect CBF (Graphs 23.1 and 23.2)

Graph 23.1

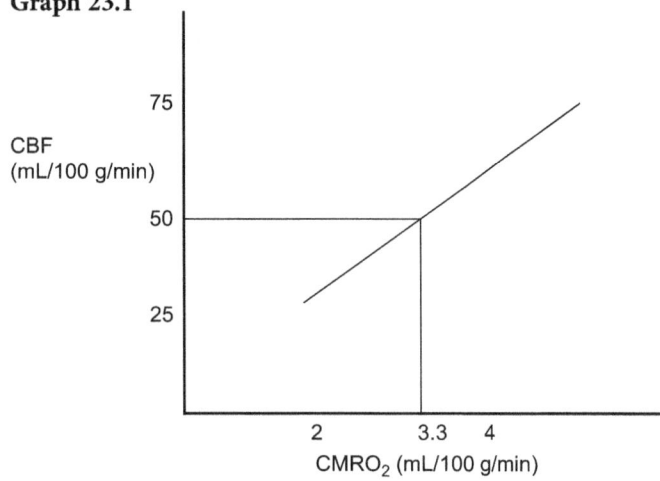

Graph 23.2

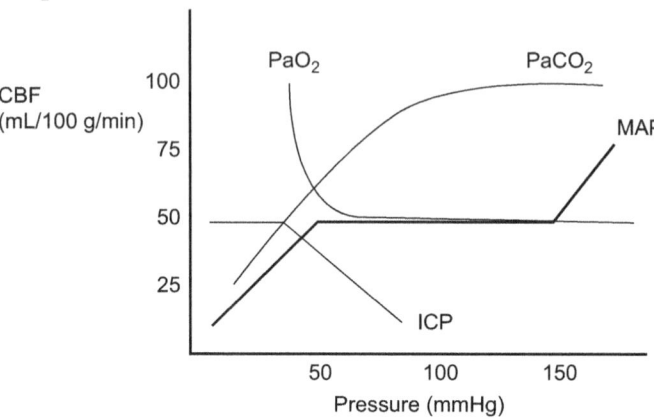

- $CMRO_2$
    - Coupled with CBF under normal conditions.
    - Increased $CMRO_2$ increases CBF.
- Autoregulation
    - Between MAP 60 and 160.
    - This range is "right-shifted" in chronic hypertension.
    - Can be impaired by brain tumor, injury or stroke. Under these conditions CBF becomes pressure-dependent. Small change in MAP can lead to profound changes in CBF.
- $PaCO_2$: 1 mmHg $PaCO_2$ decrease leads to 1–2 mL/100 g/min decrease in CBF.
- PaO_2: Only affects CBF in severe hypoxemia usually when PaO_2 < 50 mmHg.
- Energy substrates for cerebral metabolism:
    - Glucose in normal conditions.
    - Ketone bodies during starvation.

Anesthetic Effect on Cerebral Blood Flow

- Desflurane, isoflurane, and sevoflurane cause:
    - Impaired auto-regulation.
    - Dose-dependent vasodilation and increase in CBF:

    Desflurane > Isoflurane > Sevoflurane.

    - Dose-dependent decrease in $CMRO_2$.
    - Uncouple $CMRO_2$ and CBF.
- Nitrous oxide causes increase in $CMRO_2$ and CBF from vasodilation.
- *Circulatory steal phenomenon*: Volatiles increase blood flow in the normal area of the brain, but not in the ischemic

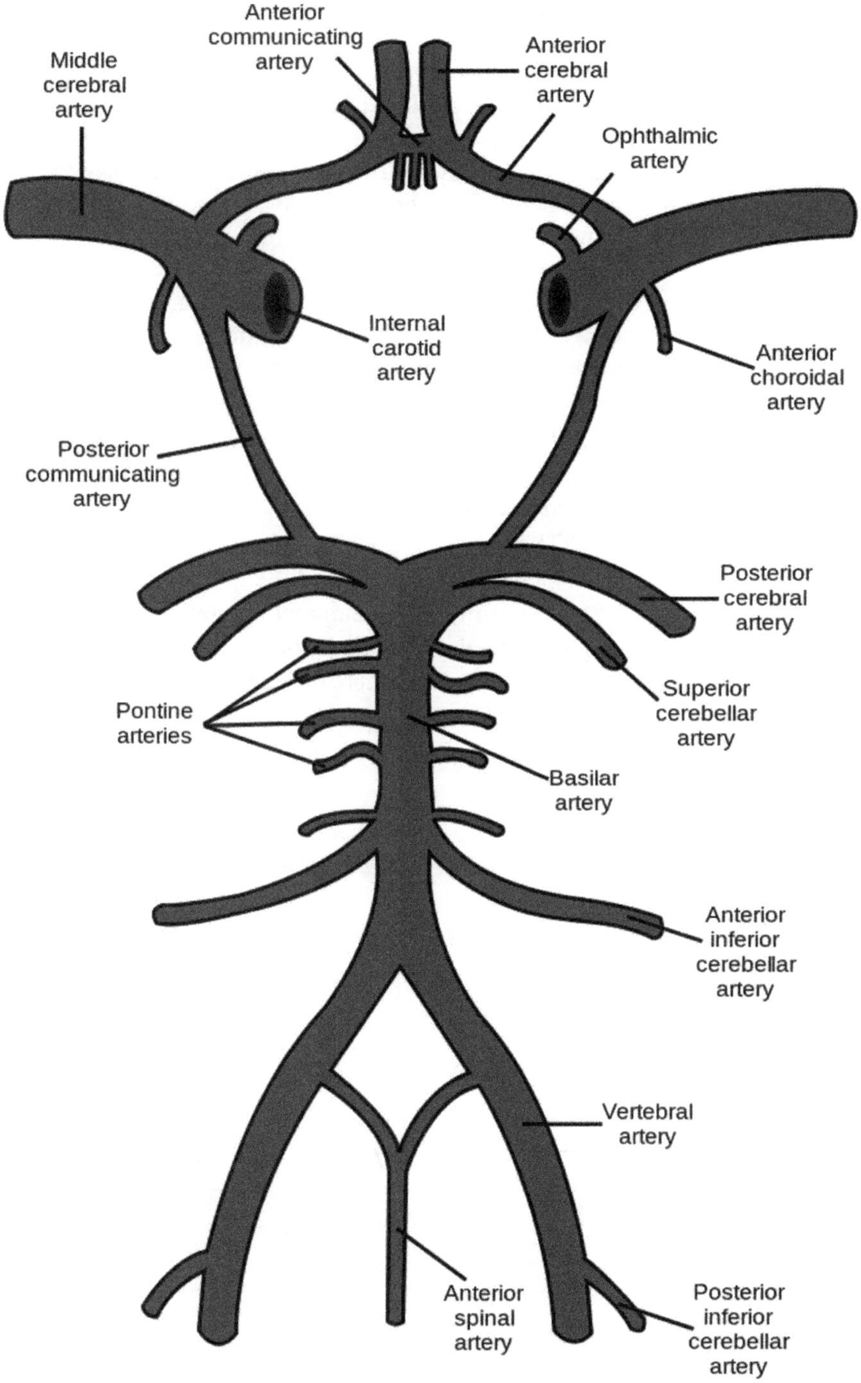

Figure 23.1 Circle of Willis.

areas, results in redistribution of blood away from the ischemic area.

- *Reverse steal phenomenon* (Robin Hood): Barbiturates cause cerebral vasoconstriction in normal area and allow blood to redistribute to ischemic area.
- Anesthetic agents effect on CBF, $CMRO_2$, and ICP (Table 23.2).

Cerebrospinal Fluid and Cerebral Protection

- Visceral pain carried by C fibers.

- At higher altitude CSF becomes more alkaline to offset the hypoxic ventilatory drive.
- Pathophysiology of cerebral ischemia: Decreased perfusion or glucose cause ATP depletion and ATP pump failure. Raised intracellular calcium level leads to lipase and protease activation, and neuron damage.
- Hypothermia:
  - The most effective method of cerebral protection.
    - For every $1°C$ decrease, $CMRO_2$ decreases by 6–7%.

127

○ Mild hypothermia (33°C–35°C) improves neurological function in patient with return of spontaneous circulation (ROSC).[1]

Spinal Cord

- Spinal cord (conus medullaris) ends at L1 in adults and L3 in infants.
- Anterior spinal artery provides 75% of spinal cord circulation.
  ○ Artery of Adamkiewicz from aorta arises at T9–T12 level and joins anterior spinal artery to supply lower spinal cord.
- Anterior spinal syndrome

○ Lower extremity motor temperature and pain sensation defect.
○ Intact proprioception and vibration.
- Posterior spinal cord is supplied by two posterior spinal arteries.
- Layers needle passes through to epidural space: skin, subcutaneous fat, supraspinous ligament, interspinous ligament, and ligamentum flavum.
- *Autonomic hyperreflexia*: T7 and above spinal cord injury. Stimulation below the lesion causes vasoconstriction in lower extremities and reflex vasodilation in upper extremities, which results in severe hypertension and bradycardia. Preventable by spinal anesthesia.

Spinal Cord Tracts

- Figure 23.3
- Three major sensory tracts:
  ○ Spinothalamic: Pain, temperature, touch
  ○ Spinocerebellar: Proprioception
  ○ Posterior column: touch, pressure, vibration

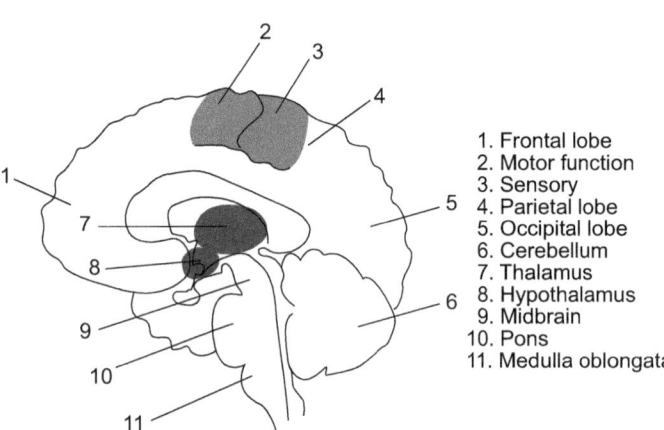

1. Frontal lobe
2. Motor function
3. Sensory
4. Parietal lobe
5. Occipital lobe
6. Cerebellum
7. Thalamus
8. Hypothalamus
9. Midbrain
10. Pons
11. Medulla oblongata

Figure 23.2 Cerebral cortex and subcortical structures.

Table 23.2 Anesthetic effects on CBF, $CMRO_2$, and ICP

	CBF	$CMRO_2$	ICP
Volatiles	↑	↓	↑ (MAC > 1)
Nitrous oxide Ketamine	↑	↑	↑
Propofol Etomidate	↓	↓	↓

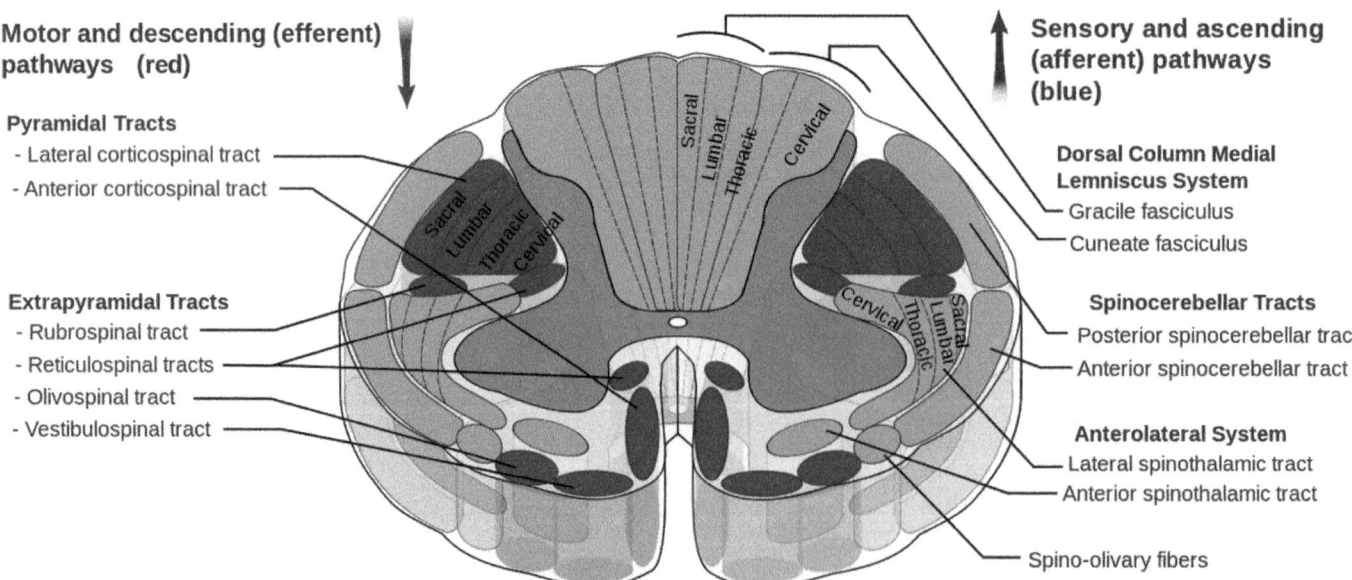

Figure 23.3 Spinal cord and spinal cord tracts. A black and white version of this figure will appear in some formats. For the color version, please refer to the plate section.

Evoked Potentials

- Anesthetic effects on evoked potential amplitude and latency (Table 23.3).
- Abnormal if amplitude decreases more than 50% or latency increases.
- In order of sensitivity to inhaled anesthetics: VEP > MEP > SSEP > BAEP (see below)[2]

Visual (VEP)	Via CN III
Motor (MEP)	Via lateral corticospinal tract
Somatosensory (SSEP)	Via dorsal column to medial lemniscus pathway
Brainstem auditory (BAEP)	Via CN VIII
	Useful for posterior fossa surgery

Neuromuscular and Synaptic Transmission

- At the neuromuscular junction (NMJ), acetylcholine (ACh) released from the presynaptic neuron binds to nicotinic ACh receptors (NAChR) on the postsynaptic muscle membrane. This leads to Na+ influx and membrane depolarization (from −90 mV to +50 mV) (Figure 23.4).
- Presynaptic ACh release is triggered by Ca^{2+} voltage-gated channel.
  - Note: Lambert–Eaton syndrome has antibody to this Ca channel.
- Postsynaptic AChR requires two ACh binding at its alpha sites to be activated.
  - Note: Myasthenia gravis has antibody to the postsynaptic AChR.

Table 23.3 Anesthetics effects on evoked potential amplitude and latency

	Amplitude	Latency
Isoflurane Sevoflurane Desflurane Propofol	↓	↑
Ketamine Etomidate	↑	↑
Opioid Benzodiazepine	No effect	No effect

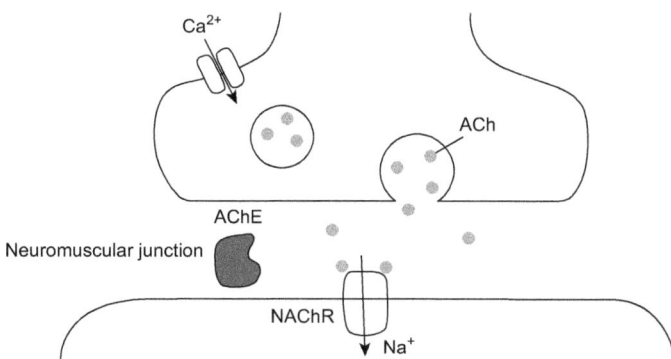

Figure 23.4 Neuromuscular junction.

- Action Potential:
  - All-or-none
  - Results from Na influx of voltage-gated Na^+ channel
- Local anesthetics inhibit Na^+ channel by binding to intracellular portion of Na^+ channel.
- Upregulation of postsynaptic receptors increases risk of hyperkalemia with succinylcholine (Box 23.1).

Skeletal Muscle Contraction

- Muscle contraction occurs by a sliding filament mechanism between actin and myosin.
- At rest, the attraction of myosin and actin filaments is blocked by troponin–tropomyosin complex.
- Action potential depolarizes muscle membrane and triggers calcium release from sarcoplasmic reticulum.
- Calcium removes the inhibitory effect of troponin–tropomyosin complex on actin and myosin and initiates contractile process.
- Energy is produced from splitting ATP by myosin head, which is also an ATPase.
- Reattachment of ATP to myosin causes myosin and actin release, after which a new cycle can start.[4]

Pain Mechanisms and Pathways

Nociceptors and Nociceptive Afferent Neurons

- Nociceptors : Pain receptors in muscle, joint and skin.
- Aβ fibers (non-nociceptive): Large diameter myelinated axons. Activated by pressure and light touch.
- Aδ fibers: Thinly myelinated axons. Activated by intense mechanical or mechanothermal stimuli, evoke sharp, intense, and tingling sensations.
- C fibers: unmyelinated axons. Respond to various nociceptive stimuli including thermal, mechanical, and chemical stimuli. Associated with prolonged burning sensation.
- Visceral pain carried by C fibers.
- In spinal cord, dorsal column nuclei and sensory nucleus process inputs from Aβ fibers. Spinal dorsal horn receives inputs from Aβ, Aδ, and C fibers.
- Wide dynamic range (WDR) neurons: second order neurons in spinal cord, concentrated in laminae III to V of dorsal horn. Respond to both innocuous (Aβ) and noxious (Aδ and C) stimuli.

Box 23.1 Conditions Causing NAChR Up-Regulation
Stroke, spinal cord injury
Burn injury (24 hours after injury up to 2 years)
Prolonged immobility
Prolonged exposure to neuromuscular blockade
Multiple sclerosis, Guillain–Barré syndrome, amyotrophic lateral sclerosis
Duchenne muscular dystrophy[3]

- Nociceptive-specific (NS) neurons: second order neurons in spinal cord, concentrated in laminae I and II. Respond to noxious stimuli.

Pain-Signaling Pathway

- Transduction: stimuli generate action potentials at the peripheral terminal of primary afferent neuron.
- Transmission: peripheral to spinal cord, synapse with second-order neurons, project to brainstem, then project to cortical sites.
- Modulation[5]
  - Spinal modulation: modulate noxious inputs at spinal level, for example, Gate-Control Theory and Wind-Up Phenomenon.
  - Gate-Control Theory: Low-threshold Aδ fibers inputs inhibit WDR response to nociceptive inputs.
  - Wind-Up Phenomenon (central sensitization): Increased neuron excitability by repeated stimulation from C fibers. Important pain processing in hyperalgesia and allodynia.
  - Supraspinal modulation: modulation of noxious input at brainstem, diencephalic, and cortical sites. Descending modulation can have inhibitory or facilitatory effect on neurons in dorsal horn.
- Perception: subjective sensation of pain.

Opioid Receptors

- Inhibitory G-protein-coupled receptors. Inhibit pain signaling when activated.
- Located throughout CNS and PNS. Concentrated in periaqueductal gray (PAG), locus ceruleus (LC), rostral ventral medulla (RVM), substantia gelatinosa (SG) of the dorsal horn of the spinal cord and peripheral afferent nerves.[6]
- Mu (μ) opioid receptors:
  - mu-1: analgesia and dependence
  - mu-2: euphoria, dependence, respiratory depression, miosis, constipation
  - mu-3: vasodilation
- Kappa (κ) opioid receptors: analgesia, diuresis, and dysphoria.
- Delta (δ) opioid receptors: analgesia and reduction in gastric motility.

Gender and Age Differences in Pain Perception

- No significant difference in pain reporting between boys and girls younger than 12 years old.[7]
- Prevalence of chronic pain increases in girls during puberty.
- Women are more likely than men to have fibromyalgia, migraine, TMJ, interstitial cystitis, and osteoarthritis.[8]

Autonomic Nervous System

Autonomic nervous system (ANS): Controls involuntary activities of the body.

Sympathetic Nervous System

- "Fight-or -flight" responses: mydriasis, increase in heart rate and contractility, bronchodilation, vasoconstriction, glycogenolysis, gluconeogenesis, insulin release, and renin release.[9]
- Originate from thoracolumbar region (T1–L2) of the spinal cord.
- Preganglionic cell body within gray matter of the spinal cord.
- Three types of ganglia[10]
  - Paired sympathetic chain:
- Presynaptic nerve fiber leaves spinal cord via anterior nerve root, enters ganglion through white ramus (myelinated).
- Postsynaptic fiber leaves ganglia through gray ramus (unmyelinated) to spinal nerve.
- Stellate ganglion formed by inferior cervical ganglion and first thoracic ganglion.
  - Unpaired prevertebral ganglia plexus: celiac, superior mesenteric, and inferior mesenteric ganglia. Innervate abdomen and pelvis.
  - Terminal ganglia: adrenal medulla, chromaffin cells.

Parasympathetic Nervous System

- "Rest and digest" responses: miosis, decrease in heart rate, and bronchoconstriction.
- Arises from cranial nerve III, VII, IX, X, and sacral segments.
- CN X (vagus nerve) transmits majority of parasympathetic nervous activities to heart, lungs, and GI tract.

Reflexes: Afferent and Efferent Limbs

- Corneal reflex: V1 of trigeminal n. (CN V) → facial n. (CN VII)
- Oculocardiac reflex: V1 of trigeminal n. (CN V) → vagus n. (CN X)
- Pharyngeal reflex (gag reflex): glossopharyngeal n. (CN IX) → vagus n. (CN X)

Temperature Regulation

- Process of thermoregulation: Afferent thermal sensing, central regulation and efferent response
- Cold travels primarily via Aδ fibers.
- Warm travels via C fibers.
- Temperature information travels in anterior spinal cord.
- Central control primarily by hypothalamus.
- Efferent response to cold: Vasoconstriction, non-shivering thermogenesis (primarily in infants) and shivering.
- Response to heat: Sweating and vasodilation.
- Core temperature measuring sites: Pulmonary artery, distal esophagus, tympanic membrane and nasopharynx.

Heat Loss

- Primary preoperative heat loss via convection and radiation.
- Anesthesia impairs thermoregulation, causes hypothermia
- Temperature decreases by 0.5–1.5°C in the first hour of anesthesia (redistribution). Then decrease slowly, plateau after 3–4 hours of anesthesia.[11]
- Redistribution hypothermia can be prevented by preoperative forced-air warming to increase peripheral temperature.

Effect of Drugs/Anesthetic Technique on Temperature Regulation

- General anesthesia decreases vasoconstriction and shivering thresholds by 2–3°C.
- Neuraxial anesthesia decreases vasoconstriction and shivering threshold by approximately 0.6°C above the level of the block.
- Mild hypothermia: Impairs coagulation, increases surgical bleeding and need of transfusion, increases risks of advert myocardial event and wound infection, and prolongs postoperative recovery.
- Forced air-warming: Most common and cost-effective method to maintain normothermia during anesthesia.

References

1. Butterworth JF IV, Mackey DC, Wasnick JD. Neurophysiology & anesthesia. In *Morgan & Mikhail's Clinical Anesthesiology*, 5th ed. McGraw-Hill Education, 2013; chapter 26, pp 575–592.

2. Barash PG, Cullen BF, Stoelting RK, et al., editors. Anesthesia for neurosurgery. In *Clinical Anesthesia*, 7th ed. Lippincott Williams & Wilkins, 2013; chapter 36, pp 996–1029.

3. Murray MJ, Harrison BA, Mueller JT, et al. Physiology of neuromuscular transmission. In Brull SJ, editor. *Faust's Anesthesiology Review*, 4th ed. Saunders, 2014; chapter 44, pp 98–100.

4. Hall JE. Contraction of skeletal muscle. In Hall JE, editor. *Guyton and Hall Textbook of Medical Physiology*, 13th ed. Elsevier, 2016; chapter 6, pp 75–88.

5. Ringkamp M, Dougherty PM, Raja SN. Anatomy and physiology of the pain signaling process. In Benzon HT, Raja SN, Liu SS, et al., editors. *Essentials of Pain Medicine*, 4th ed. Elsevier, 2017; chapter 1, pp 3–10.

6. Dhaliwal A, Gupta M. Physiology, opioid receptor. [Updated 2022 Jul 25]. In *StatPearls* [Internet]. StatPearls Publishing, 2022 Jan–. Available from: www.ncbi.nlm.nih.gov/books/NBK546642/

7. Fillingim RB, King CD, Ribeiro-Dasilva MC, et al. Sex, gender, and pain: a review of recent clinical and experimental findings. *J Pain* 2009;**10**(5):447–485.

8. Mogil JS. Sex differences in pain and pain inhibition: multiple explanations of a controversial phenomenon. *Nat Rev Neurosic* 2012;**13**(12):859–866.

9. Click DB. The autonomic nervous system. In Miller RD, Cohen NH, Ericsson LI, et al., editors. *Miller's Anesthesia*, 8th ed. Saunders, 2014; chapter 16, pp 346–386.

10. Murray MJ, Harrison BA, Mueller JT, et al. Autonomic nervous system; The sympathetic nervous system: anatomy and receptor pharmacology; The parasympathetic nervous system: anatomy and receptor pharmacology, In Hannon JD, editor. *Faust's Anesthesiology Review*, 4th ed. Saunders, 2014; chapters 39–41, 85–93.

11. Sessler DI. Temperature regulation and monitoring. In Miller RD, Cohen NH, Ericsson LI, et al., editors. *Miller's Anesthesia*, 8th ed. Saunders, 2014; chapter 54, pp 1622–1646.

Pain Mechanisms and Pathways

James Yeh and Yury Khelemsky

Introduction

Pain is "an unpleasant sensory and emotional experience associated with actual or potential tissue damage," as defined by the International Association for the Study of Pain.[1] Other important pain-related definitions are listed in Table 24.1.

In the neurophysiological classification, pain is divided into three categories based on mechanism:[2]

1. Inflammatory
   - Caused by tissue damage and the resultant inflammatory response
2. Pathological
   - The result of a dysfunctional nervous system. This includes:
     - Neuropathic pain, which is a result of damage to the nervous system (e.g., diabetic neuropathy)
     - Dysfunctional pain, which occurs in the absence of nerve damage or inflammation (e.g., fibromyalgia)
3. Nociceptive
   - Caused by the activation of specific neural pathways by potentially harmful stimuli
   - Serves as a warning for impending or current tissue damage

Pain can also be classified temporally:[2]

- Categorized as chronic or acute based on the duration of symptoms

Table 24.1 Definitions for commonly encountered vocabulary in pain medicine[1,2]

Allodynia	Perception of a non-noxious stimulus as painful
Analgesia	Absence of pain in response to a normally painful stimulus
Anesthesia dolorosa	Pain in an area without sensation
Dysesthesia	An unpleasant abnormal sensation, with or without stimulus
Hyperalgesia	Increased pain in response to a noxious stimulus
Hyperesthesia	Increased sensitivity to sensory stimuli (includes allodynia and hyperalgesia)
Hyperpathia	An abnormally painful response to a stimulus, especially a repetitive one, and an increased threshold
Hypoalgesia	Decreased pain in response to a noxious stimulus
Hypoesthesia	Decreased sensitivity to sensory stimuli
Paresthesia	An abnormal sensation, with or without stimulus

- The cutoff is arbitrary; however, 3 months and 6 months are the most commonly used values to define acute and chronic pain, respectively.

Nociceptors and Nociceptive Afferent Neurons

Nociception involves four complex processes:

1. **Transduction** is the conversion of the noxious stimuli to an electrical impulse.
2. **Transmission** involves the conduction of this signal from its origin into the central nervous system (CNS).
3. **Modulation** of the pain signal can occur in the spinal cord via various inhibitory pathways.
4. **Perception** is the end result of this pathway and involves the subjective experience of noxious stimuli.

Nociceptors

- Specialized receptors located at the terminals of afferent neurons
- They convert mechanical, thermal, and chemical stimuli into action potentials that are carried into the CNS.[3] These receptors include:
  - Mechanonociceptors – respond to pinch and pinprick
  - Silent nociceptors – respond to inflammation
  - Polymodal mechanoheat nociceptors – the most common; stimulated by extremes of pressure or temperature and certain noxious compounds, including bradykinin, histamine, prostaglandins, and capsaicin[4]

Transmission of the pain signal from the site of stimulation to the cortex involves:

- **First-order neurons**, with cell bodies in the dorsal root ganglia
- **Second-order neurons**, with cell bodies in the dorsal horn of the spinal cord
- **Third-order neurons**, with cell bodies in the thalamus

Dorsal Horn Transmission and Modulation, Wind-Up Phenomenon

1. Signals from nociceptors are transmitted by first-order neurons into the dorsal horn of the spinal cord.
   - *First-order neurons are composed of myelinated A delta and unmyelinated C fibers.*
2. These synapse selectively with *second-order neurons* in the *ipsilateral dorsal horn*, which is composed of Rexed laminae I–VI.

○ *Rexed lamina II*, also known as the *substantia gelatinosa*, is notable for having large numbers of interneurons and opioid receptors and likely plays a significant role in the modulation of pain.[5]

○ Second-order neurons are composed of:

■ Wide dynamic range (WDR) neurons, which respond to the full range of noxious and non-noxious stimuli

■ Nociceptive specific neurons, which respond only to painful stimuli

3. These fibers then cross midline and ascend in the *contralateral spinothalamic tract* to the *thalamus*.

4. They then synapse with third-order neurons, which project to the *postcentral gyrus* and *superior wall of the sylvian fissure*.[4,6]

5. The *spinoreticular tract* is responsible for the transmission of signals from the spinal cord to the *reticular formation* and may play a role in the motivational and emotional components of pain.[7]

Wind-Up Phenomenon

• Occurs in spinal cord neurons and is implicated in the *development of chronic pain*

• When exposed to the same stimulus repeatedly, WDR neurons have a progressive increase in their response per stimulus.

• The neurotransmitters *glutamate and aspartate*, as well as *NMDA receptors*, are believed to be involved in this process.[4]

Spinal and Supraspinal Neurotransmission and Modulation

Pain may be modulated by inhibitory mechanisms at multiple different levels throughout its pathway from the periphery to the cortex.

• In the periphery, tissue damage results in the release of endogenous opioid peptides by leukocytes, which interact with peripheral opioid receptors, resulting in attenuation of the pain response.[3]

• In the spinal cord, non-noxious sensation transmitted by afferent fibers can disrupt the transmission of the pain signal by WDR neurons and the spinothalamic tract.

○ This contributes to the "gate theory" of pain processing and is mediated by *glycine and GABA*.[4]

Supraspinal pathways are involved in the inhibition of pain transmission in the spinal cord.

• Inhibitory pathways interact with primary afferent neurons and interneurons.

○ Utilizes *alpha-2 adrenergic, serotonergic, and opioid-mediated mechanisms*

• This inhibitory signal originates in the *periaqueductal grey area* and *reticular formation*, is conducted to the *nucleus raphe magnus* and *medullary reticular formation*, and is then transmitted to the *dorsal horn neurons*.[4]

Autonomic Contributions to Pain

Areas of the nervous system involved in the processing of pain can overlap with areas dedicated to the regulation of the autonomic nervous system (ANS).

• Altered ANS function can contribute to pain syndromes, such as complex regional pain syndrome (CRPS).[8]

• The sympathetic nervous system has been shown to play roles in neuropathic, vascular, and visceral pain.

• Many interventional pain procedures specifically target the sympathetic nervous system. Commonly performed procedures include:[9]

○ Stellate ganglion blocks for upper extremity pain

○ Celiac plexus blocks for abdominal pain

○ Hypogastric plexus blocks for pelvic pain

○ Ganglion Impar blocks for perineal pain

○ Lumbar sympathetic blocks for lower extremity pain

Psychological Influences on Pain Perception

The experience of pain is not solely limited to the physiological processes of nerves and neurotransmitters. Psychological and cognitive factors can greatly influence a patient's perception of pain and impact treatment outcomes.[10]

• Fear: The threat of pain or re-injury may prevent patients from pursuing beneficial physical therapy

• Loss of control: The feeling that pain is uncontrollable can lead to decreased motivation in seeking out new management strategies

• Depression: Common in chronic pain, with an estimated prevalence of at least 50% of patients in specialized pain centers

○ While depression is generally thought to be a result of chronic pain, it has also been identified as a risk factor for developing chronic pain.

Gender and Age Differences in Pain Perception

Gender and Pain

Gender can influence the perception of pain and there is some evidence of differential responses to pain depending on gender, but results have been inconsistent.

• Women have been shown to have greater pain sensitivity, greater use of pain relieving medication, and be at increased risk for chronic pain.

○ The reason for this is thought to be multifactorial, involving psychological, social, and physiological elements.[11]

Aging and Pain[12]

• Aging is associated with the development of chronic painful conditions:

○ Arthritis, back pain, neuropathies, previous fractures

- There are numerous age-related changes in pathways involved in the processing of pain:
  - *Damage* or degeneration of *sensory fibers*
  - Lower levels of neurotransmitters of primary sensory nerves

- There is an increase in pain thresholds in the elderly, which has been shown to be a result of decreased sensitivity to low intensity pain.
  - Subsequently, the elderly may be at increased risk for tissue damage.[13]

References

1. IASP Terminology. 2012. Available from: www.iasp-pain.org/resources/terminolgy/

2. Nagda JV, Bajwa ZH. Definitions and classification of pain. In Bajwa ZH, Wootton RJ, Warfield CA, editors. *Principles and Practice of Pain Medicine*, 3rd ed. McGraw-Hill Education, 2016; chapter 6.

3. Stein C, Kopf A. Anesthesia and treatment of chronic pain. In Miller RD, editor. *Miller's Anesthesia*, 8th ed. Elsevier/Saunders, 2015; pp 1898–1918.

4. Rosenquist RW, Vrooman BM. Chronic pain management. In Butterworth JF, Mackey DC, Wasnick JD, editors. *Morgan & Mikhail's Clinical Anesthesiology*, 5th ed. McGraw-Hill, 2013; chapter 47.

5. Kleiner JS. Substantia gelatinosa. In Kreutzer JS, DeLuca J, Caplan B, editors. *Encyclopedia of Clinical Neuropsychology*. Springer New York, 2011; pp 2432–2433.

6. D'Mello R, Dickenson AH. Spinal cord mechanisms of pain. *Br J Anaesth* 2008;**101**(1):8–16.

7. Cohen RI. Anatomy and physiology of pain. In Bajwa ZH, Wootton RJ, Warfield CA, editors. *Principles and Practice of Pain Medicine*, 3rd ed. McGraw-Hill Education, 2016; chapter 2.

8. Gill JS. Sympathetic blocks. In Bajwa ZH, Wootton RJ, Warfield CA, editors. *Principles and Practice of Pain Medicine*, 3rd ed. McGraw-Hill Education, 2016, chapter 83.

9. Menon R, Swanepoel A. Sympathetic blocks. *Continuing Education Anaesth Crit Care Pain* 2010;**10**(3):88–92.

10. Turk DC, Okifuji A. Psychological aspects of chronic pain. In Bajwa ZH, Wootton RJ, Warfield CA, editors. *Principles and Practice of Pain Medicine*, 3rd ed. McGraw-Hill Education, 2016; chapter 14.

11. Bartley EJ, Fillingim RB. Sex differences in pain: a brief review of clinical and experimental findings. *Br J Anaesth* 2013;**111**(1):52–58.

12. McCarberg W. Pain in the elderly. In Bajwa ZH, Wootton RJ, Warfield CA, editors. *Principles and Practice of Pain Medicine*, 3rd ed. McGraw-Hill Education, 2016; chapter 67.

13. Lautenbacher S, Peters JH, Heesen M, Scheel J, Kunz M. Age changes in pain perception: a systematic-review and meta-analysis of age effects on pain and tolerance thresholds. *Neurosci Biobehav Rev* 2017;**75**:104–113.

Autonomic Nervous System

Joseph Park, Nakiyah Knibbs, and Jeffrey Ciccone

Sympathetic System

- **Receptors:** Sympathetic receptors are G protein coupled with two main groups: α and β. Dopamine receptors also play a role in sympathetic stimulation.
  - There are two types of α receptors, α1 (Gq-coupled receptor) and α2 (Gi-coupled receptor).
  - There are three types of β receptors, β1, β2, and β3, all of which are Gs-coupled. β2 receptors are mainly stimulated by epinephrine. All increase level of cAMP, the second messenger.
  - Dopamine receptors are sympathetic receptors found on blood vessels and are also G protein-coupled.[1]
- **Transmitters:** Sympathetic preganglionic neurons originating from T1 to L2–L3 of spinal cord travel to ganglia and release acetylcholine (ACh). Upon being stimulated by the ACh in the ganglia (usually paravertebral or prevertebral ganglia), the nicotinic postganglionic receptor causes the release of:
  - Norepinephrine (NE)
  - Dopamine (from the kidneys)
  - Acetylcholine (from sweat glands)
  - Epinephrine (from chromaffin cells in the adrenal medulla, which preganglionic neurons synapse directly with)

  These neurotransmitters activate target tissues, which leads to the effects seen with the sympathetic nervous system (Table 25.1).[2]
- **Synthesis:** Sympathetic neurotransmitters are synthesized from tyrosine as follows: Tyrosine → DOPA → dopamine → NE → epinephrine. The first step is the rate-limiting step, catalyzed by tyrosine hydroxylase.
  - All of these steps, except for the transformation from NE to epinephrine, occur in the *postganglionic sympathetic nerve ending.*
  - NE transforms to epinephrine in the adrenal medulla. They are stored in vesicles until postganglionic nerve is stimulated.[1,2]
- **Release:** Once the nicotinic postganglionic nerve or adrenal medulla is stimulated, storage vesicles containing NE, ACh, dopamine, or epinephrine merge with cell membrane and release contents into synapse and the receptors located on target organs are activated.[1]
- **Responses** (Table 25.1)

- **Termination of Action:** Most NE and epinephrine is removed from synaptic cleft *via reuptake* into storage vesicles. The small amount not taken up by vesicles enters circulation where it is *metabolized by monoamine oxidase (MAO), catechol-o-methyl transferase (COMT),* or both in the blood, liver, and kidney. About 25% of *NE is removed by the lungs,* whereas dopamine and epinephrine are not affected.[3]

Parasympathetic System

- **Receptors:** There are five types of muscarinic receptors: M1, M2, M3, M4, M5. Of these, M2 and M3 receptors affect the patients' hemodynamics.
  - M2 receptors are Gi-coupled receptors found on the heart.
  - M3 receptors are Gq-coupled receptors located in various parts of the body that lead to increased intracellular calcium.[4]

  (The location and action of these receptors are detailed in Table 25.1.)
- **Transmitters:** The main neurotransmitter used in the parasympathetic system is acetylcholine (ACh). Parasympathetic preganglionic neurons originating from brainstem nuclei CN III, VII, IX, and X as well as sacral levels S2–S4 travel to ganglia (usually located on target organ) where it releases ACh. This ACh acts on nicotinic postganglionic receptors, which also release ACh, activating target tissues and leading to effects seen with the parasympathetic nervous system (Table 25.1).
- **Synthesis:** ACh is synthesized in the preganglionic and postganglionic neurons from the compounds choline and acetyl coenzyme A (acetyl-CoA) by the enzyme choline acetyltransferase (ChAT).[4]
- **Release:** Acetylcholine is located within vesicles of preganglionic and postganglionic neurons until its release into the synapse. The influx of calcium stimulates the docking, fusion, and ultimately release of ACh-containing vesicles.[4,5]
- **Responses:** See Table 25.1.
- **Termination of Action:** ACh is inactivated within the synapse by the enzyme acetylcholinesterase (AChE), which hydrolyzes the ACh into its component choline and acetic acid.[4]

Table 25.1 Autonomic responses of target organs

Organ		Sympathetic response		Parasympathetic response		Dominant response
		Response	Receptor	Response	Receptor	
Heart	Force of contraction	Increase	β1	Decrease	M2	P
	Rate of contraction	Increase	β1	Decrease	M2	P
Blood vessels	Arteries	Vasoconstriction	α1 (α2)			
	Veins	Vasoconstriction	α2 (α1)			S
	Skeletal muscle	Vasodilation	β2			S
Bronchial tree		Bronchodilation	β2	Bronchoconstriction	M3	P
Splenic capsule		Contraction	α1			S
Uterus		Contraction	α1	Variable		S
Vas deferens		Contraction	α1			S
Gastrointestinal tract		Relaxation	α2	Contraction	M3	P
Eye	Radial muscle (iris)	Contraction (mydriasis)	α1			S
	Circular muscle (iris)			Contraction (miosis)		P
	Ciliary muscle	Relaxation	β2	Contraction (accommodation)	M3	P
Kidney		Renin secretion	β1			S
Bladder	Detrusor	Relaxation	β2	Contraction	M3	P
	Trigone and sphincter	Contraction	α1	Relaxation	M3	Neither
	Ureter	Contraction	α1			S
Pancreas – Insulin release		Decrease	α2			S
Fat cells – lipolysis		Increase	β1/β3			S
Liver glycogenolysis		Increase	α1/β2			S
Hair follicles, smooth muscle		Contraction (piloerection)	α1			S
Nasal secretion		Decrease	α1/α2	Increase		P
Salivary glands		Increase secretion	α1	Increase secretion		P
Sweat glands		Increase secretion	α1	Increase secretion		P

S = sympathetic, P = parasympathetic.

Source: Adapted from *Brody's Human Pharmacology: Molecular to Clinical* (Table 9–2), by L. Wecker, L. M. Crespo, T. M. Brody, G. Dunaway, C. Faingold, 2010, Philadelphia, PA: Mosby/Elsevier. Copyright Year 2010 by Mosby/Elsevier.

- **Pharmacological Agents:** Two classes of medications that manipulate the PNS with anesthetic relevance are *muscarinic antagonists and cholinesterase inhibitors.*
  - *Muscarinic Antagonists:* Compete with acetylcholine specifically at muscarinic receptors. Used for their chronotropic, sedative, and anti-sialogogue effects. For example, glycopyrrolate is usually paired with an anticholinesterase to mitigate bradycardia during neuromuscular blockade reversal.
    - These anti-muscarinics exhibit similar efficacy in receptor blockade with some notable differences in the robustness of response (Table 25.2). For example, atropine causes a greater heart rate response, whereas scopolamine has increased sedative effects. As an exception, glycopyrrolate (a quaternary ammonium compound) does not cross the blood–brain barrier and therefore has no CNS or ophthalmic effects.

Table 25.2 Comparative pharmacological characteristics of muscarinic antagonists

	Atropine	Scopolamine	Glycopyrrolate
Antisialogogue effect	++	+++	+++
Bronchodilation	++	+	++
Sedation	+	+++	0
CNS toxicity	+	+++	0
Cycloplegia/ mydriasis	+	+++	0
Increased heart rate	+++	+	++

0, none; +, mild effect; ++, moderate effect; +++, marked effect.

- Due to their tertiary amine structure, atropine and scopolamine both cross the blood–brain barrier and their use could potentially lead to CNS toxicity, evidenced by altered mental status. This can be treated with the anticholinesterase, physostigmine, that can also cross the blood–brain barrier.
  - *Cholinesterase Inhibitors:* Used for the reversal of neuromuscular blockade and the diagnosis and treatment myasthenia gravis. These medications reversibly bind the cholinesterase enzyme, rendering it inactive and increasing the amount of acetylcholine available to bind at both nicotinic and muscarinic receptors.[1]
    - The use of these drugs (neostigmine, physostigmine, pyridostigmine, edrophonium) leads to bradycardia, bronchospasm, salivation, increased GI motility, and miosis.

Ganglionic Transmission

- **Sympathetic**: Sympathetic preganglionic neurons, which are *relatively shorter,* arise from T1 to L2 of spinal cord and travel to paravertebral ganglion (or prevertebral ganglion for the celiac, superior mesenteric, and inferior mesenteric ganglia).
  - Here they synapse with postganglionic neurons, which are relatively longer. At the synapse, ACh is released by the preganglionic neurons that activate the nicotinic acetylcholine receptors on the postganglionic neurons.
  - The postganglionic neurons will then release their neurotransmitters, primarily NE but also epinephrine, dopamine, or ACh, which then affects the target organ.
- **Parasympathetic**: Parasympathetic preganglionic fibers, which are *relatively longer* originate, arise from cranial nuclei or the sacral plexus (S2–S4 of spinal cord) and travel to small ganglia located near the target organ.
  - Here they synapse with postganglionic neurons, which are relatively shorter. At the synapse, ACh is released by preganglionic neurons that activate the nicotinic acetylcholine receptors (much like the sympathetic system).
  - The postganglionic neurons will then release Ach, which then affects the target organ.[6]

Reflexes

- **Afferent Limbs:** Sensory neurons that receive input from viscera have cell bodies located in the sensory ganglia of either a cranial nerve for parasympathetic fibers or a paravertebral ganglion versus a prevertebral ganglion for sympathetic fibers. These project to the central nervous system and initiate the efferent portion of the reflex.
- **Efferent Limbs:** Starts with the preganglionic neuron cell body, which for the sympathetic system is located in the T1–L2 region of the spinal cord and for the parasympathetic system is located in the cranial nuclei or sacral plexus. This axon extends to ganglia where it synapses with the postganglionic neuron that projects to the smooth muscles of the target organ or cardiac muscle. The effect on the organ will depend on which system, sympathetic or parasympathetic is predominating at the time.[7]

Temperature Regulation

Temperature Sensing: Central, Peripheral

The process of thermoregulation is controlled by multiple distinct tissue types and thermally sensitive cells throughout the body in three distinct phases:

- **Afferent Thermal Sensing**
  - Cold signals travel typically along A delta fibers and increase action potential and firing with decreased temperatures while warm signaling is transmitted via unmyelinated C fibers.
    - C fibers also transmit pain, which is why it is not possible to distinguish high temperature from sharp pain.
  - Thermal input transmitted diffusely across spinothalamic tract of anterior spinal cord[8]
- **Central Regulation**
  - The hypothalamus receives afferent thermal input from skin surfaces, deep tissues and the central nervous system.
    - It appears that thermal information is processed within the spinal cord and central nervous system to a certain degree prior to reaching the hypothalamus, which is why in animal studies and patients with high spinal cord transections are still able to regulate core body temperature.[9]
- **Efferent Response**
  - Changes in both peripheral and core temperature elucidate an autonomic response that alters both metabolic heat production and environmental heat loss.
    - Typically, the body attempts to conserve both heat and energy maximally by employing energy efficient techniques such as vascular tone modulation (vasoconstriction or vasodilation) prior to metabolically taxing activities such as shivering/sweating.
  - Even in response to inhibition of various thermoregulatory techniques (shivering inhibited by muscle relaxant administration), core body temperature will remain normal unless other temperature regulating techniques unable to compensate.
  - Illness, medications, and advanced age all diminish the efficacy of the thermoregulatory response.[8]

Temperature-Regulating Centers: Concept of Set Point

- **Hypothalamus** responsible for maintaining core body temperature within narrow range known as the interthreshold range (range that does NOT induce an autonomic response).
  - Core body temperature that rises above *interthreshold range* will induce peripheral vasodilation and sweating.
  - Core body temperature that falls below this range will induce vasoconstriction and shivering.[10]
  - Exact mechanism that maintains the temperature threshold remains unknown, although it is believed to be mediated by a complex interaction of various neurotransmitters (NE, dopamine, 5-hydroxytryptamine, ACh, PGE-1, various other neuropeptides)
    - Response controlled primarily by thermal input from core structures and tissues (up to 80%)
  - Circadian rhythm (times of day), sex, age (marginally impaired in older adults), menstrual phase, exercise, nutritional intake, endocrine conditions such as hyper/hypothyroidism, and drugs (anesthetics, alcohol, CNS stimulants/depressants) all constantly modify the *interthreshold range*.[8]

Heat Production and Conservation

- Decreases in central core temperature below the *interthreshold range* will first induce energy efficient temperature conservation by inducing **vasoconstriction** prior to shivering thermogenesis.
  - Vasoconstriction mediated by α-adrenergic sympathetic nerves decrease metabolic heat loss by mitigating convection and radiation (primary source of heat loss) from surface skin.
  - Capillaries (up to 10 μm in diameter) compose the nutritional component of blood flow to the skin that are not affected by thermoregulation and provided blood flow independent of thermoregulatory response.
    - Arteriovenous shunts (up to 100 μm) are the predominant thermoregulatory vasculature component. It can hold up to 10,000 times as much blood in comparison to an equal length of capillary.
    - Sympathetic activation induces vasoconstriction of AV shunts thereby returning more warm blood to core tissues and organs.
- **Non-Shivering Thermogenesis:** Mechanism whereby skeletal muscle and brown fat increase metabolic heat production without producing mechanical work
  - More pronounced in infants (can nearly double heat production) versus a minimal increase in heat production in adults.
  - Controlled primarily by NE release from adrenergic nerve terminals

- **Shivering Thermogenesis:** Centrally mediated rapid tremor and unsynchronized muscular activity that can increase metabolic heat production by 50–100% in adults.
  - Does not occur in infants, and mechanism not entirely developed until 7 years of age[8]

Heat Loss: Mechanisms

- **Radiation:** Heat loss to the environment that occurs anytime the temperature of the patient is above absolute zero (always).
  - Most significant portion of total heat loss (up to 67%) in certain studies[11]
  - Proportional to the temperature difference between any two sources raised to the fourth power.
- **Convection:** Heat loss secondary to air movement
  - Mechanism by which forced air warming devices and blankets protect from intraoperative convection heat loss.
- **Conduction:** Heat loss that occurs through to direct contact
  - Use of table padding with foam or rubber on the operating room table will insulate the patient and minimize heat loss via conduction.
- **Evaporation:** Sweating is suppressed under general anesthesia and therefore a minor contributor to heat loss.

Body Temperature Measurement: Sites, Gradients

- Temperature monitoring is indicated for all general and neuraxial anesthetics extending beyond 30 minutes. It detects intraoperative hypothermia, hyperthermia, and possible incidence of malignant hyperthermia.
  - Temperatures vary greatly throughout body and each reading has its own distinct physiological and practical significance.
- Core temperatures are typically more uniform and higher when compared to peripheral skin temperatures, and are most useful when used to detect malignant hyperthermia or quantify hypothermia.
  - Core body temperature should be maintained > 36°C whenever possible, unless hypothermia (cerebral/cardiovascular protection during cardiopulmonary bypass) is indicated.
  - True core body temperature sites: Tympanic membrane, pulmonary artery catheter, distal esophagus, and nasopharynx should be used whenever possible.
    - Oral, axillary, bladder, rectal temperatures, all provide reasonable estimations of core temperature
  - Skin temperature will be lower in comparison to central core temperatures and may be used as an estimate of core temperature, but values must be interpreted with caution.
    - Especially during cases with large, rapid swings in temperature (i.e., cardiopulmonary bypass),

skin temperature readings are of minimal utility when used to guide intraoperative thermal management.[8]

Effect of Drugs/Anesthesia on Temperature Regulation

- **Redistribution:** Occurs during both general anesthesia (secondary to pharmacological effects of anesthetic agents) and during neuraxial anesthesia (secondary to loss of sympathetic tone)
  - Phase 1: Thermal energy (warm blood volume) from "central" compartments such as abdomen and thorax to the extremities and peripheral tissues secondary to anesthetic-induced vasodilation.
    - 1–2°C decrease during first hour of general anesthesia
    - Forced-air warming devices used preoperatively to warm patient may mitigate this phase of heat loss by neutralizing central-peripheral temperature gradient.[12]
  - Phase 2: Continued heat loss to environment over next 3–4 hours of general anesthesia
    - Much more gradual than Phase 1
    - Also minimized with the use forced air warming devices, increasing ambient temperature of operating room environment, and warmed IV fluids.
  - Phase 3: Steady state where the production of heat is approximately equal to metabolic heat production (> 4 hours from anesthesia induction)[12]
- **Central Thermoregulation Inhibition:** Anesthetic agents inhibiting reflexive responses from hypothalamus that maintain the interthreshold range.
  - For each percentage of inhaled isoflurane, there is approximately a 3°C decrease in the temperature threshold that induces vasoconstriction.[3]
    - Primarily occurs under general anesthesia, although occurs to some degree during neuraxial techniques, which is thought to be due to altered perception of the hypothalamus to temperature of the anesthetized dermatomes[12]

- Shivering generally absent while under general anesthesia especially with co-administration of paralytics.
- **Postoperative Shivering**
  - Occurs as a result of the direct neurological effect secondary to general anesthetic agents.
    - More common with longer surgery duration and greater volatile anesthetic concentrations used during surgery[12]
  - Actual hypothermia upon reactivation of the interthreshold range by the hypothalamus.
  - Increased risk of myocardial ischemia during severe shivering, as this may increase oxygen consumption 5× that of a normothermic patient[12]
  - Very common during the postpartum period.
    - Thought to be a combination of central heat redistribution secondary to peripheral vasodilation and interruption of sympathetic tone.
    - Also may be attributed possible hormonal response in the immediate postpartum period, which is why up to 23–44% of patients exhibit shivering even after natural child birth without neuraxial anesthesia.[13]

- **Harmful Effects of Hypothermia in Intraoperative and Postoperative Period**
  - Increased incidence of myocardial ischemia secondary to shivering, increased oxygen consumption and increased vascular resistance
  - Cardiac arrhythmias
  - Decreased oxygen release by RBCs due to leftward shift of hemoglobin–oxygen saturation curve
  - Coagulopathy and possibly increased transfusion requirements
    - Mild hypothermia (1–2°C below 37°C) can increase need for allogenic transfusions by 20%
  - Potentiation of neuromuscular blockade
  - Delayed wound healing and increased infection risk (up to 3× wound infection rate)
  - Decreased drug metabolism and anesthetic requirements[8]
    - Minimum alveolar concentration (MAC) reduced by approximately 5% per °C below 35°C[14]

References

1. Brody TM, Larner J, Minneman KP, Wecker L, editors. Introduction to the autonomic system. In *Brody's Human Pharmacology: Molecular to Clinical*, 4th ed. Elsevier Mosby, 2005; chapter 9, pp 93–106.

2. Philipson LH. beta-Agonists and metabolism. *J Allergy Clin Immunol* 2002 Dec 31;**110**(6):S313–S317.

3. Glick DB. The autonomic nervous system. In Miller RD, Eriksson LI, Fleisher LA, et al., editors. *Miller's Anesthesia*, 7th ed. Elsevier/ Saunders, 2009; chapter 16, pp 346–386.

4. Taylor P, Brown JH. Acetylcholine. In Siegel GJ, Agranoff BW, Albers RW, et al., editors. *Basic Neurochemistry: Molecular, Cellular and Medical*

Aspects, 6th ed. Lippincott-Raven, 1999; pp 186–207.

5. Wessler I. Acetylcholine release at motor endplates and autonomic neuroeffector junctions: a comparison. *Pharmacol Res* 1996 Feb 29;**33** (2):81–94.

6. David G, Hirst S, Bramich NJ, Edwards FR, Klemm M. Transmission

at autonomic neuroeffector junctions. *Trends Neurosci* 1992 Feb 29;**15** (2):40–46.

7. Binder MD, Hirokawa N, Windhorst U, editors. Autonomic reflexes. In *Encyclopedia of Neuroscience*. Springer, 2009; pp 272–281.

8. Miller RD, Eriksson LI, Fleisher LA, et al., editors. *Miller's Anesthesia*, 8th ed. Churchill Livingstone/Elsevier, 2015.

9. Simon E. Temperature regulation: the spinal cord as a site of extrahypothalamic thermoregulatory functions. *Rev Rhysiol Biochem Pharmacol* 1974;**71**:1–76.

10. Butterworth JF, Mackey DC, Wasnick JD, editors. *Morgan & Mikhail's Clinical Anesthesiology*, 5th ed. McGraw-Hill, 2013.

11. Sessler DI. Mild perioperative hypothermia. *N Engl J Med* 1997;**336** (24):1730–1737.

12. Sessler DI. Perioperative heat balance. *Anesthesiology* 2000;**92** (2):578–596.

13. Harper RG, Quintin A, Kreynin I, et al. Observations on the post partum shivering phenomenon. *J Reprod Med* 1991;**36**:803–807.

14. Eger EI, Johnson BH. MAC of I-653 in rats, including a test of the effect of body temperature and anesthetic duration. *Anesth Analg* 1987;**66**:974–976.

Central Nervous System: Anatomy

Kenneth John, Devon Flaherty, and Jonathan Gal

Monro–Kellie Doctrine: The intracranial space is a fixed space composed of: (1) brain parenchyma, (2) cerebrospinal fluid, and (3) blood. An increase in the volume of one must result in a decrease in one or both of the remaining two volumes.[1]

The Brain

Cerebral hemispheres have three components: cerebral cortex (gray matter), subcortical white matter, and the basal ganglia (also gray matter).

- **Primary motor cortex** – Located on the precentral gyrus. Critical for voluntary motor movement of the contralateral side of the body. Stimulated with transcranial motor evoked potentials. Organized into a motor homunculus. See Figures 26.1 and 26.2.

- **Primary somatosensory cortex** – Located on the postcentral gyrus. Receives sensory information from the contralateral side of the body. Stimulation is monitored with somatosensory evoked potentials.

Basal Ganglia
- Composed of three nuclei: caudate nucleus, putamen, and globus pallidus interconnected by the internal capsule.
- Essential for motor control.
- Functionally they work with the *substantia nigra, subthalamic nuclei,* and other midbrain structures to form the *extrapyramidal system.*
- *Parkinson's disease:* Loss of dopaminergic neurons in the substantia nigra
- *Huntington's disease:* Neuron loss in the caudate and putamen.[2]

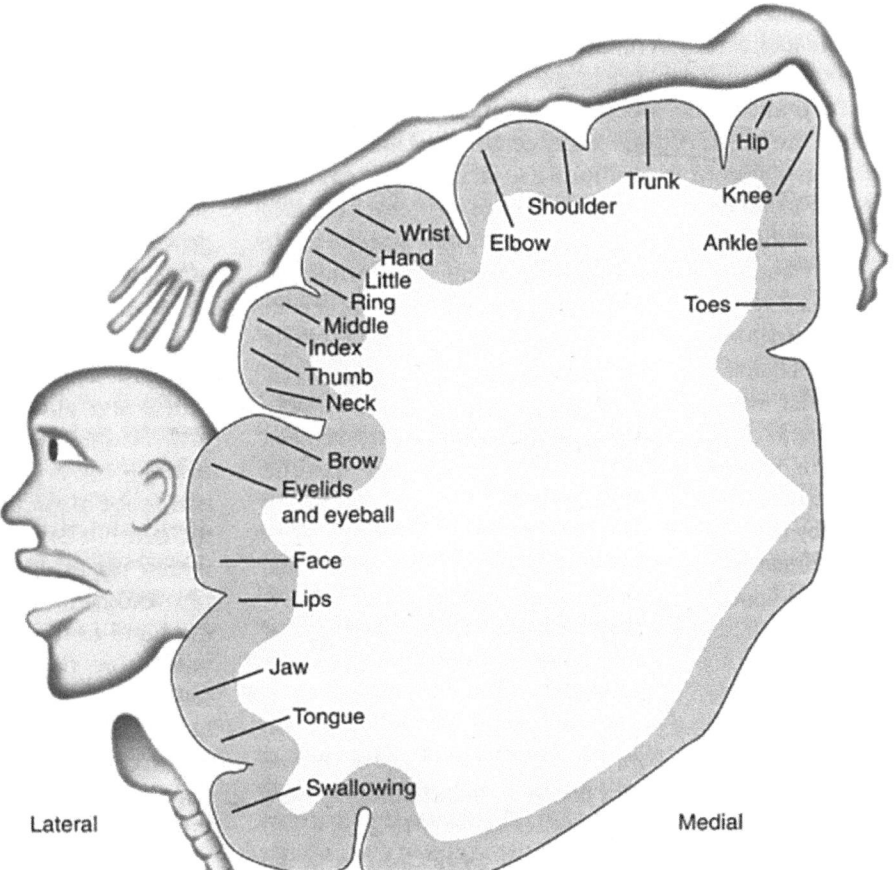

Figure 26.1 Homunculus – lower extremity is represented medially, followed by upper extremity and head as you move more laterally along the gyrus.

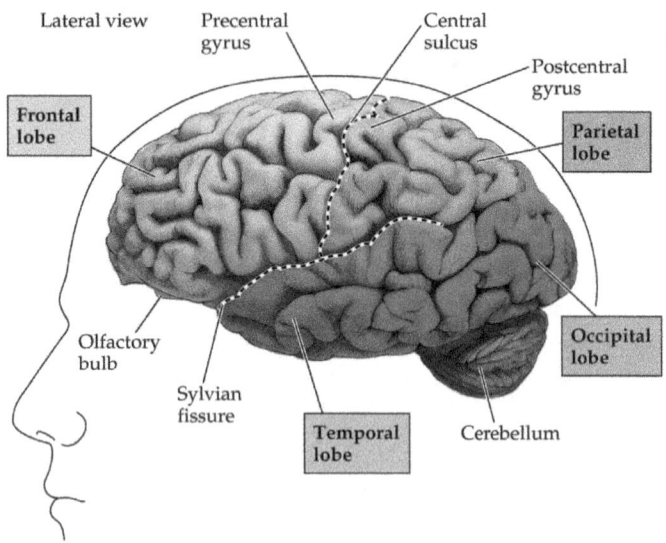

Lateral view · Precentral gyrus · Central sulcus · Postcentral gyrus · Frontal lobe · Parietal lobe · Occipital lobe · Olfactory bulb · Sylvian fissure · Temporal lobe · Cerebellum

Figure 26.2 Lobes of the cortex – the brain is divided into four lobes (frontal, parietal, occipital, and temporal). The precentral and postcentral gyri are separated by the central sulcus. The frontal and temporal lobes are separated by the lateral sulcus. By Allan Ajifo [CCBY2.0 (http://creativecommons.org/licenses/by/2.0), via Wikimedia Commons.

Brainstem

The brainstem consists of the *midbrain, pons, and medulla.*

The *reticular formation* (reticular-activating system) – constellation of nuclei located in the tegmentum of the brainstem, lateral hypothalamus, and thalamus. It functions to regulate consciousness and arousal.

Area postrema (medulla) – A chemoreceptor trigger zone for emesis. Lacks blood–brain barrier and is a direct interface between parenchyma, blood, and cerebrospinal fluid (CSF).

Nausea/vomiting impulses can also come from the vestibular system, midbrain, and cerebral cortex.[3,4]

How Is Respiration Controlled?

1. **Primary respiratory center** (medulla) – Also known as "medullary respiratory center" is comprised of dorsal and ventral respiratory groups
   a. **Dorsal respiratory group** – Initiates inspiration. Downstream effects activate phrenic and intercostal nerves. Active during quiet breathing. Stimulated either by intrinsic pacemaker function, or possibly by extrinsic pacing by the *Pre-Botzinger complex.*
   b. **Ventral respiratory group** – Both inspiratory and expiratory neurons. Stimulated by intense activity in the dorsal respiratory group. Inactive during quiet breathing, but functions during active exhalation.
2. **Apneustic center** (pons, reticular formation) – Modulates signals from the primary respiratory center. Stimulates inspiratory neurons, inhibits expiratory neurons.
3. **Pneumotaxic center** (pons, nucleus parabrachialis, and Kolliker–Fuse nucleus) – Modulates signals from the primary respiratory center. Inhibits inspiratory neurons or apneustic center.
   ○ Respiratory centers contain chemoreceptors that detect pH levels and adjust ventilation accordingly. Peripherally, aortic and carotid bodies contain chemoreceptors that increase ventilation in response to decreased pH, increased $PaCO_2$, and decreased PaO_2.
   ○ **Aortic body** afferent impulses transmitted along *the vagus nerve.*
   ○ **Carotid body** afferent impulses transmitted along *the glossopharyngeal nerve.*
   ○ Many drug classes such as opioids and sedative/hypnotic agents inhibit transmission in the dorsal respiratory group of the primary respiratory center causing respiratory depression.[5]

Cerebral Circulation

Major vessels course through the subarachnoid space before entering the brain parenchyma. A ruptured aneurysm in these vessels will lead to subarachnoid hemorrhage rather than parenchymal hemorrhage.

Arterial System

Circle of Willis – Allows for anastomosis and collateral blood flow between both sides of the brain and is composed of the anterior communicating artery, anterior cerebral arteries, internal carotid arteries (right and left), posterior communicating arteries, posterior cerebral arteries, and the basilar artery.
   ○ Highly variable anatomy, only ~ 25% of the population has a complete vascular ring.[6]
   ○ Following clamping of the internal carotid artery during a carotid endarterectomy, the arterial blood pressure is intentionally elevated to increase perfusion of the contralateral brain tissue via the circle of Willis.
   ○ Vertebral artery injection can be implicated in local anesthetic systemic toxicity following brachial plexus, stellate ganglion, and cervical plexus blocks.

Venous System

- Internal regions of the brain are drained by the internal cerebral veins, which empty into the great cerebral *vein of Galen.*
- All other regions of the brain are drained by *venous sinuses*, which are enveloped within the layers of dura and ultimately drain into the *internal jugular veins or pterygoid plexus.* Venous sinuses in the skull are kept patent by connections to the dura and surrounding osseous structures allowing for the entrainment of air and the possibility of venous air embolism when open sinuses are exposed to atmospheric air (i.e., craniotomy in sitting position).

Bridging veins traverse the dura and can be torn with applied traction (e.g., trauma or CSF drainage after a spinal tap), which can lead to a subdural hematoma.

The Spinal Cord

Spinal cord blood supply:
- One anterior spinal artery
  - Gets contributions from the *radicular arteries* – branches from intercostal arteries (T1–L1, highly variable).
  - *Artery of Adamkiewicz* is the largest radicular artery, usually arises at T9–T12 (highly variable) and supplies the lower half of the anterior spinal cord.
  - Two posterior spinal arteries
  - Supply dorsal white columns and dorsal gray matter

Notable tracts:
- Ascending tracts
  - **Spinothalamic tract** – Carries *pain and temperature input.*
    - First-order neurons with cell bodies in *dorsal root ganglion* (DRG) are stimulated via their peripheral free nerve endings.
    - Axons travel through Lissauer's tract to synapse on to second-order neurons in the dorsal horn *(substantia gelatinosa or nucleus proprius).*
    - Secondary neurons' axons decussate within 1 to 3 vertebral levels via the *ventral white commissure* and travel to the contralateral *ventral posterolateral nucleus of the thalamus.*
    - Third-order neurons send impulses along the internal capsule to the somatosensory cortex.
  - **Dorsal column/medial lemniscus** – Carries tactile discrimination, proprioception, form recognition, and vibratory input.
    - First-order neurons are in the DRG. They ascend ipsilaterally, until they synapse with second-order neurons in the medulla.
    - Fibers of the second-order neurons decussate, forming the *medial lemniscus* and synapse on to the *contralateral ventral posterolateral nucleus of the thalamus.*
    - Third-order neurons send axons along the posterior limb of the internal capsule to the *somatosensory cortex.*
- Descending tracts
  - **Corticospinal tracts**: Voluntary control of skeletal muscle to the body.
    - Originate from upper motor neurons in the primary motor cortex. Decussate in the medulla. Synapse onto lower motor neuron in ventral horn of spinal cord. Lower motor neuron interacts directly with skeletal muscle.

  - **Corticobulbar tract**: Voluntary control of skeletal muscle to regions of the body controlled by cranial nerves.
    - Originates in the primary motor cortex (upper motor neurons), travels down the internal capsule, crosses to contralateral side in the brainstem to innervate motor nuclei of cranial nerves (innervates some cranial nerves bilaterally).[7]

The Spine

Important Landmarks:
- Chassaignac's tubercle – C6 transverse process
- Vertebra prominens – C7
- Inferior angle of the scapular – T7
- Lower rib margin – T10
- Tuffier's line – Imaginary line between iliac crests, estimates L4 vertebral body or L4/5 interspace
- Posterior iliac spines – S2
- Sacral cornu – S5

Key Locations:
- Spinal cord extends from skull base to conus medullaris ~ L1/2 in adults, L3 in infants
- Dural sac extends from foramen magnum to S2 in adults and S3/4 in infants
  - Dermatomal blockade at certain anatomical sites can be used to assess adequacy of block height (Table 26.1).

Regional Differences in Vertebral Morphology:
- In general, vertebral bodies are larger in the more caudal regions of the spine. The thoracic spinal processes are sharply angled in a caudal fashion, while the lumbar spinous processes are almost perpendicular to the neuraxis.

Table 26.1 Dermatomal sensory blockade with anatomical landmark correlate, as required for different types of surgery

Sensory level	Landmark	Surgery/site
T4	Nipple	Entire peritoneum, cesarean section, upper abdominal
T6	Xiphoid process	Hernia repair, lower abdominal surgery (gynecologic, urologic)
T10	Umbilicus	Hip surgery, TURP, labor/vaginal delivery
L1	Inguinal ligament	Thigh/knee surgery
L2	Knee	Ankle and foot surgery
S1	N/a	Perineal and anal surgery

Atlantoaxial Instability: Associated with Down syndrome, long-standing rheumatoid arthritis, trauma, and ankylosing spondylitis.

Paravertebral Space
- Borders: Parietal pleura (anterolateral), superior costotransverse ligament (posterior), vertebral body/disk, and intervertebral foramina (medial)
- Contains spinal nerves that can be affected by paravertebral nerve blocks.

Facet Joints – See Figure 26.3.
- Small stabilizing joints between vertebrae. Often implicated as a source of axial back pain.
- Innervated by the *medial branch of the posterior division* of spinal nerves. Can be blocked by a "medial branch block."
- A single facet joint is only sufficiently blocked if both the above and below branches are blocked.

Meninges

Three layers of meninges are dura, arachnoid, and pia mater.
In general, the dura imparts structure while the arachnoid imparts impermeability.

What layers does a midline spinal needle pass through?
- Skin > subcutaneous fat > supraspinous ligament > interspinous ligament > ligamentum flavum > epidural space > dura > subdural space > arachnoid mater > subarachnoid space

What layers does a paramedian spinal needle pass through?
- Skin > subcutaneous fat/skeletal muscle > ligamentum flavum > epidural space > dura > subdural space > arachnoid mater > subarachnoid space

What are the borders of the epidural space?
- Superiorly – Foramen magnum (a "high epidural" wouldn't block the cranial nerves)
- Inferiorly – Sacrococcygeal ligament

- Anteriorly – Posterior longitudinal ligament
- Posteriorly – Lamina and ligamentum flavum
- Laterally – Pedicles

What is contained in the epidural space?
- Fat, nerves, blood vessels
- *Internal vertebral plexus* (also known as Batson's plexus) – Venous drainage of the epidural space. The plexus is valveless and communicates with both the basilar plexus and deep pelvic veins.

  ○ Veins can act as a pathway for spread of infection or malignancy.
  ○ Veins are more prominent in lateral epidural space, providing an explanation for the higher rate of intravascular catheters with a paramedian epidural approach.
  ○ Patients with IVC compression or elevated intraabdominal or intracranial pressures have more distention of epidural veins leading to a higher likelihood of intravascular injection/absorption and increased spread of local anesthetic.

Cranial Nerves

Olfactory (Cranial Nerve I)

Optic (Cranial Nerve II)
- Ischemia can result in *ischemic optic neuropathy*, either anterior (affecting the optic disk) or posterior (retrobulbar optic nerve ischemia) and presents as *painless visual loss.*

Oculomotor (Cranial Nerve III)
- Controls the majority of eye motion via four extraocular muscles (see CN IV and VI for the other two).
- Patients with a palsy of this nerve have an *inferior and lateral diversion* to their pupil ("down and out"), as well as *mydriasis* ("blown pupil").

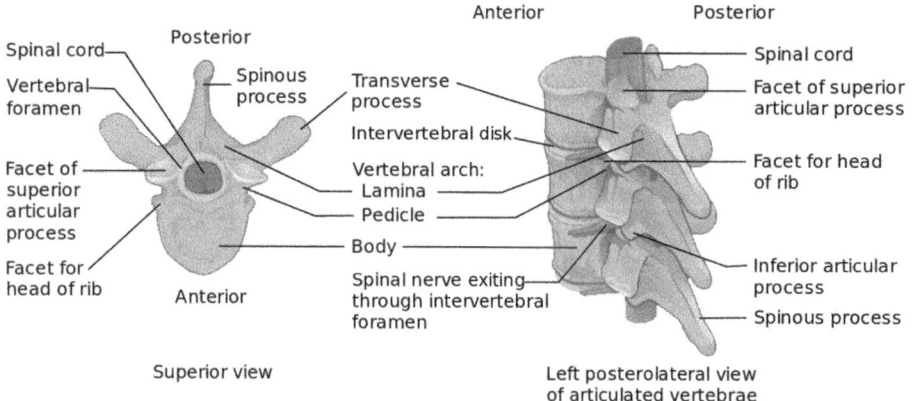

Figure 26.3 Vertebral anatomy – transverse and sagittal views of the vertebral column depicting the vertebral body, transverse processes, lamina, spinous processes, and facet joints.

- During herniation, this nerve is stretched by the medial temporal lobe leading to an ipsilateral palsy.

Trochlear (Cranial Nerve IV)

Trigeminal (Cranial Nerve V)

- Three distributions – Opthalmic (V1), maxillary (V2), and mandibular (V3)
- Controls the muscles of mastication, such as the masseter (these muscles can be directly stimulated with a peripheral nerve stimulator to give "false twitches").
- Affected in trigeminal neuralgia, most commonly V2 or V3.
- Branches can be blocked for supraorbital (V1), infraorbital (V2), greater palatine (V2), or nasopalatine (V2) nerve blocks.
- Mandibular nerve provides general sensory innervation to the anterior two-thirds of the tongue.
- Oculocardic reflex initiated by V1 due to compression of globe or traction on extraocular muscles.

Abducens (Cranial Nerve VI)

Facial nerve (Cranial Nerve VII)

- Five branches control facial muscles: (1) temporal, (2) zygomatic, (3) buccal, (4) mandible, and (5) cervical branches.
- Branches pass through but do not innervate the parotid gland. These nerve branches are often monitored intraoperatively during parotidectomies.
- Activity of orbicularis oculi via stimulation of the zygomatic branch of CN VII is often used for neuromuscular blockade monitoring.
- Taste sensation from the anterior two-thirds of the tongue is carried by the chorda tympani.

Vestibulocochlear (Cranial Nerve VIII)

- Connects to the dorsal vagal complex, allowing for nausea with ear surgeries and motion sickness.
- Aminoglycosides (e.g., gentamicin) are classic ototoxic agents.

Glossopharyngeal (Cranial Nerve IX)

- Sensory innervation of soft palate, posterior one-third of tongue, posterior oropharynx, and vallecula.
- Blocked by topicalized local anesthetic administration or injection at the base of the anterior tonsillar pillar (anesthetizes the tonsillar, lingual, and pharyngeal branches) prior to an awake fiberoptic intubation.

Vagus (Cranial Nerve X)

- Motor innervation to the larynx via the recurrent laryngeal nerve and external branch of the superior laryngeal Sensory innervation
  - Internal branch of the superior laryngeal nerve
    - Hypopharynx, vallecula (shared with CN IX), epiglottis
- Larynx at and above vocal cords
  - Recurrent laryngeal nerve
    - Below vocal cords, including trachea and lower airways
- Unilateral palsy of the recurrent laryngeal nerves leads to hoarseness and is not an airway emergency. It can result from interscalene block, thyroid/parathyroid surgery, overinflated endotracheal tube cuff, or aortic arch surgery.
- Bilateral complete palsy of recurrent laryngeal nerves leaves vocal cords flaccid and rarely results in complete airway obstruction.
- Bilateral incomplete palsy of the recurrent laryngeal nerves leaves the vocal cords with unopposed adduction forces resulting in complete airway obstruction. This is an airway emergency.
  - Posterior cricothyroid muscle is the only muscle that can abduct the vocal cords.
- CN X provides parasympathetic innervation diffusely including the respiratory tract (bronchoconstriction and secretions).
  - Opposing sympathetic innervation is provided from T1 to T4 (cardioaccelerator fibers).[8]

Spinal Accessory (Cranial Nerve XI)

Hypoglossal (Cranial Nerve XII)

- Innervates all intrinsic and extrinsic muscles of the tongue except for palatoglossus (CN X)
- Very rare unilateral lesions have been described after oral airway, LMA, and orotracheal tube placement (Table 26.2).

Table 26.2 Cranial nerve reflexes

Reflex	Afferent nerve	Efferent nerve
Corneal	V_1	VII
Oculocardiac	V_1	X
Lacrimation	V_1	VII
Pupillary	II	III
Gag	IX	X

References

1. Mokri B. The Monro–Kellie hypothesis: applications in CSF volume depletion. *Neurology* 2001;**6**:1746–1749.

2. Jacobson S, Marcus EM. Motor system II: basal ganglia. In *Neuroanatomy for the Neuroscientist*, 2nd ed. Spinger Science + Business Media, 2011; pp 207–224.

3. Waxman SG The brain stem and cerebellum. In Waxman SG, editor. *Clinical Neuroanatomy*, 27th ed. McGraw-Hill, 2013; chapter 7.

4. Hornby PJ. Central neurocircuitry associated with emesis. *Am J Med* 2001;**111**(8):106–112.

5. Balofsky A., George J., Papadakos P. Neuropulmonology. *Handb Clin Neurol* 2017;**140**(2006):33–48. doi:10.1016/B978-0-444-63600-3.00003-9

6. Waxman SG. Vascular supply of the brain. In Waxman SG, editor. *Clinical Neuroanatomy*, 27th ed. McGraw-Hill, 2013; chapter 12.

7. Waxman SG. The spinal cord. In Waxman SG, editor. *Clinical Neuroanatomy*, 27th ed. McGraw-Hill, 2013; chapter 5.

8. Monkhouse SU. General considerations. In *Cranial Nerves: Functional Anatomy*. Cambridge University Press, 2006; chapter 1.

Respiratory System: Physiology

Maria Castillo

Lung Volumes and Capacities

Tidal Volume (TV): Volume inspired and expired during quiet breathing cycle (~ 500 mL)

Residual Volume (RV): Volume left in lungs after maximum expiratory effort (~ 2 L)

Expiratory Reserve Volume (ERV): Maximal volume that can be forcibly exhaled from end-expiratory position of a tidal volume

Inspiratory Reserve Volume (IRV): Volume that can be inspired with maximal effort above the normal resting end-expiratory position of a tidal volume

Total Lung Capacity (TLC): Volume in lung after maximum inspiration (6–8 L); TLC increased in COPD; decreased in restrictive lung disease

$$\textbf{TLC} = \textbf{IRV} + \textbf{ERV} + \textbf{TV} + \textbf{RV} = \textbf{VC} + \textbf{RV}$$

See Figure 27.1.

Vital Capacity (VC): Maximum volume that can be exhaled after maximal inspiration (4–6 L); VC decreased in both restrictive and obstructive lung disease

$$\textbf{VC} = \textbf{TLC--RV} = \textbf{IRV} + \textbf{ERV} + \textbf{TV}$$

Functional Reserve Capacity (FRC): Volume in lungs after an ordinary expiration (3–4 L); FRC increased with increased height and age; decreased in pregnant women, obese patients, supine position and general anesthesia.

$$\textbf{FRC} = \textbf{ERV} + \textbf{RV}$$

Inspiratory Vital Capacity (IVC): Maximal volume inhaled from the point of maximum expiration

Time Constants (Tau) τ: Describes the rapidity of change in an exponential curve

$\tau =$ time required to inflate lung (τ = 63%; 2τ = 87%; 3τ = 95%; 4τ = 99%)

$\tau = $ **Total compliance × Airway resistance**

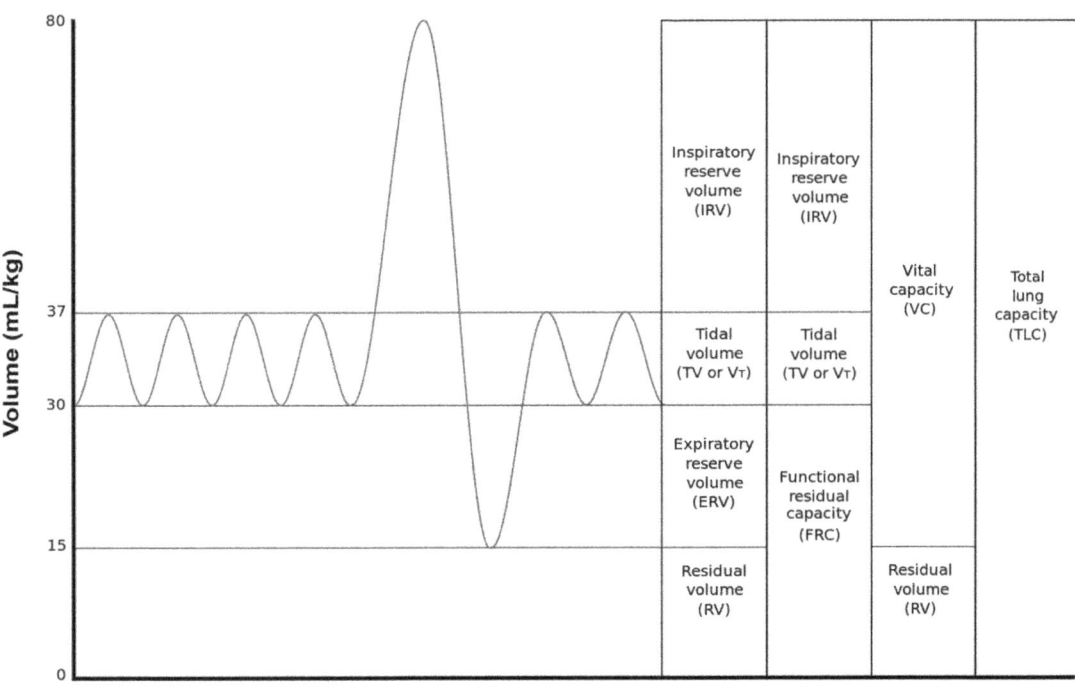

Figure 27.1 Lung volumes.

Spirometry: Measures lung function, volume, flow, and breathing pattern

FEV$_1$ (Forced expiratory volume in 1 second)–volume exhaled by the end of the first second of forced expiration

FVC (Forced vital capacity) – vital capacity determined from a maximally forced expiratory effort

Dead Space (physiological): The volume of gas ventilating the conducting airways and unperfused alveoli (anatomical dead space ~ 2 mL/kg)

Closing Capacity: Volume at which small airways lacking cartilaginous support begin to close in dependent parts of the lung. Highly dependent on lung volume and the radial traction of the surrounding lung tissue to keep open. Increases with age, meaning small airways will collapse at higher volume than in younger people.

Methods of Measurement of Lung Volumes

Nitrogen Washout: Patient breathes O_2 for several minutes to eliminate N_2; then, the quantity of N_2 eliminated is measured. Thus, if 2 L of N_2 are eliminated, and initial alveolar concentration was 80%, then the initial volume of the lung was 2.5 L.

Helium: Use as a tracer gas. If 50 mL of helium is introduced to lungs and concentration is measured to be 1%, then the lung volume is 5 L.

Plethysmograph: Gas-tight box in which changes in the volume of the body can be determined as a change in pressure within the box

O_2 Uptake: Oxygen diffuses into erythrocytes down the pressure gradient, O_2 partial pressure of atmosphere = 160 mmHg; in alveolus = 150; in pulmonary arterial blood in capillaries ~ 20–40 mmHg. Increasing FIO_2 to 100% increases alveolar partial pressure, increasing gradient, aiding O_2 diffusion.

Increased O_2 Uptake: Caused by left-shift, transfusion, increased alveolar ventilation, and increased FIO_2

Decreased O_2 Uptake: Caused by anemia, blood dyscrasias, dead space, V/Q mismatch, COPD, and diffusion limitations

CO_2 Production: Parallels O_2 consumption according to respiratory quotient. Only 80% as much CO_2 is produced as O_2 is consumed.

Respiratory Quotient (RQ): CO_2 produced/O_2 consumed, which under normal conditions is 0.8. It indirectly indicates whether proteins, carbohydrates, or fats are primary being used for energy consumption. When RQ is > 0.8, carbohydrates are being metabolized. When < 0.8, lipids are being metabolized. At 0.8, a combination of proteins, lipids and carbohydrates are metabolized.

Exercise Testing: Heart rate and ventilation plotted against O_2 consumption

Excessive increase in heart rate – primarily cardiac causes of exercise limitation
Excessive increase in ventilation – primarily respiratory causes of limitation
Both are increased – likely pulmonary vascular disease

Lung Mechanics

$$\text{Compliance} = \Delta V/\Delta P$$

Dynamic Compliance: Volume change divided by the <u>peak</u> inspiratory trans-thoracic pressure

Static Compliance: Volume change divided by the <u>plateau</u> inspiratory trans-thoracic pressure

Total compliance is lung and chest wall together, defined as:

$$1/C_{total} = 1/C_W + 1/C_L$$

Pleural Pressure Gradient: Due to lung density, gravity, and conformation of the lung within the thorax, which predominates in the basal lung tissue, pleural pressure is less negative at the base than at higher portions of the lung.

Flow-Volume Loops: Plot of y-axis = rate of airflow; x-axis = total volume inspired or expired during maximally forced inspiratory and expiratory maneuvers (Figure 27.2).

Hysteresis: Pressure–volume curves of the lung compliance during inflation and deflation, which are different due to additional energy required during inspiration to recruit alveoli

Surfactant: Secreted by type II alveolar epithelial cells; profoundly lowers surface tension of the alveolar lining fluid, increasing compliance of the lung, decreasing work of expanding the lung, inhibiting transudation of fluid, increasing stability of alveoli, and decreasing atelectasis

LaPlace's Law: The pressure in an alveolus (P) is greater than ambient pressure by an amount dependent on the surface tension in the liquid lining (T) and the radius of the alveolus (R):

$$P = 2T/R$$

Resistance: Airway resistance $R = \Delta P/\Delta V$

For air to flow into lungs, ΔP must be developed to overcome airway resistance. ΔP depends on caliber of airway and rate and pattern of airflow.

Principles of Gas Flow Measurement

Laminar flow occurs when the gas passes down parallel-sided tubes at less than a critical velocity; the pressure drop is proportional to the flow rate as per **Poiseuille's equation:**

$$\Delta P = 8\, QL\mu/\pi r^4 \text{ otherwise written as } Q = \Delta P\pi r^4/8\, \mu L$$

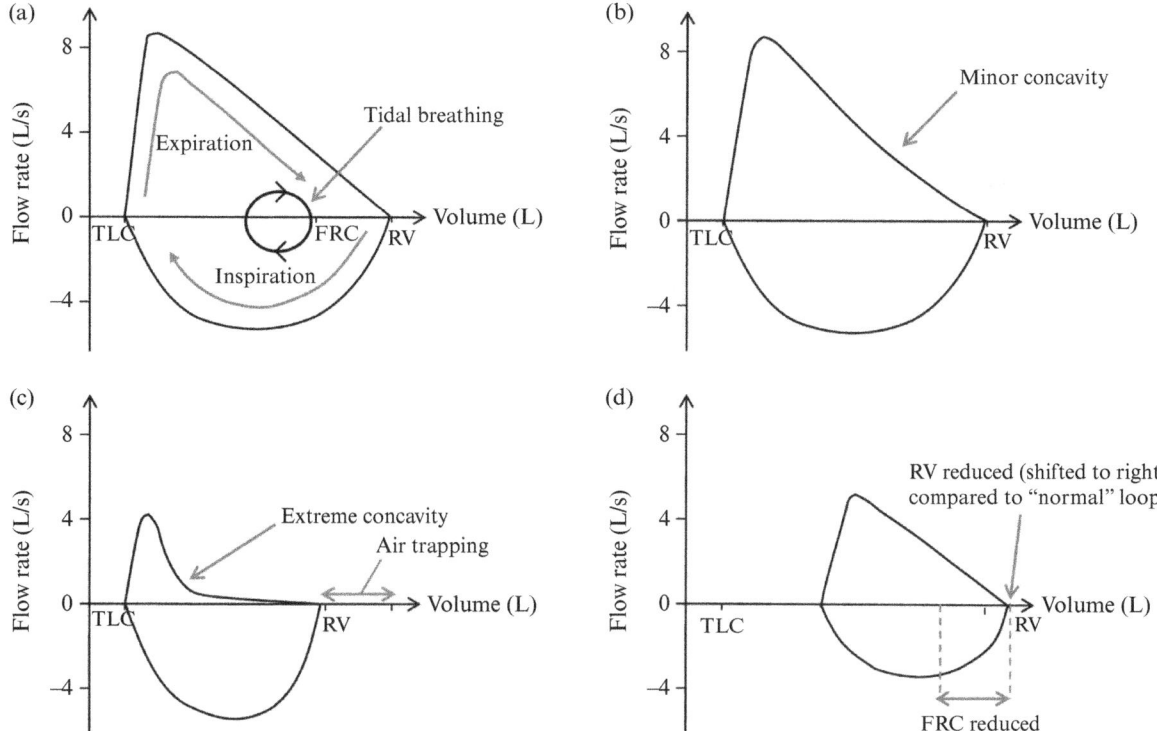

Figure 27.2 Flow-volume loop. (a) Normal flow volume loop, (b) mild obstructive disease, (c) obstructive pulmonary disease, (d) restrictive pulmonary disease.

ΔP: Pressure difference between two ends
Q: Gas flow rate
L: Length of the tube
μ: viscosity
r: Radius of the tube

Turbulent Flow: Pressure proportional to the volume of gas flow squared times a gas density constant. There is more resistance with turbulent flow, which occurs at airway branch points and airway wall irregularities.

Orific Flow occurs at severe constriction such as stenosis or obstruction of the upper airway; the pressure drop is dependent on density of the gas rather than viscosity, which is why using helium decreases resistance to flow

Note: At *low flow rates*, there is *laminar flow*, which depends on the *viscosity* of the gas. At *high flow rates*, there is *turbulent flow*, which depends on the *density* of the gas.

Work of Breathing: Potential energy is stored by the lung during inspiration and expended during expiration, thus expiration is passive.

Work against elastic resistance is increased when breathing is slow and deep; work against air flow resistance is increased when breathing is rapid and shallow

Increased elastic resistance (pulmonary fibrosis, pulmonary edema) – rapid and shallow is favored

Increased airway resistance (asthma, obstructive lung disease) – deep and slow is favored

Regulation of Airway Caliber: Neural control of airway smooth muscle and there is pharmacological modulation of this input

Acetylcholine (Ach) acts on muscarinic subtypes, especially M_3 receptors for contractile response; epinephrine and norepinephrine act on α- and β-adrenergic receptors; vasoactive intestinal peptide (VIP), nitric oxide (NO), substance P, and neurokinin A act via second messenger cascades

Ventilation–Perfusion

Distribution of Ventilation: In low flow states, distribution is determined by compliance. In high flow states, distribution is determined by resistance. In upper, more expanded regions of the lung, resistance is lower, so flow rate is increased, equalizing distribution of ventilation

Distribution of Perfusion: Determined by gravity and hydrostatic pressure; decreased blood flow to apex; with positive pressure ventilation, apical alveoli can compress surrounding capillaries, preventing blood flow

Zones

Zone 1 – Alveolar pressure P_A > arterial P_a > venule P_v, creating decreased transmural pressure causing collapse of blood vessels and minimal blood flow. Includes apical area of lungs.

Zone 2 – Transition region below Zone 1, where P_a > P_A > P_v, resulting in resistance to flow during most but not all of the respiratory cycle

Zone 3 – Dependent region where $P_a > P_v > P_A$, thus blood flow is unimpeded and gas exchange happens continuously; includes most of the lung

Zone 4 – Atelectatic portion of the lung.

Hypoxic Pulmonary Vasoconstriction: Adaptive vasomotor response to alveolar hypoxia, which redistributes blood to optimally ventilated lung segments by an active process of vasoconstriction, thereby improving ventilation–perfusion matching

$$\textbf{Alveolar Gas Equation: PAO}_2 = [\text{FiO}_2 \times (\text{Patm} - \text{PH}_2\text{O})] - \text{PaCO}_2/\text{RQ}$$

PAO_2 = Alveolar O_2 tension
FiO_2 = Inspired oxygen fraction
Patm = Ambient barometric pressure
PH_2O = Partial pressure of water
$PaCO_2$ = Partial pressure of CO_2
RQ = respiratory quotient

Diffusion

Pulmonary Diffusion Capacity: Amount of gas that can diffuse across a membrane in a given period

    Diffusing Capacity of Lung for Carbon Monoxide (DLCO) is determined by the surface area of gas exchange, the membrane thickness, the pressure gradient between the gas phase in the alveolus and the plasma in the capillary, the molecular weight and solubility

> CO used as the test gas, inhaled at a small concentration to TLC just after a maximal expiration, held, then deeply exhaled to RV; inhaled CO – exhaled CO = quantity either taken up by the blood or remaining in the lung (RV); RV can be determined if an insoluble gas is administered with CO.

Apneic Oxygenation: Diffusion of oxygen to alveoli in absence of ventilation

    Diffusion Hypoxia: When nitrous oxide is discontinued, large quantities cross from the blood into the alveolus down its concentration gradient, diluting the O_2 and CO_2 in the alveolus, causing a decrease in the partial pressure of oxygen resulting in hypoxia; can be avoided by increasing fractional inspired O_2 concentration.

Blood Gas

O_2 Transport: As RBC passes alveolus, O_2 diffuses into the plasma, increasing PaO_2; as PaO_2 increases, O_2 diffuses into the RBC and combines with hemoglobin (Hb).

O_2 Physical Solubility: Oxygen exists in dissolved form or combined with Hb.

Oxyhemoglobin (Hb–O_2) Saturation: Each Hb consists of four heme molecules attached to a globulin molecule; each heme consists of glycine, α-ketogluteric acid, and iron in the ferrous form. Each ferrous ion can bind loosely to one oxygen molecule; as they bind, the Hb becomes saturated.

Hb–O_2 Dissociation Curve: Relates the saturation of Hb to the PaO_2

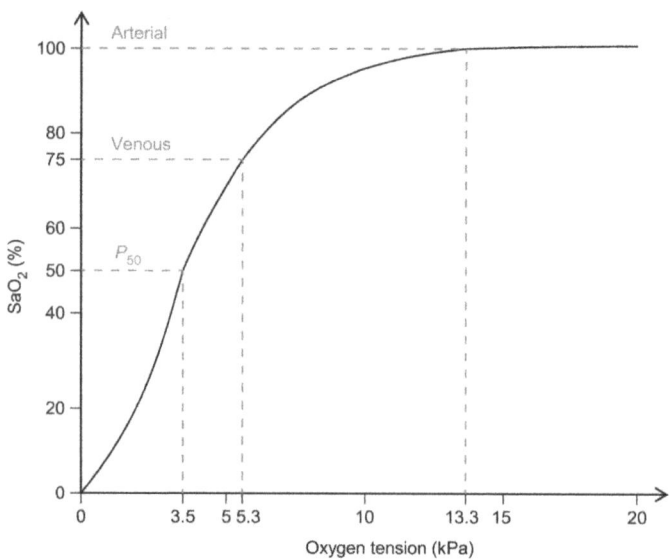

Figure 27.3 Hemoglobin–oxygen dissociation curve.

Hb is fully saturated at 700 mmHg; the flat part of the curve signifies 95–98% saturation and $PaO_2 \sim$ 90–100 mmHg; when $PaO_2 < 60$, saturation falls steeply. PaO_2 of 60 is roughly a saturation of 90% (Figure 27.3).

Rightward shift means increased oxygen unloading at a given PO_2; can be caused by increased temperature, increased H+, increased PCO_2, and increased 2,3-DPG.

2,3-Diphosphoglycerate (2,3-DPG): An end-product of red blood cell metabolism

Shifts O_2 dissociation curve to the right; increased in chronic hypoxia and chronic lung disease

P_{50}: PO_2 at which Hb is 50% saturated; $\sim$ **26.7 mmHg**

Blood O_2 Content: In arterial blood, 98% is oxyhemoglobin, < 2% is dissolved in plasma.

$$\textbf{CaO}_2 = (\textbf{Hgb} \times \textbf{1.39} \times \textbf{SaO}_2\%) + (\textbf{PaO}_2 \times \textbf{0.003})$$

1.39 mL = amount of O_2 bound per gram Hb at 1 atmosphere
0.003 mL = amount of dissolved O_2 in blood

Respiratory Enzymes: Oxidases catalyze the transfer of electrons from its substrate to molecular oxygen.

CO_2 Transport: CO_2 and O_2 move between the systemic capillary blood and tissue cells, and between the capillary blood and alveolar gas in the lungs by *passive diffusion*.

CO_2 diffuses 20 times faster than O_2.
In plasma, CO_2 exists in physical solution and hydrated to *carbonic acid* (H_2CO_3) and as *bicarbonate* (HCO_3^-); in erythrocytes, CO_2 combines with Hb as *carbaminohemoglobin* (Hb–CO_2).

Carbonic Anhydrase: Speeds up first part of reaction inside RBCs

(a)

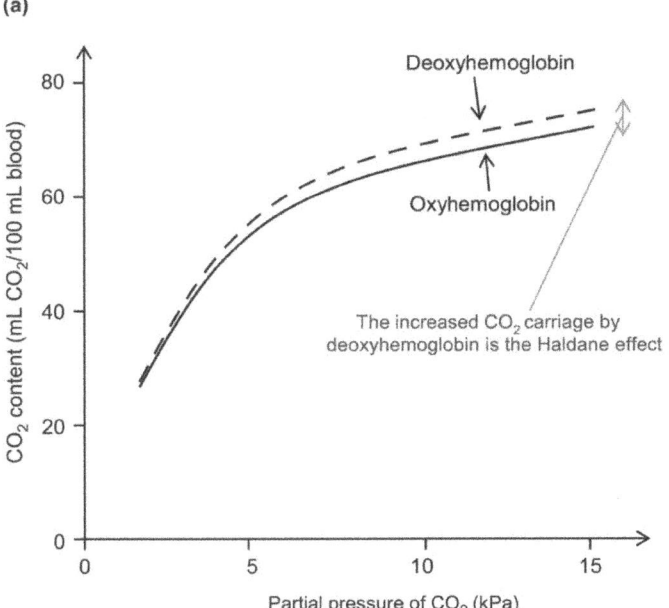

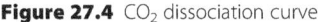

(b)

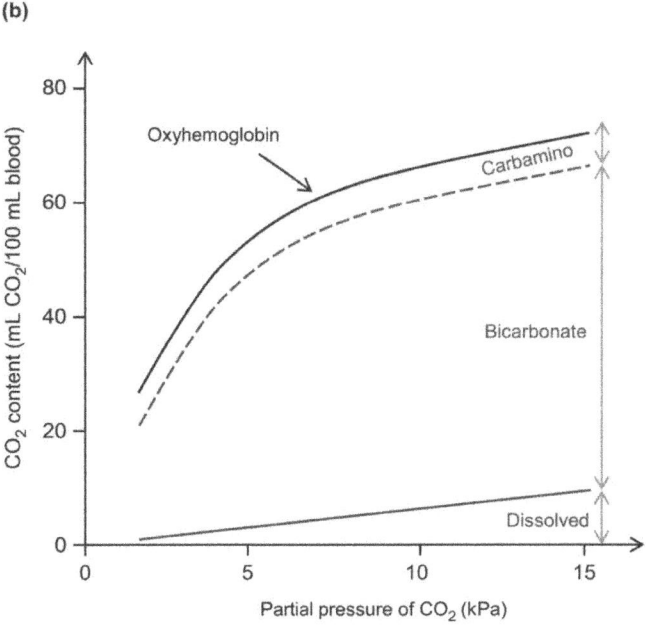

Figure 27.4 CO_2 dissociation curve.

HCO_3^- diffuses out of the cell more easily than H^+, so Cl^- ions diffuse into the cell (chloride shift); some of the H^+ ions bind to Hb due to the fact that reduced Hb is less acidic than the oxygenated form.

Reduced Hb in peripheral blood helps with loading of CO_2, while oxygenation in pulmonary capillaries assists with unloading

$$CO_2 + H_2O \Leftrightarrow H_2CO_3 \Leftrightarrow H^+ + HCO_3^-$$

Hemoglobin (Hb) as a buffer: H^+ is then buffered by Hb.

$$H^+ + Hb \Leftrightarrow HHb$$

CO_2 Dissociation Curve: Total CO_2 is plotted against the PCO_2, illustrating the amount of each form of CO_2 in the blood (Figure 27.4).

Bohr Effect: Shift of the Hb–O_2 dissociation curve caused by changes in CO_2 or pH

Shift is to the right in systemic capillaries where PCO_2 is higher and pH is lower, increasing offloading of O_2 to tissues.

Shift is to the left in pulmonary capillaries where CO_2 is lower, increasing O_2 binding to Hb.

Haldane Effect: Deoxygenation of blood increases its ability to carry CO_2; the lower the saturation of Hb with O_2, the larger the CO_2 concentration for a given PCO_2.

Systemic Effects of Hypercarbia and Hypocarbia

Hypercarbia: Restlessness, tremor, slurred speech, mood changes, increased cerebral blood flow (CBF) leading to headache, increased CSF pressure, papilledema, increased catecholamine release, $\uparrow$ HR, $\uparrow$ BP

Hypocarbia: decreased CBF, decreased cerebral blood volume, decreased cerebral oxygen delivery, decreased ICP, decreased myocardial oxygen supply, increased coronary vascular resistance, increased risk of coronary artery spasm, increased coronary micro-vascular leakage, increased myocardial oxygen demand, increased intracellular calcium concentration, increased platelet count and aggregation

Systemic Effects of Hyperoxia and Hypoxemia/Hypoxia

Hyperoxia: Increased production of cytotoxic oxygen free radicals that can cause damage to the alveolar-capillary membrane, increased mucous plugging and atelectasis, increased risk of ARDS, retrolental fibroplasia, nausea, vomiting, numbness, twitching, dizziness, possibly seizures.

Hypoxia: Increased catecholamine release, $\uparrow$ HR, decreased CBF, headache, somnolence, mental status changes, heart failure, renal function impairment, sodium retention, proteinuria, shock, V fib, asystole

Basic Interpretation of Arterial Blood Gas: Normal room air PO_2 = ~100, PCO_2= ~40

Respiratory acidosis: $\uparrow$ PCO_2 $\rightarrow$ $\downarrow$ HCO_3^-/PCO_2 ratio; $\downarrow$ pH

Respiratory alkalosis: $\downarrow$ PCO_2 $\rightarrow$ $\uparrow$ HCO_3^-/PCO_2 ratio; $\uparrow$ pH

Metabolic acidosis: $\downarrow$ HCO_3^-/PCO_2 $\rightarrow$ $\downarrow$ pH

Metabolic alkalosis: $\uparrow$ HCO_3^-/PCO_2 $\rightarrow$ $\uparrow$ pH

If PCO_2 cannot account for value of pH, compensatory changes may be creating a mixed picture

Control of Ventilation

Respiratory Center

Dorsal Medullary Respiratory Group – receives afferent visceral input from CN IX and X; regulates timing of the respiratory cycle; inspiration-intrinsic periodic firing generates repetitive bursts of action potentials

Ventral Medullary Respiratory Group – Expiration-quiescent during normal breathing but become active during exercise and then begin firing expiratory cells; control over musculature of pharynx, larynx, and tongue

The cortex, the apneustic center in lower pons, the pneumotaxic center in upper pons, the limbic system, and the hypothalamus can also affect breathing pattern.

Central Chemoreceptors: Located near ventral surface of medulla, surrounded by brain extracellular fluid (ECF); increased H^+ or dissolved CO_2 stimulates breathing, decreases inhibition.

Peripheral Chemoreceptors: Carotid bodies – located at the bifurcation of the common carotids; aortic bodies- located above and below aortic arch; respond to decreased arterial PO_2 and pH as well as increased arterial PCO_2

Proprioceptive Receptors: Pulmonary stretch receptors inhibit further inspiration and slow respiratory frequency; juxtacapillary "J" receptors respond to engorgement of capillaries, respond via vagus nerve.

Respiratory Muscles, Reflexes, Innervation

Diaphragm: Thin, dome-shaped sheet of muscle attached to lower ribs and spine; innervated by the phrenic nerves (C3–5)

External Intercostal Muscles: connect adjacent ribs; slope downward and forward causing increased lateral and anteroposterior diameters of the thorax when they contract; innervated by intercostal nerves of the same level

Internal Intercostal Muscles: Pull ribs downward and inward, decreasing thoracic volume

Abdominal Wall (rectus abdominis, internal and external obliques, transversus abdominis): Raise intra-abdominal pressure by contracting, pushing diaphragm upward

Accessory Muscles of Inspiration: Scalene muscles elevate first two ribs; sternomastoids raise the sternum.

CO_2 and O_2 Response Curves: Central and peripheral chemoreceptors sensing an increase in H+ activate a negative feedback loop to change rate of ventilation.

Opioids cause a right-shift in the response curve, while hypoxemia causes a left-shift Benzodiazepines and propofol decrease the slope of the curve, while volatile anesthetics decrease the slope and cause a right-shift.

Nonrespiratory Functions of the Lungs

Metabolic: Pulmonary endothelial cells metabolize endogenous substances and can affect pharmacokinetics

"First-Pass" Uptake – Amount of substance removed from blood on first cycle through the lungs

Lungs have substantial concentrations of P_{450} isoenzymes as well as a high concentration of angiotensin-converting enzyme (**ACE**).

Mast cells and neuroendocrine cells can produce serotonin (**5-HT**), and the lungs can extract from blood and metabolize 5-HT to 5-HIAA.

Lungs also metabolize leukotrienes, cyclo-oxygenase, prostaglandins, thromboxane, and prostacyclin.

Immune: Cytoplasmic vesicles and caveolae are involved in endocytosis.

Airway surface film has antimicrobial properties.

Respiratory epithelium contains *ciliated columnar cells* that help move out mucous and particles and goblet cells that secret mucous.

Other cells include submucosal secretory cells, Clara cells, which produce detoxifying proteins, mast cells, macrophages, monocytes, and alveolar epithelial cells, which also produce surfactant.

Lungs are also a vascular reservoir due to the capacity of the pulmonary vessels, a physical filter for particles and pathogens, and humidify inhaled air.

Perioperative Smoking

Physiological Effects

Nicotine stimulates nicotinic acetylcholine receptors, affecting the sympathetic nervous system, causing hypertension, tachycardia, and increased risk of tachyarrhythmias.

Carbon monoxide takes the place of oxygen on the Hb molecule (binds with 300-fold greater infinity), shifting the Hb–O_2 dissociation curve to the left, decreasing oxygen availability in the tissues.

Smoking increases mucus production, increases mucous viscosity, damages cilia, impairs clearing of secretions, irritates bronchial tree, and inhibits immune function.

Cessation of Smoking

48–72 hours – May have more reactive airways and increased secretions; less hypertension and tachycardia, less carbon monoxide, thus less carboxyhemoglobin, less tissue hypoxia, increased ciliary function.

2–4 weeks – Decreased mucus production, less reactive airways.

4–6 weeks – Immune functions normalize.

< 8 weeks – Possibly an increase in complications.

> 8 weeks – Decreased postoperative morbidity and mortality.

Further Reading

Barash PG, Cullen BF, Stoetling RK, editors. *Clinical Anesthesia*, 7th ed. Lippincott Williams & Wilkins, 2013.

Benumof JL. *Anesthesia for Thoracic Surgery*, 2nd ed. W. B. Saunders, 1995.

Butterworth JF, Mackey DC, Wasnick JD, editors. *Morgan & Mikhail's Clinical Anesthesiology*, 7th ed. McGraw-Hill, 2022.

Carrick MA, Robson JM, Thomas C. Smoking and anaesthesia. *BJA Educ* 2019;**19**(1):1–6.

Cohen E. *Cohen's Comprehensive Thoracic Anesthesia*. Elsevier, 2022.

Gropper MA, Eriksson LI, Fleisher LA, et al., editors. *Miller's Anesthesia*, 9th ed. Elsevier, 2019.

Katznelson R, Beattie WS. Perioperative smoking risk. *Anesthesiology* 2011;**114**:734–736.

Slinger PD. *Principles and Practice of Anesthesia for Thoracic Surgery*, 2nd ed. Springer, 2019.

West JB. *Pulmonary Physiology and Pathophysiology: An Integrated, Case-Based Approach*. Lippincott Williams & Wilkins, 2001.

Respiratory System: Anatomy

Samuel Hunter and Daniel Katz

Nose

- Structure – Cartilage and bone; divided by septum into similar halves.
  - External nares → nasal conchae → nasopharynx
- Blood Supply – Dual supply from internal carotid and external carotid
  - Majority of epistaxis from anterior nose, Kiesselbach's plexus
  - Posterior bleeds are less common, harder to control
- Innervation – Cranial nerves (CN) V_1 (ophthalmic branch) and V_2 (maxillary branch)
- Clinical Relevance: Most airway resistance in nasal passages
  - Nasal approach to fiberoptic intubation
    - Topical anesthesia to V_1 and V_2
    - Topical vasoconstrictor for decreased bleeding

- Sinus surgery
  - Controlled hypotension to optimize surgical field
  - Regional Nerve Blocks – Infraorbital nerve block for V_2, sphenopalatine block for nasal mucosal anesthesia and vasoconstriction

Pharynx

- Anatomy – Nasopharynx, oropharynx, laryngopharynx
- Innervation
  - Nasopharynx – Maxillary branch of trigeminal (V_2)
  - Oropharynx – Glossopharyngeal (CN IX): posterior one-third of tongue, superior epiglottis, gag reflex (Figure 28.1)

Larynx

- Sensory Innervation
  - Internal branch of superior laryngeal nerve (X): Inferior epiglottis to cords

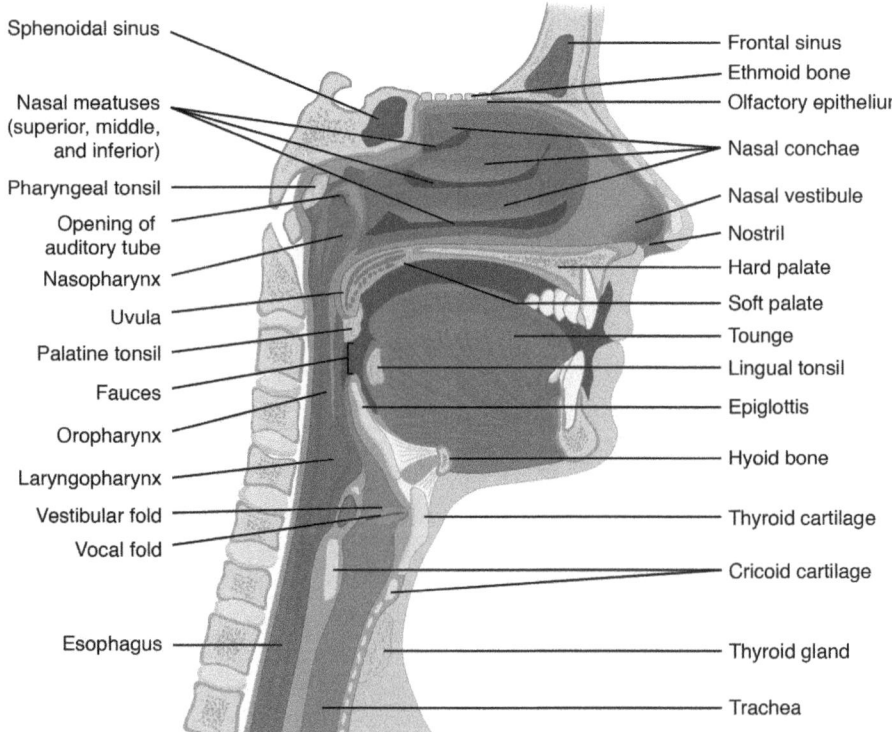

Sphenoidal sinus

Nasal meatuses (superior, middle, and inferior)

Pharyngeal tonsil

Opening of auditory tube

Nasopharynx

Uvula

Palatine tonsil

Fauces

Oropharynx

Laryngopharynx

Vestibular fold

Vocal fold

Esophagus

Frontal sinus

Ethmoid bone

Olfactory epithelium

Nasal conchae

Nasal vestibule

Nostril

Hard palate

Soft palate

Tounge

Lingual tonsil

Epiglottis

Hyoid bone

Thyroid cartilage

Cricoid cartilage

Thyroid gland

Trachea

Figure 28.1 Pharynx. A black and white version of this figure will appear in some formats. For the color version, please refer to the plate section.

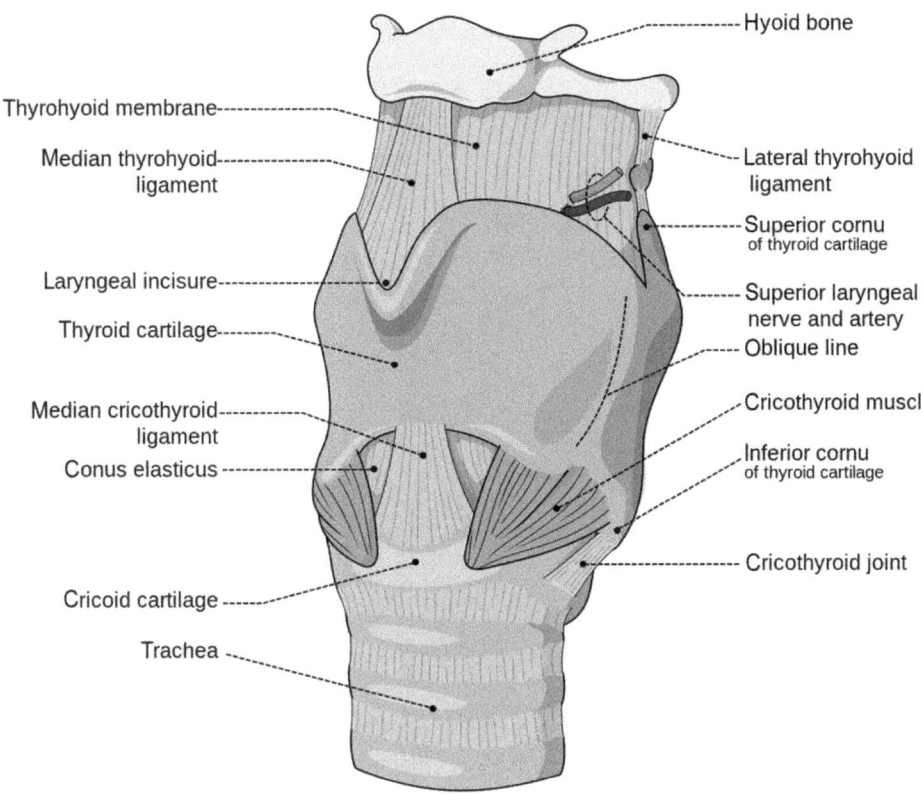

Hyoid bone

Thyrohyoid membrane

Median thyrohyoid ligament

Lateral thyrohyoid ligament

Superior cornu
of thyroid cartilage

Laryngeal incisure

Superior laryngeal nerve and artery

Thyroid cartilage

Oblique line

Cricothyroid muscle

Median cricothyroid ligament

Inferior cornu
of thyroid cartilage

Conus elasticus

Cricothyroid joint

Cricoid cartilage

Trachea

Figure 28.2 Larynx.

- Block inferior to the greater cornu of the hyoid bone within the thyrohyoid membrane for awake intubation
  - Recurrent Laryngeal Nerve (CN X): Mucosa below cords
    - Transtracheal block through cricothyroid membrane for awake intubation
- Motor Innervation
  - External branch of superior laryngeal nerve (SLN; CN X): Cricothyroid muscle
  - Recurrent laryngeal nerve (CN X): All other laryngeal muscles
- Notable Muscles
  - Cricothyroid – Vocal cord tensor and adductor; only muscle innervated by SLN
  - Posterior cricoarytenoid – Only pure abductor of cords (Figure 28.2)
- Bones and Cartilages
  - Hyoid bone – Most superior
  - Thyroid cartilage – Most prominent, "Adam's apple"
  - Cricoid cartilage – Most inferior, only complete ring of cartilage
    - Margin of safety with percutaneous access, as posterior cartilage protects other neck structures

- Nerve Injury Patterns
  - Superior laryngeal nerve injury – Fixed partially abducted cords leading to hoarseness and vocal fatigability, aspiration risk
  - Partial recurrent laryngeal nerve injury – Complete adduction of cords due to unopposed cricothyroid action, loss of abductor function
    - Bilateral partial injury may lead to stridor and complete airway obstruction
  - Complete recurrent laryngeal nerve injury – Partial adduction of cords into a fixed position, hoarseness (Figure 28.3)

Trachea

- Connects larynx to lungs; anterior to esophagus in the neck
- Approximately 20 cartilaginous partial rings with posterior muscle and connective tissue
  - 2nd through 4th rings covered by thyroid isthmus
- Jugular veins run anterolateral; common carotid arteries run posterolateral
- Posterior to aorta and superior vena cava in mediastinum
  - Innominate artery adjacent to trachea, can predispose to tracheoinnominate fistulas in context of tracheostomies

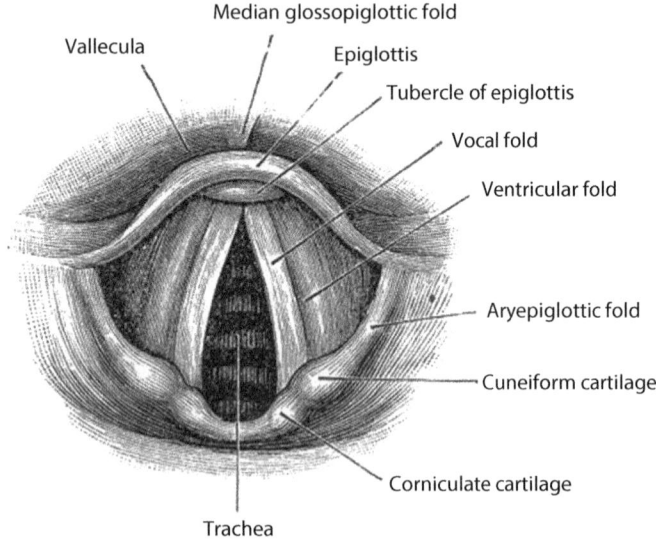

Figure 28.3 Vocal cord.

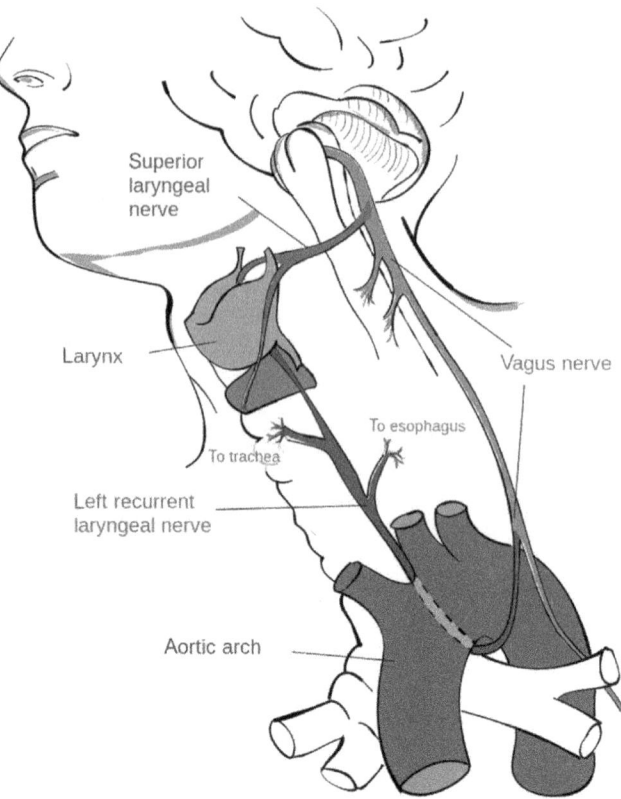

Figure 28.4 Recurrent laryngeal nerve.

- Left main bronchus crosses directly under aortic arch
  - Left bronchus can be compressed by aortic aneurysms.
  - Left recurrent laryngeal can be compromised by aortic dissection or aneurysm (Figure 28.4)
- Neck: Highly vascular area with intricate muscle and nerve anatomy
  - Location of major anatomy in neck from medial → lateral: Recurrent laryngeal n. → carotid artery → vagus n. → internal jugular vein → phrenic n.
  - Important to be aware of neck anatomy for procedures including central line placement, stellate ganglion blocks, and cervical plexus blocks
  - Thoracic Duct: Lymphatic vessel, containing chyle, that runs from T12 to root of neck and drains into systemic circulation at junction of left subclavian and internal jugular veins. Left-sided thoracic duct is bigger in diameter than right.
    - Concern for damage to left thoracic during left-sided central venous line placement resulting in chylothorax.
  - Subclavian Artery and Vein: Travel alongside each other above the 1st right rib but below the clavicle, putting them at risk for compression in pathologies resulting in thoracic outlet syndrome
    - Subclavian artery: Located between the two heads of the anterior scalene muscle
    - Subclavian vein: Located anterior to the anterior scalene muscle
  - Brachial Plexus: Located between the anterior and middle scalene muscle

Lung

- Nerve Innervation: Parasympathetic innervation to lung provided by the vagus nerve, and sympathetic by T1–4 nerves through the stellate ganglion

- Blood Supply:
  - Pulmonary Circulation: Pulmonary artery → pulmonary capillaries → pulmonary veins
  - Bronchial Circulation: Left heart → bronchial artery supplying airway → pulmonary circulation (as above)
  - "Onion Effect": Blood flow greater in hilum (inner) than in periphery (outer)
- Structure: Right bronchus take-off is 2 cm below carina with a steep angulation which is the reason for more foreign body obstructions on right rather than left.
  - Right Lung: Three lobes (upper, middle, lower) with approximately 53% of the ventilation
  - Left Lung: Two lobes (upper, lower) with approximately 47% of the ventilation
- West's Zones of the Lung: Conceptual organization of pulmonary hemodynamics based on gravity
- Zone 1: Airway pressures (P_a) > pulmonary artery (P_A) pressure > pulmonary venous pressure (P_v)
  - With this pressure gradient there is no blood perfusion despite ventilation, which normally does not exist. However, with high positive end-expiratory pressure (PEEP) or low P_a pressure such as with general anesthesia Zone 1 may occur.
- Zone 2: $P_A > P_a > P_v$
  - Blood flow is proportional to difference between P_a and P_A.

- Zone 3: $P_A > P_v > P_a$
  - Blood flow is proportional to the difference between P_A and P_v.
  - Body positioning can also be used to decrease blood flow to abnormal areas of the lung such as in unilateral pneumonia encouraging patient to lie on nondiseased side.
  - In an upright position, Zone 3 falls in the most dependent portion of the lung and thus, there is both increased ventilation and perfusion with increased gravity.
- Pneumocytes (alveolar cells): Line the alveoli in the lungs
  - Type I Cell: Thin cells that line 97% of the alveolar surface, ideal for gas diffusion
  - Type II Cell: Line 3% of the alveolar surface, secrete pulmonary surfactant to decrease the alveolar tension
- Muscles of Respiration
  - Diaphragm
  - Innervated by phrenic nerve
  - "C3, 4, 5 keeps the diaphragm alive."
  - Contraction moves diaphragm down, decreasing intrathoracic pressure and causing inspiration.
  - Mostly type 1, slow-twitch muscle – Prevents fatigue. Neonatal diaphragms proportionally more type 2 fast-twitch, predisposing to respiratory fatigue.
  - Openings in the diaphragm allow passage to the abdominal cavity:
    - Vena cava at T8
    - Esophagus at T10
    - Aorta at T12
  - Intercostals
  - External intercostals aid inspiration
  - Internal intercostals aid exhalation
  - Accessory muscles of respiration – More prominently utilized in respiratory fatigue
  - Sternocleidomastoid
  - Scalene muscles
  - Minor – Pectorals, trapezius, latissimus dorsi, serratus muscles
  - Exhalation – Passive during normal breathing
  - Forceful exhalation aided by abdominal wall and internal intercostals.
- Pediatric Airway
  - Funnel-shaped larynx and trachea
  - Anteriorly slanted vocal cords
  - More cephalad larynx – C4 in infants vs. C6 in adults
  - Narrowest portion at cricoid cartilage in infants vs. at vocal cords in adults
  - Infants have a long, floppy, omega-shaped epiglottis, which is more difficult to lift indirectly with a Macintosh blade
  - Relatively larger tongue and occiput predispose to obstruction

Further Reading

Koeppen B, Hansen J. *Netter's Atlas of Human Physiology*. Icon Learning Systems, 2002.

Pawha P, Jiang J, Shpilberg K, Luttrull M, Govindaraj S. Gross and radiographic anatomy In DeMaria S Jr, editor. *Anesthesiology and Otolaryngology*. Springer, 2013; pp 3–33.

Respiratory System: Pharmacology

Kyle James Riley and Daniel Katz

Bronchodilators

Overview

Bronchodilators relax smooth muscle and expand the airways.[1,2] Beta-2 agonists and anticholinergics are the two bronchodilators most commonly used for this purpose.[3,4]

Typical route of administration: inhaler or nebulizer, but for some medications, oral and injection choices are available.[4]

- Basic inhalation options:
  - Metered dose inhaler (MDI)[5]
  - Dry powder inhaler (DPI)[5]
  - Soft mist inhaler (SMI)[6]
  - Nebulizer[5]

Beta-2 agonists

Beta-2 agonists stimulate the beta-2 receptors in the airway muscles, relaxing the muscles, thereby widening constricted airways.[7]

Bronchoconstriction Mechanism

Increased rhythmic Ca^{2+} concentration oscillations activate myosin light-chain kinase (MLCK) phosphorylation. This increases the contractile interaction of actin and myosin,[8] resulting in increased bronchoconstriction.[9–11]

Beta-2 Agonists Effects

Beta-2 agonists reduce Ca^{2+} concentration through beta-2 receptor stimulation of the cAMP-PKA (protein kinase A) pathway resulting in increasing bronchodilation.[9–11]

Some beta-2 agonists can indirectly decrease bronchospasm by other mechanisms that include:

- Inhibiting the release of acetylcholine by action at cholinergic nerve presynaptic beta-2 receptors[12]
- Preventing the release of inflammatory mediator from human lung mast cells[13]

Although many of these medications are receptor specific, at high doses their specificity may be decreased, resulting in crossover reactions. For example, high doses of albuterol may cross react with beta-1 receptors to cause tachycardia.

Beta-2 Agonists Drug Examples

Short-acting beta agonists (SABAs): albuterol and fenoterol[4]

Long-acting beta agonists (LABAs): salmeterol and formoterol[3,4]

Combined Agonist Drug Examples

Short-acting combined agonist: epinephrine

Acting on both alpha- and beta-adrenergic receptors, epinephrine is a potent bronchodilator and is utilized in both inhaled and intravenous (IV) forms as means to reverse severe bronchoconstriction, often from allergy type-mediated reactions.

Anticholinergics

Anticholinergics act on cholinergic nerve signal transmission, including the parasympathetic nervous system, by blocking the binding of the neurotransmitter acetylcholine to its receptors.[14]

Bronchoconstriction Mechanism

In the smooth muscle cells of the bronchi and bronchioles, increases in cytoplasmic Ca^{2+} results in contraction of the muscle cells leading to bronchoconstriction.[14]

Postganglionic parasympathetic neurons release acetylcholine → activate smooth muscle cell muscarinic M_3 receptors → activate a Gq class protein → up-regulate the phospholipase C pathway → release inositol trisphosphate (IP3) into cellular cytoplasm[14,15] → IP3 molecules bind to sarcoplasmic reticulum Ins3P receptors on a Ca^{2+} channel → sarcoplasmic reticulum release of Ca^{2+} → increase concentration of cytoplasmic Ca^{2+} → increase in contractile interaction of actin and myosin → bronchoconstriction.[15,16]

Anticholinergics Effects

Muscarinic anticholinergics will bind to the muscarinic M3 receptors, which reduces the binding of acetylcholine to the same M3 receptors. The reduced binding allows natural cellular pathways to reduce the concentration of cytoplasmic Ca^{2+}, resulting in bronchodilation.[14]

These medications can act systemically, especially if given via the IV or intramuscular (IM) route and may produce other anticholinergic side effects such as tachycardia, dry mouth, and confusion if the medication crosses the blood–brain barrier (e.g., atropine).

Anticholinergics Drug Examples

Short-acting anticholinergic medications: Ipratropium and oxitropium[7]

Long-acting anticholinergic drugs also known as long-acting muscarinic agents (LAMAs): Tiotropium[4]

Anti-Inflammatory Medications

The following classes of anti-inflammatory medications have been shown to be effective treatments in controlling asthma symptoms and attacks:[17,18]

- Corticosteroids
- Leukotriene modifiers
- Mast cell stabilizers
- Immunoglobulin E (IgE) blockers
- Phosphodiesterase-4 inhibitors

Corticosteroid Effects

Corticosteroids, specifically glucocorticosteroids, work in responsive cells by activating glucocorticoid receptors to directly and indirectly regulate the transcription of target genes.[19]

Glucocorticosteroids can increase the levels of anti-inflammatory proteins.

- Glucocorticoid receptor dimers bind to DNA at sites in the promoter region of steroid-responsive anti-inflammatory genes, usually increasing transcription with resulting increase in anti-inflammatory protein synthesis.

Glucocorticosteroids inhibit gene transcription of inflammatory mediator proteins. Many of the genes for inflammatory mediator proteins are up-regulated in asthmatic airways by transcription factors like nuclear factor-kappaB (NF-kappaB).

Corticosteroids and beta-2 agonists can also have mutually synergistic effects.

- Corticosteroids → increase the transcription of the beta-2 receptor gene → restoring G-protein/beta-2 receptor coupling → inhibiting beta-2 receptor down-regulation.[20]
- Beta-2 agonists → increase the nuclear translocation of glucocorticoid receptors → enhancing the suppression of the transcription of inflammatory genes.[21]

Corticosteroid Drug Examples

Inhaled glucocorticosteroids: Budesonide and fluticasone[4]
Oral systemic corticosteroids: Prednisone and methylprednisolone[3,4]

Leukotriene Modifier Effects

Leukotrienes, a family of eicosanoid inflammatory mediators, are synthesized in a number of different immune system cells, including eosinophils, leukocytes, and mast cells.[22]

- Leukotrienes activate G protein-coupled receptors found in structural cells including glandular epithelium, smooth muscle cells, and in inflammatory cells like basophils, eosinophils, and neutrophils.[23]
- Cysteinyl leukotrienes primary effect is through their binding to cysteinyl leukotriene receptor 1 (CysLTR1). CysLTR1 activation causes: airway

bronchoconstriction, edema, influx of eosinophils and neutrophils, smooth muscle proliferation, mucin secretion by goblet cells, and respiratory epithelial cell hypertrophy.

Leukotriene modifier drugs (or antileukotrienes) function either as:

- 5-lipoxygenase pathway inhibitors – inhibiting the formation of both cysLTs and LTB4
- Cysteinyl leukotriene receptor CysLTR1 antagonists, blocking the actions of cysLTs on target cells like bronchial smooth muscle cells[23]

Leukotriene Drug Examples

Oral leukotriene receptor antagonists (LTRAs): Montelukast and zafirlukast[3]
Oral 5-lipoxygenase inhibitor: Zileuton[3]

Mast Cell Stabilizer Effects

The degranulation of mast cells and eosinophils release potent inflammatory mediators including histamine and leukotrienes.[24] Mast cell stabilizers work by stabilizing the plasma membranes of eosinophils and mast cells through the blocking of a calcium channel essential for cell degranulation. The blockade prevents the release of inflammatory mediators from the cell granules.[24]

Mast Cell Stabilizer Drug Example

Mass cell stabilizer nebulizer: Cromolyn[3]

Immunoglobulin E (IgE) Blocker Effects

Immunoglobulin E antibodies can increase the levels of an individual's proinflammatory mediator proteins:

1. Production of allergen-specific immunoglobulin E (IgE) antibodies is triggered by an atopic person's initial exposure to the allergen.[25]
2. These IgE molecules can then become attached to inflammatory cells including basophils, macrophages, and especially mast cells, through its Fc portion linking with the cell Fc receptors.
3. Release of proinflammatory mediators, including histamine, leukotrienes, and cytokines, is triggered by subsequent allergen exposure where cross-bridging between IgE on the inflammatory cells' surface and the allergen provokes cell degranulation.[25,26]

IgE blockers work by blocking the binding of IgE to an inflammatory cell's Fc receptors by binding to the IgE molecules Fc portion themselves. This prevents IgE from attaching to inflammatory cells and being able to cause a cell's degranulation when exposed to allergens.[25]

IgE Blockers Drug Example

Immunomodulators subcutaneous injection: Omalizumab[3]

Phosphodiesterase-4 Inhibitor Effects

Phosphodiesterase-4 inhibitors (PDE4 inhibitor) block the degradative action of PDE4 on cyclic adenosine monophosphate (cAMP).[27]

1. Phosphodiesterase occurs in many areas of the body; however, the PDE4 family is found in immune cells primarily.[27]

2. The increase in cAMP activity is responsible for anti-inflammatory effects.[28]

3. NOT bronchodilators, commonly used to treat chronic obstructive pulmonary disease to reduce exacerbation rate

Phosphodiesterase-4 Inhibitor Example

PDE-4 Inhibitor tablet: Roflumilast[27]

References

1. CDC/National Center for Health Statistics. Asthma. 2017. Available at: www.cdc.gov/nchs/fastats/asthma.htm (accessed February 28, 2017).

2. National Center for Chronic Disease Prevention and Health Promotion, Division of Population Health. Chronic obstructive pulmonary disease (COPD). 2016. Available at: www.cdc.gov/copd/index.html (accessed February 28, 2017).

3. National Heart, Lung, and Blood Institute, National Institutes of Health. Asthma Care Quick Reference. Guidelines from the National Asthma Education and Prevention Program. Expert Panel Report 2. 2012. Available at: www.nhlbi.nih.gov/files/docs/guidelines/asthma_qrg.pdf (accessed February 27, 2017).

4. Rabe KF, Hurd S, Anzueto A, et al. Global strategy for the diagnosis, management, and prevention of chronic obstructive pulmonary disease: GOLD executive summary. *Am J Respir Crit Care Med* 2007;**176**(6):532–555.

5. Ram FS, Sestini P. Regular inhaled short acting beta2 agonists for the management of stable chronic obstructive pulmonary disease: Cochrane systematic review and meta-analysis. *Thorax* 2003;**58**(7):580–584.

6. Buhl R, Maltais F, Abrahams R, et al. Tiotropium and olodaterol fixed-dose combination versus mono-components in COPD (GOLD 2-4). *Eur Respir J* 2015;**45**(4):969–979.

7. Cooper CB, Tashkin DP. Recent developments in inhaled therapy in stable chronic obstructive pulmonary disease. *BMJ* 2005;**330**(7492):640–644.

8. Pfitzer G. Invited review: regulation of myosin phosphorylation in smooth muscle. *J Appl Physiol (1985)* 2001;**91**(1):497–503.

9. Bai Y, Sanderson MJ. Airway smooth muscle relaxation results from a reduction in the frequency of Ca2+ oscillations induced by a cAMP-mediated inhibition of the IP3 receptor. *Respir Res* 2006;7:34.

10. Perez-Zoghbi JF, Karner C, Ito S, et al. Ion channel regulation of intracellular calcium and airway smooth muscle function. *Pulm Pharmacol Ther* 2009;**22**(5):388–397.

11. Delmotte P, Sanderson MJ. Effects of albuterol isomers on the contraction and Ca2+ signaling of small airways in mouse lung slices. *Am J Respir Cell Mol Biol* 2008;**38**(5):524–531.

12. Rhoden KJ, Meldrum LA, Barnes PJ. Inhibition of cholinergic neurotransmission in human airways by beta 2-adrenoceptors. *J Appl Physiol (1985)* 1988;**65**(2):700–705.

13. Scola AM, Loxham M, Charlton SJ, Peachell PT. The long-acting beta-adrenoceptor agonist, indacaterol, inhibits IgE-dependent responses of human lung mast cells. *Br J Pharmacol* 2009;**158**(1):267–276.

14. Gosens R, Zaagsma J, Meurs H, Halayko AJ. Muscarinic receptor signaling in the pathophysiology of asthma and COPD. *Respir Res* 2006;7:73.

15. Penn RB, Benovic JL. Regulation of heterotrimeric G protein signaling in airway smooth muscle. *Proc Am Thorac Soc* 2008;**5**(1):47–57.

16. Jude JA, Wylam ME, Walseth TF, Kannan MS. Calcium signaling in airway smooth muscle. *Proc Am Thorac Soc* 2008;**5**(1):15–22.

17. Barnes PJ, Chung KF, Page CP. Inflammatory mediators of asthma: an update. *Pharmacol Rev* 1998;**50**(4):515–596.

18. Busse WW, Lemanske RFJ. Asthma. *N Engl J Med* 2001;**344**(5):350–362.

19. Barnes PJ. How corticosteroids control inflammation: Quintiles Prize Lecture 2005. *Br J Pharmacol* 2006;**148**(3):245–254.

20. Mak JC, Hisada T, Salmon M, Barnes PJ, Chung KF. Glucocorticoids reverse IL-1beta-induced impairment of beta-adrenoceptor-mediated relaxation and up-regulation of G-protein-coupled receptor kinases. *Br J Pharmacol* 2002;**135**(4):987–996.

21. Eickelberg O, Roth M, Lorx R, et al. Ligand-independent activation of the glucocorticoid receptor by beta2-adrenergic receptor agonists in primary human lung fibroblasts and vascular smooth muscle cells. *J Biol Chem* 1999;**274**(2):1005–1010.

22. Radmark O, Werz O, Steinhilber D, Samuelsson B. 5-Lipoxygenase: regulation of expression and enzyme activity. *Trends Biochem Sci* 2007;**32**(7):332–341.

23. Peters-Golden M, Henderson WR Jr. Leukotrienes. *N Engl J Med* 2007;**357**(18):1841–1854.

24. Finn DF, Walsh JJ. Twenty-first century mast cell stabilizers. *Br J Pharmacol* 2013;**170**(1):23–37.

25. Gould HJ, Sutton BJ, Beavil AJ, et al. The biology of IGE and the basis of allergic disease. *Annu Rev Immunol* 2003;**21**:579–628.

26. Fahy JV, Fleming HE, Wong HH, et al. The effect of an anti-IgE monoclonal antibody on the early- and late-phase responses to allergen inhalation in asthmatic subjects. *Am J Respir Crit Care Med* 1997;**155**(6):1828–1834.

27. Parikh N, Chakraborti A. Phosphodiesterase 4 (PDE4) inhibitors in the treatment of COPD: promising drug candidates and future directions. *Curr Med Chem* 2016;**23**(2):129–141.

28. Li H, Zuo J, Tang W. Phosphodiesterase-4 inhibitors for the treatment of inflammatory diseases. *Front Pharmacol* 2018;**9**:1048.

Cardiovascular Physiology

Jessica Brodt and Kaitlin Flannery

Cardiac Cycle

The cardiac cycle consists of a series of electrical and mechanical (valvular and pressure) events during one cycle of contraction (systole) and relaxation (diastole).

Wiggers diagram (Figure 30.1) displays synchronicity between electrical, mechanical, valvular, and pressure events of the cardiac cycle and corresponding heart sounds.

Electrical Events

Impulse propagation: SA node (cardiac pacemaker) → Atrial internodal tracts → AV node → Bundle of His → Bundle branches → Purkinje fibers[1]

The cartilaginous skeleton of the heart electrically isolates the atria from the ventricles. Electrical conduction must move through the AV node, unless accessory pathways exist.[2]

Two distinct action potentials occur within the cells of the heart. Fast action potentials within the myocytes and slow action potentials within the SA and AV nodes. The action potentials are divided into phases outlined below. Knowledge of the action potential phases facilitates understanding the mechanism of action of anti-arrhythmic medications.[2]

Fast Action Potential

Phase 0: Fast inward flow of Na^+ ions causing depolarization

Phase 1: Slight repolarization from outward flow of K^+ ions

Phase 2: Plateau to maintain contraction caused by inward flow of Ca^{2+} ions via L-type (slow) channels

Phase 3: Repolarization to resting potential from outward flow of K^+ ions

Phase 4: Resting potential

Slow Action Potential

This action potential excludes phases 1 and 2. The rate of depolarization in phase 4 sets the heart rate.

Phase 0: Inward flow of Ca^+ ions causing depolarization

Phase 3: Repolarization from outward flow of K^+ ions

Phase 4: Inward flow of Na^+ ions causing spontaneous depolarization

The autonomic nervous system moderates heart rate by controlling the rate of depolarization of the SA node. Acetylcholine

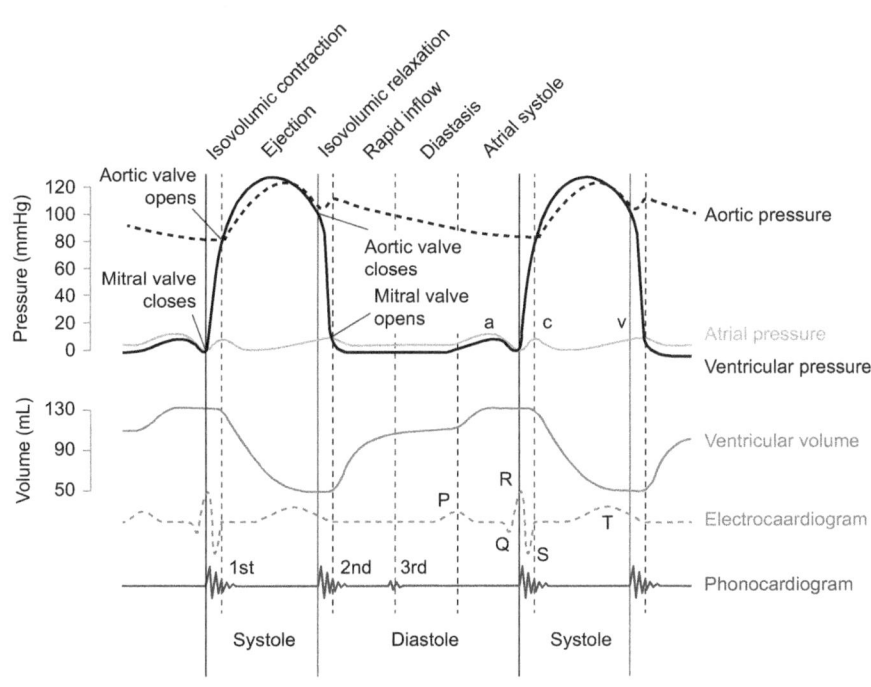

Figure 30.1 Wiggers diagram. Cardiac cycle demonstrating electrical, mechanical, valve, pressure, and heart sound synchronicity during systolic and diastolic events. A black and white version of this figure will appear in some formats. For the color version, please refer to the plate section.
From https://en.wikipedia.org/wiki/Wiggers_diagram

binding to muscarinic receptors on the SA node causes outward flow of K^+ ions, hyperpolarizing the cell and slowing the heart rate. The sympathetic nervous system increases heart rate through release of epinephrine and norepinephrine.[2]

Intrinsic rates (in beats per minute): SA node 60–100, AV node 40–60, bundle of His 40, and Purkinje fiber 15–20

Systole: Isovolumetric contraction is electrically identified by QRS complex. Bundle branch conduction slows electrical conduction and widens the QRS complex. Systolic ejection phases are identified as ST segment period.

Diastole: Isovolumetric relaxation is electrically identified by T wave. Diastole is complete at conclusion of atrial systole marked by P wave.

Mechanical Events

Ventricular systole and diastole can be represented by an LV pressure–volume loop (Figure 30.2) displaying four mechanical phases of the cardiac cycle: ventricular filling, isovolumic contraction, ventricular ejection, and isovolumic relaxation.[2]

Systole technically consists of three phases: *isovolumetric contraction*, *rapid ejection*, and *slower ejection phases*.

Isovolumetric contraction is the time between mitral valve closure (responsible for S_1 heart sound, c wave on venous waveform) and aortic valve opening during which LV volume remains constant.

LV ejection occurs when ventricular pressure exceeds aortic pressure, the aortic valve opens, and blood is ejected. Systole ends when ventricular pressure falls below aortic pressure leading to closure of the aortic valve (S_2 heart sound). During inspiration, increased venous return and prolonged RV ejection may cause physiological splitting of S_2 due to the aortic valve closing slightly before the pulmonic valve.

Diastole technically consists of four phases: *isovolumetric relaxation*, *early (rapid) filling*, *diastasis*, and *atrial systole*.

Isovolumetric relaxation is the time between aortic valve closure and mitral valve opening during which LV volume remains constant. This is an active process that requires energy and is marked by the v wave on the venous waveform.

Early or rapid filling phase occurs when ventricular pressure falls below atrial pressure, the mitral valve opens, and blood enters the ventricle (y descent of venous waveform). Diastasis (slower ventricular filling) and atrial systole (a wave on CVP waveform) complete ventricular diastole (Figure 30.3).

Early filling provides 70–75% of end diastolic volume, diastasis 3–5%, and atrial systole 15–25%. Loss of the "atrial kick" due to loss of sinus rhythm significantly decreases the end diastolic volume and may reduce stroke volume and cardiac output.[3,4]

Ventricular Function[4]

CO: Cardiac output

SV: Stroke volume

HR: Heart rate

SVR: Systemic vascular resistance

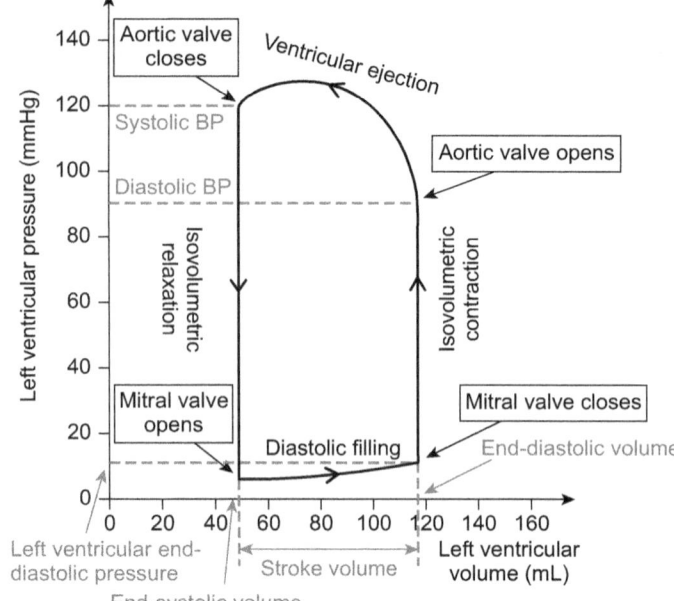

Figure 30.2 Stylized LV pressure–volume loop demonstrating a normal ventricle through four phases: isovolumetric contraction (no change in volume, increase in pressure), ventricular ejection, isovolumetric relaxation (no change in volume, decrease in pressure), ventricular diastole. A black and white version of this figure will appear in some formats. For the color version, please refer to the plate section.
From Chambers D, Huang C, Matthews G. Cardiac pressure–volume loops. In *Basic Physiology for Anaesthetists*. Cambridge University Press, 2019; pp 136–140. doi:10.1017/9781108565011.034.

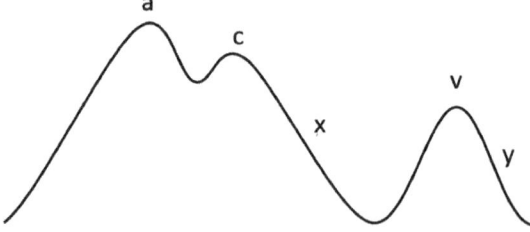

Figure 30.3 CVP waveform. Usually measured at SVC–RA junction. Consists of three peaks and two descents. a wave: atrial contraction; c wave: isovolumetric contraction causes tricuspid valve to bulge into RA and increase RA pressure; x descent: atrial relaxation; v wave: venous return and passive filling of RA; y descent: tricuspid valve opens and atria empties into the ventricle. Created by J. Brodt.

$CO = HR \times SV$

$SV = EDV - ESV$ (End diastolic volume – End systolic volume)

SV depends on preload (~ EDV), contractility and afterload (~ SVR)

SV is generally between 50 and 100 mL producing a CO of about 4–5 L/min

Preload: Determined by fluid status, intrathoracic pressure, venous return. End diastolic volume. Fixed restriction in mitral stenosis.

Frank–Starling mechanism = ↑ venous return → ↑ myocardial fiber stretching → ↑force of contraction → ↑ SV (Figure 30.4)

Contractility: Determined by actin–myosin cross-bridge coupling, increased mainly by raising intracellular calcium.

Afterload: Determined mostly by SVR and aortic pressure. Increases in afterload decrease SV.

Increased in hypertension, aortic stenosis or by α_1 agonists. Decreased in sepsis, neurogenic shock or by α antagonists.[2]

Fick Principle: This can be utilized to calculate cardiac output. Under steady states, the total uptake of a substance by the peripheral tissues is equal to the product of the blood flow to the peripheral tissues and the arterial–venous concentration gradient of the substance.[2] Oxygen is used as the substance in typical calculations. Inaccurate in patients with altered metabolic requirements (e.g., hypothermia, sepsis, burns, shock states), morbidly obese, or with increased pulmonary consumption (e.g., pneumonia).

$$CO = VO_2 / CaO_2 - CvO_2$$

VO_2 = Oxygen consumption (difficult to directly measure, in practice an assumed value from nomogram based on age and body surface area, for example, 250 mL/min

CaO_2 = LV oxygen content = $1.36 \times Hb \times SaO_2$

CvO_2 = PA (mixed venous) oxygen content = $1.36 \times Hb \times SvO_2$

Myocardial Oxygen Supply and Demand

Coronary perfusion pressure (CPP) = diastolic blood pressure − LV end diastolic pressure (LVEDP)

LV myocardium is predominantly perfused during diastole. The RV is perfused during both diastole and systole (Table 30.1).

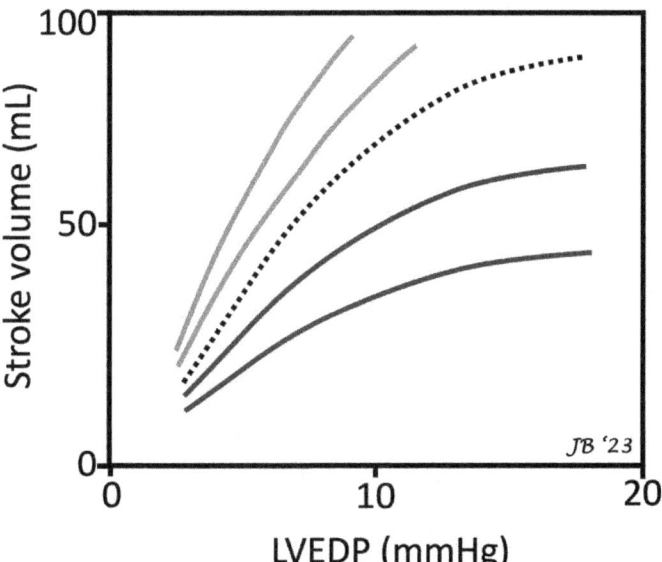

Figure 30.4 Frank–Starling curve. Relationship between LV filling, pressure, and stroke volume illustrated by family of curves. Black dotted curve represents "normal" curve where increased stroke volume is proportional to increasing LVEDP. Green curves depict hearts with reduced afterload and/or increased inotropy. Red curves depict hearts with increased afterload and/or reduced inotropy.
Created by J. Brodt. A black and white version of this figure will appear in some formats. For the color version, please refer to the plate section.

Changes in heart rate have the largest effect on the balance of myocardial oxygen supply and demand as it affects both.

LaPlace's law:[2,3]

$$\sigma \propto \frac{P.r}{h}$$

(σ, wall stress; P, ventricular pressure; r, ventricular radius; h, wall thickness)

Aortic regurgitation leads to LV dilation (increasing radius) and therefore increases wall stress and oxygen demand. LV remodeling with dilated results, increasing end diastolic volume and stroke volume.

Aortic stenosis leads to increased ventricular pressure and therefore increases wall stress and oxygen demand. LV remodeling with hypertrophy results, increasing the wall thickness and decreasing wall stress.

Venous Return[3]

The flow of blood back to the heart. As the cardiovascular system is a closed loop, venous return equals cardiac output, so decreases in venous return will decrease CO and increases in venous return will increase CO.

$$V_R = P_V - P_{RA} / R_V$$

V_R = Venous return

P_V = Venous pressure

- Increased by exhalation during spontaneous ventilation, limb muscle contractions, increased blood volume, sympathetic activation
- Decreased by positive pressure ventilation

P_{RA} = Right atrial pressure (CVP)

- Increased by CHF, pulmonary HTN, positive pressure ventilation
- Decreased with inspiration during spontaneous ventilation

R_V = Venous vascular resistance

- Increased by Valsalva maneuver, pregnancy

Pressures and Blood Flow

Systolic blood pressure (SBP) is the maximum pressure in the arteries during ventricular contraction. Diastolic blood pressure (DBP) is the minimum pressure in the arteries and occurs during ventricular relaxation and filling.

Table 30.1 Myocardial oxygen supply and demand

Determinants of supply	Determinants of demand
Heart rate (slower = more time in diastole)	Heart rate
CPP (higher = more supply)	Contractility
Oxygen content (myocardium extracts 70–80% of oxygen)	Wall stress (further explained with LaPlace's law)
Coronary vessel diameter	

The mean arterial pressure (MAP) is the primary pressure to evaluate delivery of blood to tissues and organs ("end organ perfusion").

$$MAP = 2/3\ DBP + 1/3\ SBP = CO \times SVR$$

A MAP > 60 mmHg is generally considered necessary to adequately perfusion end organs in adults. However, evaluation of the equation will show situations where this may not be true. For example, in cardiogenic shock a patient may have a low CO and a high SVR, resulting in a normal MAP but inadequate end organ perfusion.

Pressure Calculations

Pulse Pressure (PP) = SBP – DBP

SVR = (MAP – CVP) * 80/CO Normal = 800 – 1,200 dynes/sec/cm^5

PVR = (MPAP – PCWP) * 80/CO Normal = 60 – 200 dynes/sec/cm^5 (Table 30.2)

Poiseuille's law shows that blood flow (Q) is determined by the pressure gradient (ΔP) and resistance (R) in the vessel. Resistance is determined by three primary factors: vessel length (L), fluid viscosity (n), and vessel radius.

$$Q = \Delta P/P \qquad\qquad Q = \Delta P * \pi r^4/8nL$$

As radius is to the fourth power, it has the most effect on flow. Putting this into the clinical context, IV fluids will run faster if the catheter radius is larger, catheter length is shorter, the pressure gradient is higher (raising the IV pole), and the viscosity of the fluid is lower (crystalloid vs. colloid solution).

Cardiac Reflexes

The carotid sinus and aortic arch baroreceptors are mechanoreceptors that control acute changes in blood pressure through negative feedback reflexes. Afferent signals travel via Hering's (branch of glossopharyngeal) and vagus nerves to the nucleus tractus solitaries with efferent signal through the vagus nerve. When pressure increases, the baroreceptors are stretched, resulting in increased afferent signals. The efferent effect is decreased heart rate and vasodilation to reduce blood pressure.[4]

The atrial stretch reflex (Bainbridge reflex) is mediated by baroreceptors in the wall of the right atrium. Stretching of

Table 30.2 Normal pressures in mmHg

CVP	0–8
RAP	0–8
RVDP	0–8
RVSP	15–25
PAP systolic	15–25
PAP diastolic	8–15
PAP mean	10–20
PCWP	6–14
MAP	65–90

these baroreceptors from increased venous return results in increases in heart rate. This reflex causes sinus arrythmias. Heart rate increases during inspiration when venous return to the heart increases and decreases during expiration.[4]

The Bezold–Jarisch reflex is mediated by both chemoreceptors and mechanoreceptors in the left ventricle. Noxious stimuli conducted via the vagus nerve result in bradycardia, hypotension, and coronary vasodilation. This reflex may be a protective mechanism in coronary ischemia, as the bradycardia will decrease myocardial oxygen demand and coronary vasodilation will increase supply. Clinically, neuraxial anesthesia can elicit this reflex, which may result in circulatory collapse.[5]

Microcirculation

The microcirculation consists of arterioles, capillaries, and venules and is where oxygen, carbon dioxide, nutrients, and waste are exchanged. Fluid movement across the capillary membrane is driven by the Starling pressures described by the following equation:

Fluid movement = $K_f (P_c - P_i) - (\pi_c - \pi_i)$

P_c is the capillary hydrostatic pressure (increases with heart failure, venous constriction, arteriolar dilation).

P_i is the interstitial hydrostatic pressure

π_c is the capillary oncotic pressure (decreases with nephrotic syndrome, liver failure, malnutrition).

π_i is the interstitial oncotic pressure.

K_f is the filtration coefficient (increases with burns, inflammation).

Blood flow through capillaries is controlled by oxygen and nitric oxide (NO). Nitric oxide is released by endothelial cells, causing vasodilation and increasing oxygen delivery. Increased oxygen in the microcirculation causes vasoconstriction,[3] which may be a protective mechanism against oxidative stress.

The Fahraeus–Lindqvist effect occurs in small vessels (< 0.3 mm) where RBCs move to the middle of the vessel and a cell-free plasma layer forms at the vessel walls.[6] This leads to decrease blood viscosity and increased blood flow.

Mixed Venous Oxygen Saturation

Mixed venous oxygen saturation (SvO$_2$) measures the oxygen saturation of blood returning to the heart from the systemic circulation. S_vO_2 is measured by sampling blood from the pulmonary artery, allowing mixing of blood returning from the superior vena cava, inferior vena cava, and coronary sinus. It is used as a surrogate to interpret oxygen consumption and delivery. Measurement of blood from a central line in the SVC, central venous oxygen saturation ($S_{cv}O_2$), may be used as an alternative, less invasive option.[4]

$$SvO_2 = SaO_2 - [(VO_2)/(Hb \times 1.36 \times CO)]$$

VO$_2$: Oxygen consumption

SvO_2: Venous oxygen saturation

SaO_2: Arterial oxygen saturation

Normal S_vO_2 is 70% with a range of 60–80%.

High SvO_2
- *Increased oxygen delivery*: Increased inspired oxygen, hyperbaric oxygen, high flow states like hyperthyroidism
- *Decreased oxygen consumption*: Hypothermia, anesthesia

Low SvO_2
- *Decreased oxygen delivery*: Anemia, decreased oxygen supply, low flow state like heart failure
- *Increased oxygen consumption*: Sepsis, hyperthermia, shivering, pain, seizures

Regional Blood Flow and Regulation

Blood flow to an organ is regulated by arteriolar resistance via either local control (intrinsic) or neural control (extrinsic). Below are unique features of blood flow to different organs.[3]

Coronary: 5% of CO

Blood flow is regulated locally by adenosine and hypoxia. Extraction of oxygen from myocytes is 75–80% at baseline, so increases in oxygen delivery must come from increased flow.

Cerebral: 15% of CO

Cerebral autoregulation maintains steady cerebral blood flow between MAPs from 60 to 150 mmHg. Changes in CO_2 can inhibit autoregulation. CO_2 is a vasodilator.

Pulmonary: 100% of CO travels to the lungs from the right heart

Blood flow is regulated by the partial pressure of O_2 in alveolar gas. Hypoxic pulmonary vasoconstriction shunts blood away from poorly ventilated areas towards well-ventilated areas.

Renal: 25% of CO

Blood flow is autoregulated via a combination of the myogenic regulation of afferent arterioles (increased pressure on stretch receptors in renal afferents results in vasoconstriction of afferents to decrease blood flow) and tubuloglomerular feedback (decreased chloride filtration monitored by chemoreceptors results increased blood flow).

Hepatic: 25% of CO

There are two sources of blood flow to the liver: the portal vein and the hepatic artery. Each contributes about half of the oxygen utilized by the liver. Portal blood flow is determined by pressure gradients. Hepatic artery flow is regulated by adenosine. Decreased in hepatic blood flow leads to accumulation of adenosine, which causes hepatic artery dilation.

Skeletal Muscle

Blood flow is regulated both by local metabolites and sympathetic nervous system. At rest, blood flow is regulated primarily by sympathetic innervation. During exercise, blood flow is increased due to metabolites like lactate, adenosine, and potassium.

Uterine: Not pregnant, 2% of CO; term pregnancy, 10% of CO

No significant autoregulation. Blood flow is directly related to arterial pressure and inversely related to uterine vascular resistance.[7]

Hormonal Control

Renin–Angiotensin–Aldosterone System: Regulates both *blood pressure and volume.*

Low arterial pressure and blood volume causes the release of renin from the kidneys. Renin catalyzes the conversion of angiotensinogen to angiotensin I. Angiotensin I is then converted to angiotensin II by angiotensin-converting enzyme (ACE), primarily in the lungs.

Angiotensin II: Regulates *blood pressure and volume.*
- Increases SVR by arteriolar vasoconstriction via AT1 receptors.
- Decreases sodium excretion by increasing sodium reabsorption by proximal tubules of the kidney.
- Releases aldosterone from the adrenal cortex.
- Releases AVP from the posterior pituitary gland.
- Augments norepinephrine (NE) release from sympathetic nerves and sensitizes vascular smooth muscle to NE.

Arginine Vasopressin (AVP): Regulates *blood pressure and volume.*

AVP is released by the posterior pituitary gland controlled by the hypothalamus. It is released in response to increased plasma osmolality or stress. It acts on renal collecting ducts via V2 receptors to increase water reabsorption, and via V1 receptors on vascular smooth muscle to cause vasoconstriction.

Atrial Natriuretic Peptide (ANP): Regulates *blood volume.*

ANP is stored in the atrial muscle cells and released into the bloodstream when the atria are stretched. By increasing sodium excretion, it decreases blood volume. It also inhibits release of renin, aldosterone, and AVP.

Erythropoietin: Regulates *blood volume (and red blood cell mass).*

Erythropoietin is a released by the kidneys in response to hypoxia and reduced hematocrit. It causes bone marrow to increase production of red blood cells, raising the total mass of circulating red blood cells.

References

1. Crystal GJ, Assaad SI, Heerdt PM. Cardiovascular physiology: integrative function. In Hemmings HC, Egan TD, editors. *Pharmacology and Physiology for Anesthesia*, 2nd ed. Elsevier, 2019; chapter 24.

2. Pagel P, Freed J. Cardiac physiology. In Kaplan JA, Augoustides JGT, Manecke GR, Maus T, Reich DL, editors. *Kaplan's Cardiac Anesthesia*, 7th ed. Elsevier, 2017; pp 143–178.

3. Costanzo LS. Cardiovascular physiology. In *Physiology*, 4th ed. Saunders Elsevier, 2010; chapter 4.

4. Cardiovascular physiology & anesthesia. In Butterworth JF IV,

Mackey DC, Wasnick JD. editors. *Morgan & Mikhail's Clinical Anesthsiology*, 7th ed. McGraw-Hill, 2022; chapter 20.

5. Warltier DC, Campagna JA, Carter C. Clinical relevance of the Bezold-Jarisch reflex. *Anesthesiology* 2003;**98**:1250–1260.

6. Ascolese M, Farina A, Fasano A. The Fahraeus-Lindqvist effect in small blood vessels: how does it help the heart? *J Biol Phys* 2019;**45**(4):379–394.

7. Page SM, Rollins MD. Physiology and pharmacology of obstetric anesthesia. In Hemmings HC, Egan TD, editors. *Pharmacology and Physiology for Anesthesia*, 2nd ed. Elsevier, 2019; chapter 37.

Chapter 31

Basics of Cardiopulmonary Resuscitation, Medications, Defibrillators, and Advanced Cardiac Life Support Algorithms

Ishu Kant and Paul Shekane

The initial assessment of an unresponsive patient, the sequence of events, CPR, medications, defibrillation, and post-resuscitative care will be described in this chapter. Unless stated otherwise, all the following recommendations apply to the adult patient.

The Initial Assessment

1. **Scene safety.** You cannot save someone if it is not safe for you or the other rescuers.
2. **Check responsiveness.** In less than 10 seconds, check for breathing and pulse. If the patient is unresponsive, not breathing, and no pulse is detected, proceed below.
3. **Activate the emergency response system.** Unlike the Out-of-hospital Cardiac Arrest (OHCA) chain of survival, the in-hospital cardiac arrest (IHCA) chain of survival includes surveillance and prevention, such as rapid response teams (RRT) and medical emergency teams (MET), which have been shown to be effective (Figure 31.1). The advance cardiac life support (ACLS) guidelines were updated in 2020 with an additional **recovery process** added to both adult and pediatric out-of-hospital and in-hospital chains of survival.[1]
   - If a mobile device is available, first phone emergency services (911).
   - If you are alone with no mobile phone, first activate the emergency response system and bring the AED prior to starting CPR.

   - If you have another rescuer, start CPR right away while they activate the emergency response system and fetch the AED.
     - Per 2020 guidelines, it is recommended that laypersons initiate CPR for presumed cardiac arrest because the risk of harm to the patient is low if the patient is not in cardiac arrest.[1]

Early Defibrillation for Shockable Rhythm[2]

- If cardiac arrest was *witnessed* and an AED is *immediately* available -> defibrillate now.
- If cardiac arrest was *unwitnessed* or an AED is *not immediately* available, in infants (< 1 year, excluding newborns) and children (1 year to puberty):
  - Give 2 minutes of CPR,
  - Then leave the victim to activate emergency response system and obtain an AED.
  - Then return to the child or infant and resume CPR, using the AED as soon as possible.
- Shock energy for defibrillation in cardiac arrest:
  - **Biphasic:** 120–200 J initial dose or maximum available.
  - **Monophasic:** Less common due to newer AEDs. 360 J
- Nonshockable rhythms:
  - Asystole
  - Pulseless electrical activity (PEA)

In-Hospital Cardiac Arrest Sequence

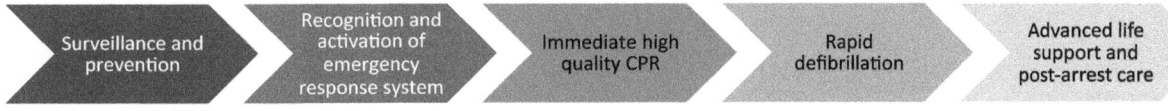

Out-of-Hospital Cardiac Arrest Sequence

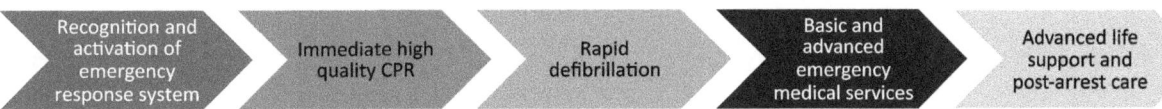

Figure 31.1 Difference between in-hospital and out-of-hospital cardiac arrest algorithm. Adapted from the ACLS *2020 Handbook of Emergency Cardiovascular Care for Healthcare Providers*. A black and white version of this figure will appear in some formats. For the color version, please refer to the plate section.[2]

- Shockable rhythms:
  - Ventricular fibrillation
  - Ventricular tachycardia
- Shock energy for unstable tachyarrhythmias without cardiac arrest:
  - 2020 guidelines suggest following the specific device's recommended energy level to maximize the success of the first shock.
- Synchronized cardioversion can range from 75 J to 150 J.
  - Wide QRS complex, irregular rhythm: defibrillation dose (not synchronized, see above)

CPR Sequence: C–A–B

- Prioritize Circulation over Airway and Breathing to avoid delays to first compression.
- Adult & Adolescent CPR:
- CPR *without* an advanced airway (endotracheal tube or supraglottic airway),[2] 1 or 2 rescuers → 30:2 compressions to breaths ratio.
- CPR *with* an advanced airway → 1 breath every 6 seconds (10 breaths/min), continuous compressions at 100–120/min
- Infant and Children CPR:
  - CPR *without* an advanced airway:
    - 1 rescuer → 30:2 compressions to breaths ratio
    - 2 or more rescuers → 15:2 compression to breaths ratio
  - CPR *with* an advanced airway → 1 breath every 2–3 seconds (20–30 breaths/min), continuous compressions at 100–120/min

High-Quality Chest Compressions

- Quickly move bulky clothes out of the way. If difficult to remove, you can still provide compressions over clothing.
- **Adequate rate:** 100–120 compressions/min
- **Adequate depth:**
  - In adults, at least 2 inches (5 cm) and no more than 2.4 inches (6 cm).
  - In children, at least 1/3 AP diameter of chest, approximately 2 inches (5 cm)
  - In infants, at least 1/3 AP diameter of chest, approximately 1.5 inches (4 cm)
- **Allow complete chest recoil after each compression:** Do not lean on the chest between compressions; allow the heart to refill.
- **Minimize interruptions:** Do not interrupt compressions for intubation, application of pads, and keep pulse checks less than 10 seconds. Maintain chest compression fraction of 80%.
- **Avoid excessive ventilation:** Avoid excessively forceful breaths.
- Rotate compressor every 2 minutes.
- Waveform capnography can be used with a bag-mask device
- $EtCO_2$ > 10 mmHg. Low $EtCO_2$ after 20 minutes of CPR is a poor prognostic sign.
- Diastolic pressure < 20 mmHg on intra-arterial pressure reflects inadequate compressions.
- Table 31.1 lists the summary of steps.

Medications

- Intravenous (IV) access is preferred, but an intraosseous (IO) access route may be considered if attempts at IV access are unsuccessful or not feasible.

Table 31.1 ACLS algorithm for the adult, pediatric, and infant patients

Recommendation	Adult patient	Pediatric patient	Infants (less than 1 year of age)
Witnessed cardiac arrest and *immediately* available AED	Defibrillate then initiate CPR		
Unwitnessed cardiac arrest or AED *not immediately* available … with 1 rescuer	1. Leave victim to activate emergency response system and obtain AED 2. Initiate CPR	1. Initiate 2 minutes of CPR 2. Leave victim to activate emergency response system, obtain AED 3. Return to victim, continue CPR, used AED as soon as it is available	
Unwitnessed cardiac arrest or AED *not immediately* available … with 2 or more rescuers	Initiate CPR while other rescuer activates emergency response system, obtains AED		
CPR *with* an advanced airway	1. Give 1 breath every 6 seconds 2. Continuous compressions at 100–120/min	1. Give 1 breath every 2–3 seconds 2. Continuous compressions at 100–120/min	
CPR *without* an advanced airway	30:2 compressions to breaths ratio	1 rescuer: 30:2 2 or more rescuers: 15:2	
CPR compression depth	At least 2 inches (5 cm)	At least 1/3 AP diameter About 2 inches (5 cm)	At least 1/3 AP diameter About 1½ inches (4 cm)

Adapted from the *2020 Handbook of Emergency Cardiovascular Care for Healthcare Providers*.[2]

- Epinephrine intravenously (IV) or intraosseous (IO) **1 mg** every 3 to 5 minutes or every 4 minutes as a midrange (every other 2-minute rhythm check)
  - Early epinephrine use is emphasized in nonshockable rhythms after starting CPR.
- For bradycardia:
  - Atropine dose changed to 1 mg with a maximum of 3 mg (previously 0.5 mg)
  - Dopamine dose changed to 5 to 20 mcg/kg/min (from 2 to 20 mcg/kg/min)
- Second-line agents amiodarone and lidocaine are equivalent for treatment. (Figure 31.2)

Tachyarrhythmias
- Algorithm:
  1. Hemodynamically stable or unstable?
  2. QRS wide or narrow?
  3. Irregular or regular ventricular rhythm
- Check a pulse.
  - No pulse → see PEA algorithm

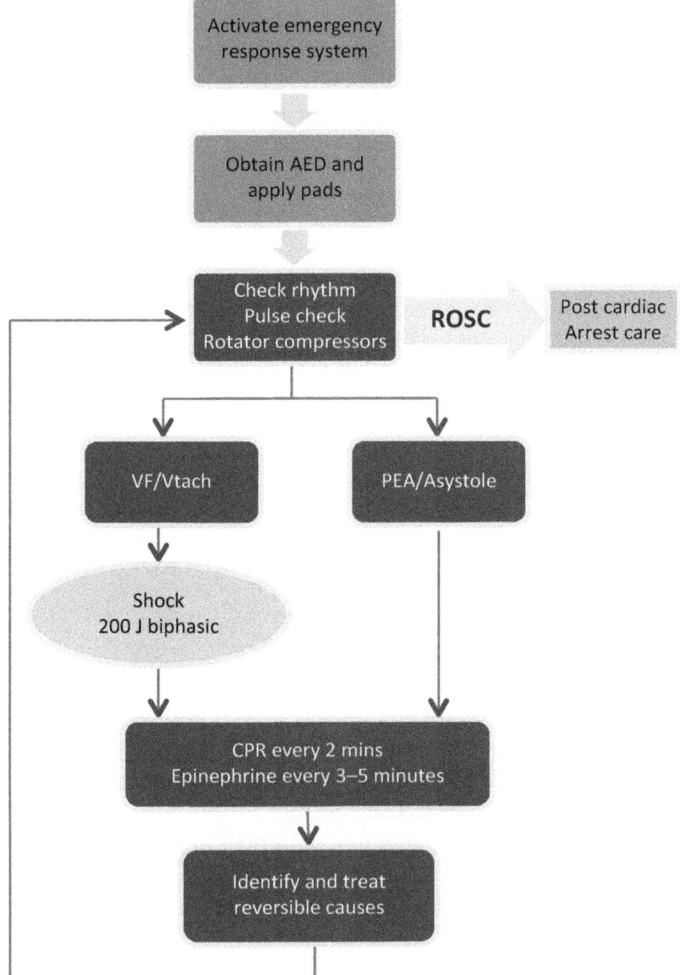

Figure 31.2 Cardiac arrest algorithm. Adapted from the *2020 Handbook of Emergency Cardiovascular Care for Healthcare Providers*. A black and white version of this figure will appear in some formats. For the color version, please refer to the plate section.[1,2]

- Pulse present:
  - Assessment using C–A–B
  - Provide oxygen
  - Hemodynamically unstable (hypotension, altered mental status, shock, acute heart failure) immediate synchronized cardioversion
  - Hemodynamically stable:
    - Establish IV access
    - 12-lead electrocardiogram (ECG)
    - Frequently check blood pressure, hemodynamic support
    - Seek expert consultation
    - Determine whether rhythm is narrow or wide, regular or irregular → see Table 31.2.

Unstable Ventricular Tachycardia and Ventricular Fibrillation
- Ventricular fibrillation (VF) is usually more resistant to shocks.
- For both, first-line treatment is to initiate CPR and give oxygen.
- Both VT and VF should be defibrillated as soon as possible with biphasic 120–200 J or monophasic 360 J.
- Maintain oxygen saturation greater than 92–98%,
- Ventricular tachycardia (VT) is divided in the following categories, each with different treatment implications:
  - **Monomorphic VT**
    - Both amiodarone and lidocaine can be used
  - **Polymorphic** VT, that is, Torsades de pointes
    - Associated with Wolff–Parkinson–White (WPW) syndrome, baseline prolongation of QT interval
    - Precipitated by electrolyte disturbances and drugs (i.e., tricyclic antidepressants, haloperidol, droperidol, type Ia antiarrhythmics)
    - Treatment: Shorten the QT interval. Magnesium, increasing heart rate with pacing or catecholamines, and for refractory rhythms, phenytoin and lidocaine
    - Note: Type Ia antiarrhythmics *prolong* the QT and are NOT helpful in Torsades de pointes

Asystole and PEA Arrest
- Start CPR and give oxygen.
- Attach monitor/defibrillator, but keep in mind that this is considered a "non-shockable" rhythm.
- Give epinephrine 1 mg every 4 minutes ASAP when IV or IO access established.
- Ventilate 1 breath every 6 seconds, maintaining oxygen saturation > 92–98%.
- Consider and address possible underlying cause(s): Hs & Ts
  - Sodium bicarbonate may be helpful in the setting of asystole caused by
    - Severe acidosis
    - Hyperkalemia
    - Tricyclic antidepressant overdose

Table 31.2 ACLS treatment algorithm for stable tachyarrhythmias[1]

QRS size	Rhythm regularity	Diagnosis	Treatment
Narrow (< 0.12 sec)	Regular	Sinus tachycardia Aflutter	– Vagal maneuvers – 6mg Adenosine IV push – If needed, follow with 12 mg adenosine – Address underlying cause such as pain, anxiety, and hypovolemia
Narrow	Irregular	Atrial fibrillation (AF) Atrial flutter (note: regular rhythm but similar treatment to Atrial fibrillation) Multi-focal atrial tachycardia	– Consider expert consultation – Consider beta-blockers, diltiazem – If becomes unstable, cardioversion
Wide	Regular	Ventricular tachycardia SVT with aberrancy	– Expert consultation – For ventricular tachycardia, consider amiodarone – Procainamide can be used until arrhythmia is suppressed – For SVT with aberrancy, consider adenosine 6mg
Wide	Irregular	Pre-excited atrial fibrillation Recurrent polymorphic VT Torsades de pointes	– Expert consultation – For pre-excited atrial fibrillation such as AF and WPW, avoid AV nodal blocking agents such as digoxin, diltiazem, verapamil

- Anesthesiologists must consider the context of PEA arrest, such as tension pneumothorax during a jet ventilation case, pericardial tamponade during a cardiac catheterization case, and so on.
- Phenytoin, lidocaine and procainamide may be useful in PEA arrest. Atropine is no longer part of the algorithm.

Reversible Causes: Treatment Options
- **Hs and Ts:**
  - Hypovolemia – volume infusion
  - Hypoxia – airway, oxygen delivery
  - Hydrogen ion (acidosis) – sodium bicarbonate
  - Hypokalemia – K replacement, Mg infusion
  - Hyperkalemia – Ca chloride, sodium bicarb
  - Hypothermia – targeted temperature management of 32–36°C
  - Tension pneumothorax – needle decompression
  - Tamponade, cardiac – pericardiocentesis
  - Toxins – antidotes, intubation
  - Thrombosis, pulmonary – embolectomy, fibrinolytic agent
  - Thrombosis, coronary – PCI, fibrinolytic agent

Unstable Bradyarrhythmias
- Causes:[3]
  - Hypoxemia
  - Vagal stimulation
  - Drug overdose (i.e., beta blocker, calcium channel blocker, cholinergic drugs, digitalis, propofol, dexmedetomidine)
  - Sinus or atrioventricular (AV) node ischemia
  - Increased intracranial pressure
- It is important to *first* assure adequate oxygenation and ventilation, then consider sympathomimetic or vagolytic drugs
- Treatment:
  - Narrow complex bradycardia from nodal failure or AV blocks → atropine (1 mg every 3 to 5 minutes, max of 3 mg)

- Atropine works by decreasing vagal tone and increasing heart rate, however, for infranodal conduction blocks, it may be ineffective and may increase the degree of block by increasing the atrial rate without increasing the ventricular rate
- For hemodynamically unstable patients and those with high degree of AV block (2nd degree type 2 to 3rd degree), initiate transthoracic pacing or transvenous pacing

Consider infusions of epinephrine 2–10 mcg/min or dopamine 5–20 mcg/kg/min while awaiting pacer or if pacer is ineffective

Postcardiac Arrest Care
- Once return of spontaneous circulation (ROSC) is achieved, an initial stabilization phase emphasizes early airway management via endotracheal tube. Obtain the following parameters:
  - Titrate FiO_2 to oxygen saturation 92–98%
  - Systolic BP > 90 mmHg or mean arterial pressure > 65 mmHg
  - Waveform capnography $PaCO_2$ 35–45 mmHg
  - New 12-lead ECG
- Awake patients should be transferred to critical care. If STEMI is present, transfer to emergency cardiac intervention.
- Emergency coronary angioplasty is recommended for patients with ST elevation, hemodynamically unstable or electrically unstable patients without ST elevation with a suspected cardiovascular lesion.
- All comatose adult patients with return of spontaneous circulation (ROSC) after VF arrest should have a targeted temperature management (TTM) target of 32–36°C maintained for at least 24 hours.
- Mild therapeutic hypothermia is beneficial for out-of-hospital VF arrest, but is unclear for out-of-hospital non-VF arrest and inpatient VF arrest. Additionally, hypothermia may exacerbate bradyarrhythmias.[4]

Other 2020 Updates to the ACLS *Guidelines*

- The medical contact-to-balloon inflation (percutaneous coronary intervention) goal is 90 minutes or less. It is recommended to bypass the emergency department if possible.
- For maternal cardiac arrest, if no ROSC is achieved in 5 minutes (instead of 4 min), consider perimortem cesarean delivery.
- For patients with suspected opioid overdose in respiratory arrest, give naloxone, and consider its administration for those in cardiac arrest.
- New stroke guidelines recommend endovascular therapy treatment window up to 24 hours (raised from previous 6 hours).
  - If indicated, both alteplase and endovascular therapy can be given/performed.
  - Suspected stroke patients may bypass the emergency department to go straight to the imaging suite for rapid initial assessment.
  - Oxygen saturation should be titrated to > 94%

Neonatal Resuscitation

- Neonatal cardiac arrest is mainly due to inadequate ventilation, so assessment of ventilation is key.
- Risk assessment:
  1. Term gestation?
  2. Good tone?
  3. Breathing or crying?
- The first minute of life, also known as the **Golden Minute**, continues to be important to assess the neonate and initiate resuscitative efforts.
  - Assess **Apgar score** (see Table 31.3):
    - Appearance (color)
    - Pulse (heart rate)
    - Grimace (reflex irritability to tactile stimulation)
    - Activity (muscle tone)
    - Respiration
- **Temperature.** Avoid hypothermia, provide warmth, and check temperature.
  - Skin-to-skin placement after birth can be effective in improving temperature control, breastfeeding, and blood glucose stability.
- **Oxygenation:**
  - Resuscitation of preterm infants less than 35 weeks should be with low oxygen (up to 30% FiO_2) and titrated to oxygen saturations
  - During CPR, use 100% FiO_2
- **Heart Rate**
  - Above 100 bpm and *no signs* of cyanosis, labored breathing →routine postnatal care
  - Above 100 bpm and signs of cyanosis, labored breathing → clear airway, monitor SpO_2, consider continuous positive airway pressure (CPAP)
  - Below 100 bpm → optimize ventilation as above, reassess

- Below 60 bpm →
  - Initiate chest compressions.
    - It is reasonable to give the initial dose of epinephrine within 5 minutes from the start of chest compressions.
  - Consider positive pressure ventilation (PPV) and intubation.
  - It is recommended that pediatric cardiac arrest survivors be evaluated for rehabilitation services.
- **Special situations:**
  - *Delayed cord clamping* for longer than 30 seconds is reasonable for healthy term neonates.
  - Meconium: In the presence of meconium-stained amniotic fluid:
    - . . . and a vigorous, pink infant → routine postnatal care and reassessment
    - . . . and poor muscle tone, inadequate breathing efforts → place the infant in a radiant warmer and begin PPV. Routine laryngoscopy with or without tracheal suctioning is not recommended.
    - However, for nonvigorous newborns who have evidence of airway obstruction during PPV, intubation and tracheal suction can be beneficial.
  - Single ventricle, pre- and postoperative Norwood/Blalock–Taussig shunt patients:
    - Lowering the systemic vascular resistance, via alpha-adrenergic antagonism and/or PDE III inhibitors, with or without oxygen use can be more useful to increase systemic oxygen delivery than addressing pulmonary vascular resistance.
    - Direct (SVC catheter) or indirect oxygen monitoring can be beneficial in management post-stage 1 Norwood palliative or shunt.
    - Use inhaled nitric oxide or prostacyclin as an initial therapy for pulmonary hypertensive crisis or secondary acute right-sided heart failure.

Table 31.3 Apgar score

Sign	0	1	2
Appearance	Blue or pale	Pink with blue extremities	Pink
Pulse	Absent	< 100/min	> 100/min
Grimace	None	Grimace only	Cry or active withdrawal
Activity	Limp	Some flexion	Active motion
Respiration	None	Weak cry, hypoventilation	Vigorous cry

Adapted from the ACLS *2020 Handbook of Emergency Cardiovascular Care for Healthcare Providers.*[2]

References

1. American Heart Association. Highlights of the 2020 American Heart Association – Guidelines Update for CPR and ECC. 2020. Available at: https://cpr.heart.org/-/media/cpr-files/cpr-guidelines-files/highlights/hghlghts_2020_ecc_guidelines_english.pdf (accessed October 15, 2022).

2. American Heart Association. *2020 Handbook of Emergency Cardiovascular Care for Healthcare Providers*. American Heart Association, 2020.

3. Marini JJ, Wheeler AP. *Critical Care Medicine: The Essentials*, 4th ed. Lippincott Williams & Wilkins, 2010; pp 361–375.

4. Oropello JM, Pastores SM, Kvetan V. *Critical Care*. McGraw-Hill Education, 2016.

Cardiovascular System: Anatomy

Claire Joseph and Diana Anca

Coronary Circulation

Coronary Arterial Circulation

Space between the aortic valve cusps and ascending aorta is referred to as aorta sinuses. The right and left aortic sinuses contain coronary ostia from which the right and left coronary arteries arise, respectively.

Left Coronary Artery (LCA) – Two Branches

- Left anterior descending (LAD) – along inter-ventricular groove and terminates at apex of left ventricle (LV) (also supplies apex of right ventricle [RV] and anterior wall of LV)
  1. Proximal LAD: From left coronary ostia to first diagonal branch.
  2. Mid LAD: From first diagonal branch to distal LAD
     Diagonal branches (supplies anterolateral heart)
     D1 = first diagonal branch of the LAD
     D2 = second diagonal branch of the LAD
  3. Distal LAD: Distal one-third of LAD
     Septal branches (supplies the anterior two-thirds of the inter-ventricular septum, bundle branches, and Purkinje system)
- Left circumflex (LCX) – along the left atrioventricular (AV) groove
  1. Obtuse marginal branches (supplies lateral LV)
     OM1 = first obtuse marginal branch of the circumflex,
     OM2 = second obtuse marginal branch of the circumflex,
  2. AVCx = AV branch of the circumflex artery
     15–25% terminate into the left PDA branch
     45% SA node blood supply from the LCX

Right coronary artery (RCA) – along the right AV groove and supplies the inferior and infero-septal walls of the LV

- Proximal RCA: Ostia until right anterior margin (RAM)
- Conus A
- SA Nodal A
- 55% SA node blood supply from the RCA
- Mid RCA: Proximal one-half segment between RAM until PDA take-off
- RAM – acute marginal branches to the anterior RV wall
- Distal RCA: distal one-half segment between RAM branch and PDA take-off.

PDA Supplies the posterior and inferior aspect of the LV and AV node (typically RCA)
AV nodal artery branch

Post LV = posterior left ventricular artery.

Supplies most of the anterior and posterior walls of RV, the RA, the upper one-half of atrial septum, the posterior one-third of the IV septum & inferior wall and posterior base of LV

Septum supplied by septal perforator branches from the RCA or the LAD.

Coronary CIRCULATION is right- or left-dominant → based on origin of PDA (RCA vs. LCX) Can be co-dominant with supply from both RCA & LCX

Papillary Muscle Blood Supply:

- Anterior papillary muscle: LCX (OM1) and LAD (D1)
- Posterior papillary muscle: RCA
  - Posterior papillary infarction/rupture more common after an MI 2/2 to single blood supply.

Anatomical Relationships between Coronary Vessels

Coronary sinus ↑↓ LCX

Great cardiac vein ↑↓ LAD and LCX

Middle cardiac vein ↑↓ PDA

Small cardiac vein ↑↓ RAM and RCA

Coronary Venous Circulation

There are two networks of myocardial venous drainage:

1. **Epicardial Coronary Veins** Distributed alongside major coronary arteries and drain into the RA via coronary sinus
   Exception – Anterior cardiac veins drain directly into RA.
2. **Thebesian Venous System** Direct venous drainage from endocardium into chambers of the heart.

Approximately 5–10% of venous drainage.

Coronary Lymphatic Drainage

Extensive lymphatic plexus in sub-endocardial connective tissue of all chambers of the heart

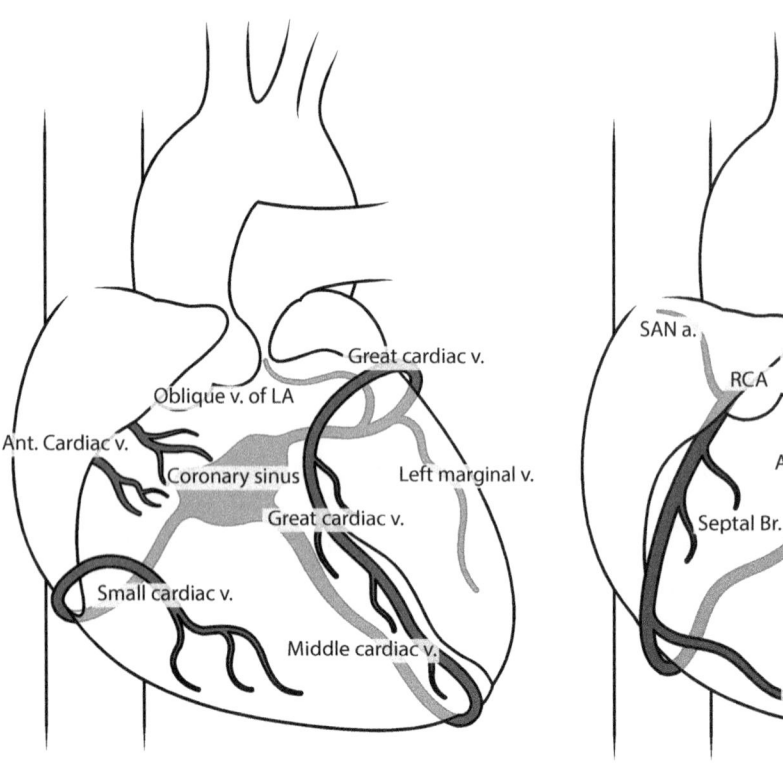

Figure 32.1 Cardiac arterial and venous circulation – anterior view.
ACx: atrial circumflex artery; AVN a.: atrioventricular nodal artery; DM1: first diagonal; D2: second diagonal; LAD: left anterior descending artery; LCA: left coronary artery; LCX: left circumflex; LM: left main coronary artery; OM1: first obtuse marginal; OM2: second obtuse marginal; PDA: posterior descending artery; Post.LV: posterior left ventricular artery; RAM: right anterior marginal; RCA: right coronary artery; SAN a.: sino-atrial nodal artery. A black and white version of this figure will appear in some formats. For the color version, please refer to the plate section.

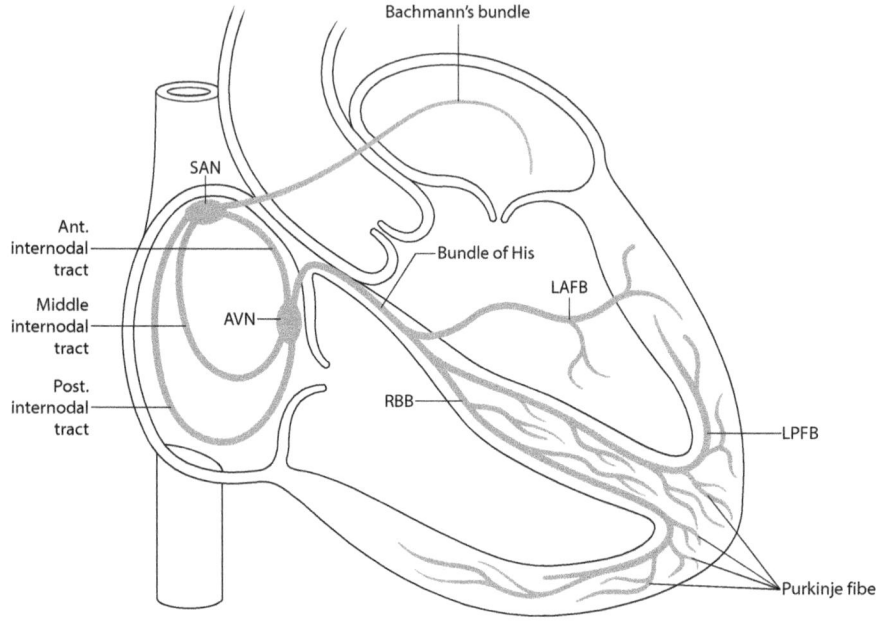

Figure 32.2 Cardiac conduction pathway.
AVN: atrioventricular node; LAFB: left anterior fascicular bundle; LPFB: left posterior fascicular bundle; RBB: right bundle branch; SAN: sino-atrial node.

Lymphatics confluence into conduit located in AV groove Coronary lymphatics drain into the mediastinal lymphatic plexus and into the thoracic duct (Figure 32.1).

Heart Conduction System

See Figure 32.2.

1. SA node: Located in the sulcus terminals of the RA.
2. Inter-nodal tracts: Anterior, middle, and posterior inter-nodal tractsBachmann's bundle

3. AV node: Located in the RA at the base of the intertribal septum, below the coronary sinus.
4. Bundle of His
5. Bundle branches:
   - Right bundle branch
   - Left bundle branch
     - Left anterior
     - Left posterior division

Purkinje Fibers

The conduction system of the heart initiates impulses and conducts them through the heart to produce the heart cycle and coordinate the contraction of cardiac chambers.

It consists of cardiac muscle cells and fibers that conduct the impulses.

Sino-atrial (SA) node is located at the junction of superior vena cava (SVC) and right atrium (RA).

The SA node is innervated with post-ganglionic adrenergic and cholinergic nerves.

Bundle of His with the AVN and goes into the membranous septum then goes into the bundle brunches, right and left.

The AVN and His bundles are innervated by adrenergic and cholinergic fibers.

Purkinje fibers connect with the ends of the bundle brunches to form networks on the endocardial surfaces of both ventricles.

Further Reading

Barash PG, Cullen BF, Stoetling RK, editors. *Clinical Anesthesia*, 7th ed. Lippincott Williams & Wilkins, 2013.

Iaizzo PA, editor. *Handbook of Cardiac Anatomy, Physiology, and Devices*. Springer, 2015.

Jain AK, Smith EJ, Rothman MT. The coronary venous system: an alternative route of access to the myocardium. *J Invasive Cardiol* 2006 Nov;**18**(11):563–568.

Kaplan JA, Reich DL, Savino JS. *Kaplan's Cardiac Anesthesia: The Echo Era*, 6th ed. Saunders, 2011.

Kenny T . *The Nuts and Bolts of Cardiac Pacing*, 2nd ed. Wiley-Blackwell, 2008.

Miller RD, Eriksson LI, Fleisher LA, et al., editors. *Miller's Anesthesia*, 8th ed. Churchill Livingstone/Elsevier, 2015.

Miller RD, Pardo M. *Basics of Anesthesia*, 6th ed. Elsevier/Saunders, 2000.

Zhu X, editor. *Surgical Atlas of Cardiac Anatomy*. Springer, 2014.

Cardiovascular System: Pharmacology

Edward R Mathney

Digoxin[1]

Mechanism of Action:

- Inotropy: Inhibition of transmembrane Na/K-ATPase → increased intracellular Na. Na/Ca exchanger results in increased intracellular calcium
- Anti-arrhythmic: Increased duration of phase 4 and phase 0 of cardiac action potential, slowed V_{max} and action potential conduction velocity, increased vagal tone to heart

Uses:

- Atrial fibrillation/flutter
- Congestive heart failure (CHF)

ECG Changes:

- Therapeutic: Prolonged PR, ST depressions, T wave inversions, "Salvador Dali moustache" ("scoop" after QRS)
- Toxicity: Frequent PVCs (bi/trigeminy), sinus bradycardia, AV blocks, Afib, VT

Side Effects/Toxicity: ECG changes (see above), GI upset, visual disturbances (yellow/green hue)

- Treatment: Digoxin immunoglobulin

Inotropes and Adrenergic Agents[2]

Phenylephrine

- Mechanism of Action: α_1 agonist
  - Vasoconstriction (α_1)
- Uses:
  - Hypotension
  - Myocardial ischemia – improved coronary perfusion pressure with increased diastolic BP
- Adverse Effects:
  - Reflex bradycardia
  - Potential decreased cardiac output due to increased afterload

Ephedrine

- Mechanism of Action: Indirect sympathomimetic resulting in catecholamine release – ↑ HR and contractility, vasoconstriction
  - Ineffective in patients with decreased catecholamine reserve (e.g., sepsis, chronically ill, shock)
- Uses:
  - Hypotension and bradycardia
- Adverse Effects:
  - Tachyphylaxis with repeated dosing
  - Concomitant use with MAOIs – exaggerated response, risk for serotonin syndrome

Norepinephrine

- Mechanism of Action: Direct adrenergic agonism (α_1, α_2, β_1)
  - Potent vasoconstrictor (α_1 – systemic and pulmonary vascular resistance)
- Uses:
  - Hypotension (gold standard in septic shock)
- Adverse Effects:
  - Worsening pulmonary hypertension
  - Potential decreased cardiac output due to increased afterload
  - Organ dysfunction and metabolic acidosis

Epinephrine

- Mechanism of Action: Direct adrenergic agonism (α_1, α_2, β_1, β_2)
  - Increased inotropy, chronotropy, automaticity (β_1)
  - Systemic vasoconstriction (α_1)
  - Bronchodilation (β_2)
  - Endocrine: Increased gluconeogenesis, glycogenolysis, lipolysis, decreased insulin secretion
- Uses:
  - Anaphylaxis
  - Heart failure (left and right)
  - Cardiac arrest
- Adverse Effects:
  - Hyperglycemia
  - Hypokalemia
  - Lactic acidosis
  - Myocardial ischemia

Dopamine

- Mechanism of Action: Agonism of α_1, β_1, and D_1 dopamine receptor
  - Dose-Dependent Effects:
    - 0.5–5.0 mcg/kg/min → D_1
      - Increased glomerular filtration rate (GFR), renal blood flow (RBF), Na^+ excretion, vasodilation
    - 5–10 mcg/kg/min → β_1
      - Increased HR, CO, BP, norepinephrine release

- 10–20 mcg/kg/min → α_1
  - Increased systemic vascular resistance (SVR)
- Uses:
  - Hypotension (better agents available)
  - Heart rate-dependent patients (e.g., infants)
- Adverse Effects:
  - Tachycardia
  - Arrhythmogenic
  - Myocardial ischemia (increased demand)
  - Bowel ischemia

Dobutamine
- Mechanism of Action: β agonist
  - Increased inotropy and chronotropy (β_1)
  - Decreased SVR (β_2)
- Uses:
  - Pharmacological stress testing
  - Treatment of low cardiac output states (e.g., post MI, post bypass)
- Adverse Effects:
  - Tachyphylaxis
  - Tachycardia
  - Arrhythmogenic
  - Myocardial ischemia (increased demand)

Isoproterenol
- Mechanism of Action: β agonist
  - Increased inotropy, chronotropy, and lusitropy ($\beta1$)
  - Decreased SVR (β_2)
- Uses:
  - Treatment of symptomatic bradycardia
  - Elicit arrhythmias in electrophysiology lab
- Adverse Effects:
  - Arrhythmogenic
  - Myocardial ischemia (increased demand) (Figure 33.1)

Phosphodiesterase Inhibitors:[2–5]

Milrinone:
- Mechanism of Action: Phosphodiesterase III inhibitor (increased cAMP)
  - Increased CO
  - Decreased SVR, PVR, LV end diastolic pressure (LVEDP)

- Uses:
  - Heart failure – especially RV failure
  - Reversal of cerebral vasospasm following subarachnoid hemorrhage (SAH)
- Adverse Effects:
  - Systemic hypotension (potentially severe)
  - Impaired platelet aggregation
- Other agents in same class – enoximone, inamrinone, olprimone, piroximone[1]

Sildenafil:
- Mechanism of Action: Phosphodiesterase V inhibitor (increased cGMP)
  - Smooth muscle relaxation
- Uses:
  - Outpatient management of pulmonary hypertension
- Adverse Effects:
  - Concomitant use with nitrates can result in severe hypotension and coronary steal
  - Headache, dyspepsia, dizziness
- Other Agents in Same Class:
  - Tadalafil

Levosimendan:[3]
- Mechanism of Action: Enhanced myocardial response to calcium resulting in increased inotropy; PDE3 inhibitor – increased inotropy; opening of potassium channels in vascular smooth muscle – vasodilation
- Uses:
  - "Inodilator" used in CHF

Anti-arrhythmics:[1]
See Figure 33.2.

Class I:
- Mechanism of Action: Na$^+$ channel blocker
- Class Ia (intermediate dissociation, including action potential duration)
  - Effects on Action Potential: Phase 0 decreased, depolarization prolonged, slowed conduction, action potential duration increased
  - Examples:
    - Quinidine: Atrial and ventricular arrhythmias.

Drug	α	β_1	β_2	CO	HR	SVR	MAP	PVR
Phenylephrine	+++	0	0	0	↓	↑	↑	↑
Ephedrine	+	+	+	↑	↑	↑	↑	0
Norepinephrine	+++	++	0	0	0	↑	↑	↑
Epinephrine	++	++	++	↑	↑	↑	↑	0
Dopamine	++	++	0	↑	↑	↑	↑	0
Dobutamine	0	+++	+	↑	↑	↓	↓	↓
Isoproterenol	0	+++	+++	↑	↑	↓	↓	0
Milrinone	0	0	0	↑	0	↓	↓	↓
Vasopressin	0	0	0	↑	0	↑	↑	0

Figure 33.1 Effects of vasoactive/inotropic agents.

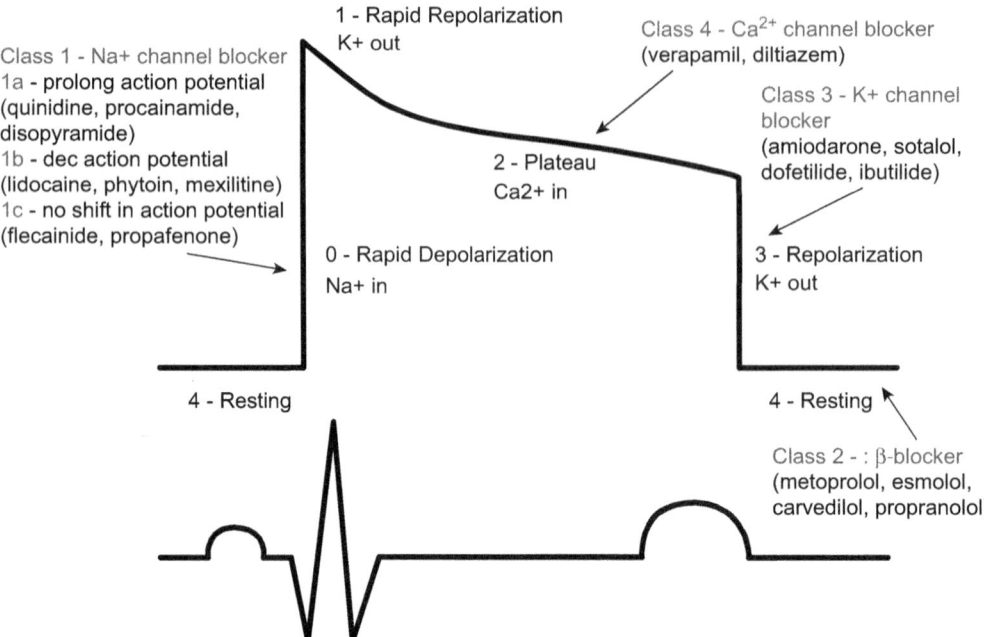

Figure 33.2 Anti-arrhythmics.

- May increase ventricular response rate in AF/flutter.
  - Adverse Effects: Prolonged QT interval →
    asystole
- Procainamide: VT/VF, PACs, Afib/Aflutter
  - Adverse Effects: Prolonged QT (less than
    quinidine), GI upset, CNS symptoms,
    agranulocytosis.
  - In setting of renal insufficiency, toxic metabolite
    N-acetylprocainamide may accumulate
- Disopyramide: SVT/VT
  - Adverse Effects: Prolonged QT interval, negative
    inotropic effects, reflex increase in SVR,
    anticholinergic side effects (GI upset, visual
    impairment, urinary retention)
- Class Ib (rapid dissociation, dec action potential duration)
  - Effects on Action Potential: Minor effects on phase 0,
    depolarization, and conduction, action potential
    duration decreased
  - Examples:
    - Lidocaine: VT/VF
      - Also exhibits local anesthetic, sedative, and
        bronchodilatory properties. Decreases
        sympathetic response to direct laryngoscopy.
      - Adverse Effects: CNS (fatigue, disorientation →
        agitation → seizures)
    - Mexiletine/Tocainide: VT/VF
      - Adverse Effects: Nausea, dysarthria, dizziness,
        paresthesia
- Class Ic (slow dissociation, no change in action potential
  duration)

- Effects on Action Potential: Phase 0 decreased, minor
  depolarization effects, slowed conduction, action
  potential duration unchanged
- Examples:
  - Flecainide: SVT, VT, Wolff–Parkinson–White
    syndrome. Can significantly alter accessory pathway
    refractory period.
    - Adverse Effects: Rare. Minimal effects on QT
      interval.
  - Propafenone: SVT, VT.
Blocks beta receptors and potassium channels as well.
    - Adverse Effects: Bronchospasm, GI upset,
      blurred vision, altered taste.

Class II
- Mechanism of Action: β-blocker resulting in decreased
  automaticity, increased action potential duration,
  decreased rate of spontaneous depolarization in SA node,
  slowed AV nodal conduction, increased effective
  refractory period
- Examples:
  - Esmolol: selective β_1 blocker
    - Short (~ 27 minutes) half-life. Metabolized by red
      blood cell esterases.
  - Metoprolol: Selective β_1 blocker
    - Adverse Effects: Like propranolol, its use can
      suppress signs of hypoglycemia.
  - Propranolol: Non-selective β blocker
    - Adverse Effects: Bronchospasm, hallucinations,
      depression, insomnia, possible withdrawal

Class III

- Mechanism of Action: Potassium channel blockade. Prolongation of repolarization and increased action potential duration/effective refractory period.
- Examples:
  - Amiodarone: SVT, VT/VF
    - Prolongs repolarization and refractory period in SA node, AV node, His–Purkinje system, and in the myocardium.
    - May decrease heart's response to T3
    - Half–life of weeks (60–142 days) with large volume of distribution (66 L/kg)
    - Adverse Effects: Hypotension, prolonged QT (chronic use), thyrotoxicity, dyspnea, apical pulmonary fibrosis
  - Sotalol: SVT, AFib, VT
    - Prolongs refractory period
    - Has beta blocking qualities
    - Adverse Effects: Prolonged QT, risk of Torsades de pointes
  - Dofetilide: AFib
    - Potassium channel blockade without slowing conduction
    - Adverse Effects: Prolonged QT
  - Dronedarone: AFib
    - Methane for iodine substitution that reduces thyrotoxicity compared with amiodarone (decreased efficacy), with a shorter half-life and smaller volume of distribution
  - Vernakalant: AFib
    - Blocks atrial sodium and potassium channels
    - More effective at higher heart rates

Class IV

- Mechanism of Action: Calcium channel blockers, decreased action potential duration, slowed AV nodal conduction
- Examples:
  - Verapamil: SVT, Afib/flutter
    - Cardiac depressive effects especially when used in the setting of inhalational anesthesia
    - Little effect on accessory pathways and therefore ineffective with antidromic reentry (ex. wide complex WPW)
    - Risk of AV block when used in conjunction with beta blockers
    - Prolongation of neuromuscular blockade
  - Diltiazem: SVT, Afib/flutter
    - Similar effects as verapamil

Others

- Adenosine
  - Very short half-life (~ 2 seconds)

- Negative chronotropic, dromotropic, and inotropic effects
- Potent AV nodal blockade used in the treatment of AV nodal reentry.
  - Exaggerated response in those with transplanted heart
- Dosing: 6 mg → 6 mg → 12 mg (q1 minute)

Anti-anginal Drugs

AHA/ACC Guideline for the Management of Patients with Non-ST-Elevation Acute Coronary Syndromes (2014)[6]

- MONA – morphine, oxygen, nitroglycerin, aspirin
- Oxygen therapy in patients with oxygen saturation less than 90%, respiratory distress, or high-risk features of hypoxemia. (Class I rec)
- Nitroglycerin (NTG):
  - Sublingual NTG q5min up to three doses (0.3–0.4 mg). (Class I rec)
  - NTG is contraindicated if a PDE inhibitor has been administered within 24 hours. (Class III – harm)
- Analgesics:
  - Morphine if chest pain persists despite maximal anti-ischemic medical therapy. (Class IIb evidence)
  - Aside from aspirin, NSAIDs have been associated with major adverse cardiac events. (Class III – harm)
- Beta blockers:
  - Beta blockers (metoprolol, carvedilol, or bisoprolol) within 24 hours if no contraindications exist. (Class I rec)
    - Contraindications include decompensated CHF, low-output states, and reactive airway disease.
  - Continue beta blocker therapy after ischemic event.
- Calcium channel blockers:
  - A non-dihydropyridine calcium channel blocker (verapamil, diltiazem) may be substituted for a beta blocker as initial therapy if a contraindication to beta blockade exists. (Class I rec)
  - Recommended for use in coronary vasospasm. (Class I rec)
- ACEI/ARB:
  - These agents should be started and continued in patients with ejection fraction less than 40% and in patients with hypertension, diabetes, or CKD. (Class I rec)
  - ARBs are a suitable substitute in patients who experience significant side effects of ACE inhibitors. (Class I rec)
  - Aldosterone antagonism is recommended in patients post myocardial infarction on both ACE inhibitors and a beta blocker without renal insufficiency.
- Antiplatelet/antithrombotic agents:
  - Aspirin therapy should be initiated in patients presenting with ACS and continued indefinitely. Initial

dose 162 or 325 mg followed by 81 mg daily thereafter. (Class I rec)

- Clopidogrel load followed by daily dose is recommended if a contraindication to aspirin therapy exists. (Class I rec)

Specific Agents[7]

- Statins:
  - Benefits extend beyond lipid-lowering effects – anti-inflammatory, improved endothelial function, plaque-stabilizing effects
- Nitrates[8] (isosorbide mono/di-nitrate):
  - Mechanism of Action: Release of nitric oxide facilitates activation of guanylyl cyclase, which results in increased levels of cGMP and both arteriolar and venous vasodilation.
    - Coronary arteries are subject to vasodilatory effects with resultant increased oxygen supply to myocardium.[9,10]
    - Decreased preload → decreased LVEDV → dec wall tension = decreased myocardial oxygen demand.
- Ranolazine:[11,12]
  - Mechanism of Action: Inhibition of late myocardial sodium current leading to decreased intracellular sodium and calcium in ischemic myocardium.
  - Little to no effect on hemodynamics
  - Adverse Effects: Constipation, nausea, dizziness

Vasodilators[1]

Nitroprusside:
- Mechanism of Action: Nitric oxide donor
- Physiological Effects:
  - Potent arterial and venous vasodilation (including pulmonary vasculature)
  - Easily titratable
- Adverse Effects:
  - Severe hypotension
  - Cyanide/thiocyanate toxicity with prolonged use especially in the setting of renal insufficiency

Nitroglycerin:
- Mechanism of Action: Conversion to nitric oxide in smooth muscle leading to production of cyclic GMP (cGMP) by way of activation of guanylyl cyclase. Smooth muscle relaxation due to myosin light chain dephosphorylation.
- Physiological Effects:
  - Preferential systemic venodilation
  - Coronary vasodilation (without coronary steal)
  - Decreased PVR
  - Increased venous pooling leading to decreased venous return and decreased preload

- Adverse Effects:
  - Hypotension
  - Headache
  - Nausea

Hydralazine:
- Mechanism of Action: Activation of ATP-dependent potassium channels
- Physiological Effects:
  - Arterial vasodilation
- Adverse Effects:
  - Reflex sympathetic activation manifesting as tachycardia, headache, flushing.

Nesiritide:
- Mechanism of Action: Analog of brain natriuretic peptide (BNP) that produces both arterial and venous vasodilation via increased cGMP.
- Physiological Effects:
  - Arterial and venous vasodilation
  - No effects on heart rate or contractility
  - To be administered to in-hospital patients only
- Adverse Effects:
  - Hypotension
  - Renal failure

Calcium Channel Blockers:
- Mechanism of Action: Binding to sites on the α-1 subunit of L-type voltage-dependent calcium channel.
- Physiological Effects:
  - Arterial vasodilation
  - Coronary vasodilation (nifedipine most potent)
- Adverse Effects:
  - Negative inotropy, dromotropy, and chronotropy
    - Hypotension, AV block, heart failure. All more likely in setting of combination therapy with beta blockade, digitalis, or in setting of hypokalemia.
  - Headache, flushing, nausea
- Specific Calcium Channel Blockers:
  - Dihydropyridine (DHP) derivatives (amlodipine, nifedipine, nimodipine, nicardipine):
    - Potent arterial dilators
    - Reflex activation of sympathetic nervous system
    - Nimodipine can cross blood brain barrier and is indicated for cerebral vascular spasm
    - Nicardipine has selectivity for coronary and cerebrovascular vessels compared to other DHPs
    - Clevidipine is inactivated by ester hydrolysis with a half-life of 1 minute
  - Phenylalkylamines (verapamil):
    - Less potent arterial vasodilation than DHPs
    - Less reflex sympathetic activation than DHPs
    - Myocardial depression

- o Benzothiazipines (diltiazem)
  - Less potent arterial vasodilation than verapamil

Alpha-Adrenergic Antagonists (phentolamine – reversible, phenoxybenzamine – irreversible):

- Mechanism of Action: Non-selective alpha-adrenergic antagonism
- Physiological Effects:
  - o Decreased SVR and PVR
  - o Positive inotropic and chronotropic effects (presynaptic α2 antagonism)
- Adverse Effects:
  - o Orthostatic hypotension
  - o Reflex tachycardia

Central Acting Alpha-Agonists (clonidine, methyldopa):

- Mechanism of Action: Reduce sympathetic outflow and SVR via agonism of central α_2-adrenergic receptors. Presynaptic α_2 agonism results in decreased release of norepinephrine at synaptic cleft
- Physiological Effects:
  - o Decreased SVR
  - o Decreased sympathetic outflow
- Adverse Effects:
  - o Rebound hypertension
  - o Sedation
  - o Dry mouth
  - o Autoimmune hemolytic anemia (methyl-dopa)

Endothelin Antagonists (bosentan, ambrisentan):

- Mechanism of Action: Antagonism of endothelin receptor, which is responsible for vasoconstriction

Angiotensin Converting Enzyme Inhibitors and Angiotensin Receptor Blockers[13]

ACE Inhibitors (ex – lisinopril, enalapril, ramipril, benazepril):

- Mechanism of Action: Prevents cleavage of angiotensin I to angiotensin II via inhibition of ACE. Angiotensin II mediates vasoconstriction, release of aldosterone, sodium retention, ventricular remodeling, and increases in sympathetic tone. ACE involved with breakdown of bradykinin. More bradykinin = vasodilation
- Uses:
  - o Hypertension
    - Increased RBF via dilation of afferent and efferent arterioles
    - Protective against development of diabetic nephropathy
  - o CHF
    - Decreased PVR and increased CO
    - Decreased sodium retention and ventricular remodeling in setting of CHF and post-MI (confers a mortality benefit)

- Adverse Effects:
  - o Cough (inc bradykinin)
  - o Hypotension
  - o Hyperkalemia (dec aldosterone)
  - o Renal insufficiency
  - o Angioedema
  - o Agranulocytosis

Angiotensin Receptor Blockers (ARB) (ex – losartan, olmesartan, valsartan):

- Mechanism of Action: Blockage of the AT_1 receptor
  - o Greater inhibition of renin-angiotensin-aldosterone system (RAAS) than ACEI
  - o No effect on bradykinin levels
- Uses: Same as ACEI
- Adverse Effects: Same as ACEI with exception of cough

Aldosterone Antagonists:

- Spironolactone
  - o Mechanism of Action:
  - o Potassium-sparing diuretic that acts as an inhibitor of the renal aldosterone-dependent Na^+/K^+ channel.
  - o Uses:
  - o Hypertension
  - o CHF (inhibits cardiac remodeling)
  - o Adverse Effects:
    - Hyperkalemia
    - Endocrine side effects (gynecomastia and oligomenorrhea)
- Eplerenone:
  - o Mechanism of Action:
    - Aldosterone receptor inhibition
  - o Uses:
    - Hypertension
    - CHF
  - o Adverse Effects:
    - Hyperkalemia

Renin Inhibitor (ex – aliskiren):[14]

- Mechanism of Action: Occupies active site of renin preventing cleavage of ATI into AT2
- Uses:
  - o Hypertension

Cardiovascular Effects of Electrolytes[3,15,16]

Calcium:

- Role:
  - o Ubiquitous second messenger

- Important role in coagulation. Links platelets to coagulation factors.
- Positive inotrope (inotropic drugs all result in including intracellular calcium)
- Peripheral vasoconstriction
- Pathological States:
  - Hypercalcemia:
    - Effects:
      - Weakness → lethargy → coma
      - Constipation, nausea/vomiting
      - Nephrogenic diabetes insipidus
      - Worsening of digitalis toxicity
    - ECG Changes:
      - Shortened QT_c
      - Prolonged PR interval
        - Osborn waves (J wave or camel-hump sign)
    - Causes:
      - Increased PTH
      - Malignancy
      - Excess vitamin D
      - Decreased renal excretion (thiazide diuretics)
      - Increased Ca^{2+} intake (milk-alkali syndrome)
    - Treatment:
      - Non-calcium-containing crystalloid
      - Loop diuretics
      - Bisphosphonates
  - Hypocalcemia
    - Effects:
      - Decreased myocardial contractility
      - Paresthesia
      - Tetany
      - Seizures
      - Chvostek sign: facial twitching from tapping on facial nerve
      - Trousseau sign: forearm spasm from inflating NIBP cuff
      - Heart block
    - ECG Changes:
      - Prolonged QT_c
      - T wave inversions
      - V fib
    - Causes:
      - Hypoparathyroidism
      - Ca^{2+} chelation (i.e., blood product administration)
      - Increased bone deposition
      - Hypoalbuminemia
    - Treatment:
      - Calcium supplementation
      - Correct coexisting electrolyte abnormalities, especially magnesium – Mg depletion can lead to hypoparathyroidism, PTH resistance, and vit D deficiency

Magnesium:
- Role:
  - Involved in ion channel activity (Ca^{2+} antagonist)
  - Vital to production of ATP, nucleotides, and proteins (DNA transcription/translation cofactor)
  - NMDA antagonist
  - Arteriolar vasodilator
  - Bronchial smooth muscle dilator
  - Tocolytic
  - Anticonvulsant
- Pathological States:
  - Hypermagnesemia:
    - Effects:
      - Prolonged effect of non-depolarizing neuromuscular blocking agents (caution in patients with myasthenia gravis and Eaton-Lambert syndrome)
      - Side effects based upon serum level:
    - 5 to 7 mg/dL: Therapeutic in treatment of pre-eclampsia
    - 5 to 10 mg/dL: Impaired cardiac conduction, nausea
    - 20 to 34 mg/dL: Sedation, reduced deep tendon reflexes, muscle weakness
    - 24 to 48 mg/dL: Hypotension
    - 48 to 72 mg/dL: Areflexia, coma, respiratory paralysis
      - ECG Changes:
        - Widened QRS
        - Prolonged PR interval
      - Causes:
        - Mostly iatrogenic
      - Treatment:
        - Non-magnesium-containing crystalloid administration
        - Diuretics
        - Renal replacement therapy
  - Hypomagnesemia
    - Effects:
      - Vertigo → weakness → seizure
      - Hypocalcemia
      - Hyperinsulinemia
      - Atherosclerosis
      - Osteomalacia
    - ECG Changes:
      - Widened QRS
      - Prolonged PR interval
      - T wave inversion
      - Ventricular arrhythmias
    - Causes:
      - Inadequate intake
      - Renal losses
    - Treatment:
      - Magnesium supplementation

- Correction other electrolyte abnormalities, especially calcium and potassium

Phosphorus:
- Role:
  - Building block for DNA, RNA, ATP, phospholipids, hydroxyapatite, 2,3-DPG
  - Phosphate buffer system
- Pathological States:
  - Hyperphosphatemia:
    - Effects:
      - Complexes with calcium leading to hypocalcemia
      - Vascular calcification leading to increased afterload and left ventricular hypertrophy[17]
    - ECG Changes:[18]
      - Prolonged QT interval
      - Ventricular tachycardia
      - Torsade de pointes
    - Causes:
      - Tumor lysis syndrome
      - Rhabdomyolysis
      - Reduced excretion (renal failure)
      - Hypoparathyroidism
      - Pseudohyperphosphatemia
  - Multiple myeloma
    - Treatment:
      - Dialysis
      - Crystalloid infusion
      - Phosphate binders
  - Hypophosphatemia:[19]
    - Effects:
      - Decreased cardiac contractility
      - Impaired respiratory function
      - Left-shift in oxygen dissociation curve
      - Seizures
      - Central pontine myelinolysis
    - ECG Changes:
      - Ventricular arrhythmia post MI
      - SVT
      - Ectopy
    - Causes:
      - Impaired intake/uptake
      - Acute respiratory alkalosis
      - Renal/GI excretion
      - Hungry bone syndrome
      - Refeeding syndrome
    - Treatment:
      - Replete cautiously to avoid causing severe hypocalcemia

Potassium:
- Role:

- Resting membrane potential (large intracellular to extracellular gradient maintained by Na+/K+/ATPase)
- Pathological States:
  - Hyperkalemia:
    - Effects:
      - Slowed conduction through AV node
      - Muscle weakness
      - Paralysis
      - Altered cardiac conduction (inc automaticity, rapid repolarization)
    - ECG changes based on serum concentration:
      - 5.5 to 6.5 mEq/L → peaked T waves
      - 6.5 to 7.5 mEq/L → prolonged PR interval
      - > 7.5 mEq/L → widened QRS
      - > 9.0 mEq/L → sine waves, bradycardia, VT, cardiac arrest
    - Causes:
      - Increased intake
      - Renal insufficiency
      - Hypoaldosteronism
      - Drugs (potassium sparing diuretics, ACEI/ARB)
      - Reperfusion of ischemic tissues
      - Acidosis
    - Treatment:
      - Calcium to stabilize cardiac membranes
      - Increase intracellular fluid K to extracellular fluid ratio (insulin, B2 agonists, bicarbonate, hyperventilation
      - Increased excretion (loop diuretics)
      - Dialysis
      - Cation exchange resins (ex – patiromer, sodium zirconium cyclosilicate, sodium polystyrene sulfonate)
  - Hypokalemia:
    - Effects:
      - Prolonged repolarization
      - Muscle weakness
    - ECG Changes:
      - T wave flattening or inversion
      - U waves
      - ST segment depression
      - Prolonged PR interval
      - Atrial and ventricular arrhythmias
    - Causes:
      - Inadequate intake
      - GI losses
      - Mineralocorticoid/glucocorticoid excess
      - Diuretics
      - Hypomagnesemia
      - Intracellular shifts (β_2 agonists, insulin, lithium overdose, acute alkalosis)
    - Treatment:
      - Oral and intravenous supplementation

Non-adrenergic Vasoconstrictors

Vasopressin:[20]

- Mechanism of Action: Synthesized in posterior pituitary gland endogenously. Released in response to increased serum osmolality, hypovolemia, pain, nausea, hypoxia, and pharyngeal stimulation.
- Receptor Effects:
  - V_1: systemic vasoconstriction with relative sparing of the pulmonary vasculature[21]
  - V_2: located in distal tubules and collecting ducts of kidney. Increased cAMP leading to insertion of aquaporin channels in collecting ducts = water retention. Also causes release of vWF and Factor VIII to facilitate clotting. Desmopressin (DDAVP) is a selective V2 agonist.
  - V_3: located in anterior pituitary and result in increased synthesis of adrenocorticohormone (ACTH).
- Uses:
  - Hypovolemic shock
  - Septic shock
  - Hepatorenal syndrome
  - Bleeding esophageal varices

- Adverse Effects:
  - Skin necrosis
  - Hyponatremia
  - Bronchospasm
  - Gut ischemia

Terlipressin: Vasopressin analog with longer half-life (6 hours vs. 24 minutes).

Methylene Blue:[22]

- Mechanism of Action: Inhibition of guanylyl cyclase and nitric oxide synthase = decreased vessel responsiveness to NO = vasoconstriction
- Uses:
  - Refractory hypotension and vasoplegia (sepsis, anaphylaxis, post-CPB, post-reperfusion syndrome)
  - Cyanide toxicity
- Adverse Effects:
  - Methemoglobinemia (high doses or G6PD deficiency)
  - Serotonin syndrome (with use of SSRIs, SNRIs, MAOIs)
  - Inaccuracies with pulse oximetry readings

References

1. Royster RL, Groban L, Locke AQ, Morris BN, Slaughter TF. Cardiovascular pharmacology. In Kaplan JA, Augoustides JGT, Maneck GR, Maus T, Reich DL, editors. *Kaplan's Cardiac Anesthesia: In Cardiac and Noncardiac Surgery*. Elsevier, 2017; pp 292–354.

2. Zimmerman J, Cahalan M. Vasopressors and inotropes. In Hemmings HC, Egan TD, editors. *Pharmacology and Physiology for Anesthesia: Foundations and Clinical Application*. Elsevier, 2013; pp 390–404.

3. Levy JH, Ghadimi K, Bailey JM, Ramsay JG. Postoperative cardiovascular management. In Kaplan JA, Augoustides JGT, Maneck GR, Maus T, Reich DL, editors. *Kaplan's Cardiac Anesthesia: In Cardiac and Noncardiac Surgery*. Elsevier, 2017; pp 1327–1357.

4. Gold Standard, Inc. Milrinone. Clinical Pharmacology [database online]. Available at: http://clinical pharmacology.com (accessed August 3, 2017).

5. Gold Standard, Inc. Sildenafil. Clinical Pharmacology [database online].

Available at: http://clinicalpharmacol ogy.com (accessed August 3, 2017)

6. Amsterdam EA, Wenger NK, Brindis RG, et al. 2014 AHA/ACC Guideline for the Management of Patients with Non-ST-Elevation Acute Coronary Syndromes. *Circulation* 2014;**130**(25):e344–e426.

7. Tarkin JM, Kaski JC. An overview of treatment guidelines: ESC/ACC-AHA /NICE. In Avanzas P, Kaski JC, editors. *Pharmacological Treatment of Chronic Stable Angina Pectoris* Ebook. Springer, 2015; pp 33–56. (overview)

8. Carro A, Avanzas P. Nitrates. In Avanzas P, Kaski JC, editors. *Pharmacological Treatment of Chronic Stable Angina Pectoris*, ebook. Springer, 2015; pp 87–114.

9. Tarkin JM, Kaski JC. Nicorandil. In Avanzas P, Kaski JC, editors. *Pharmacological Treatment of Chronic Stable Angina Pectoris*, ebook. Springer, 2015; pp 115–134.

10. Dominguez-Rodriguez A. Ivabradine. In Avanzas P, Kaski JC, editors. *Pharmacological Treatment of Chronic Stable Angina Pectoris*, ebook. Springer, 2015; pp 135–152.

11. Rosano GMC, C. Vitale C, Volterrani M. Ranolazine. In Avanzas P, Kaski JC, editors. *Pharmacological Treatment of Chronic Stable Angina Pectoris*, ebook. Springer, 2015; pp 173–188.

12. Gold Standard, Inc. Ranolazine. Clinical Pharmacology [database online]. Available at: http://clinical pharmacology.com (accessed August 3, 2017).

13. Dolinko AV, Kuntz MT, Antman EM, Strichartz GR, Lilly LS. Cardiovascular drugs. In Lilly LS, editor. *Pathophysiology of Heart Disease: A Collaborative Project of Medical Students and Faculty*. Wolters Kluwer, 2016; pp 400–455.

14. Drago J, Williams GH, Lilly LS. Hypertension. In Lilly LS, editor. *Pathophysiology of Heart Disease: A Collaborative Project of Medical Students and Faculty*. Wolters Kluwer, 2016; pp 310–333.

15. Edwards MR, Grocott MPW. Perioperative fluid and electrolyte therapy. In Miller RD, Cohen NH, Eriksson LI, et al., editors. *Miller's Anesthesia*. Elsevier, 2015; pp 1767–1810.

16. Freudzon L, Akhtar S, London MJ, Barash PG. Electrocardiographic monitoring. In Kaplan JA, Augoustides JGT, Maneck GR, Maus T, Reich DL, editors. *Kaplan's Cardiac Anesthesia: In Cardiac and Noncardiac Surgery*. Elsevier, 2017; pp 357–389.

17. Hruska KA, Mathew S, Lund R, Qiu P, Pratt R. Hyperphosphatemia of chronic kidney disease. *Kidney Int* 2008;**74**:148–157.

18. Shiber JR, Mattu A. Serum phosphate abnormalities in the emergency department. *J Emerg Med* 2002;**23**(4):395–400.

19. Geerse DA, Bindels AJ, Kuiper MA, et al. Treatment of hypophosphatemia in the intensive care unit: a review. *Crit Care* 2010;**14**:R147.

20. Kam PCA, Williams S, Yoong FFY. Vasopressin and terlipressin: pharmacology and its clinical relevance. *Anaesthesia* 2004;**59**:993–1001.

21. Currigan DA, Hughes RJA, Wright CE, Angus JA, Soeding PF. Vasoconstrictor responses to vasopressor agents in human pulmonary and radial arteries. An *in vitro* study. *Anesthesiology* 2014;**121**:930–936.

22. Nguyen L, Roth DM, Shanewise JS, Kaplan JA. Discontinuing cardiopulmonary bypass. In Kaplan JA, Augoustides JGT, Maneck GR, Maus T, Reich DL, editors. *Kaplan's Cardiac Anesthesia: In Cardiac and Noncardiac Surgery*. Elsevier, 2017; pp 1291–1310.

Anesthesiology for the Gastrointestinal and Hepatic Systems

Bryan Hill, Jeron Zerillo, Jordan Holloway, and Daphney Dorcius

Gastrointestinal (GI) System

- The wall of the GI tract consists of three layers (from outermost to innermost): serosa, muscularis (consisting of an outer longitudinal layer and circular muscular layer), submucosa, and mucosa. An individual layer of epithelial cells, the lamina propria, and the muscularis mucosae comprise the mucosal layer.[1]

- The GI tract is innervated by the sympathetic and parasympathetic autonomic nervous systems as well as the enteric nervous system. The sympathetic nervous system, coming from the T5–L2 segments, tends to cause inhibitory effects on the GI system by the neurotransmitters norepinephrine and vasoactive intestinal polypeptide (VIP). The parasympathetic system, originating from cranial and sacral regions of the spinal cord, tends to promote GI tract function utilizing acetylcholine.[1]

- The enteric system is made up of the Auerbach and Meissner plexuses and is responsive to the autonomic nervous system. The Auerbach (myenteric) plexus lies between the two muscular layers, regulating smooth muscle contraction and relaxation. The submucosa contains the Meissner (submucosal) plexus, which transmits information from the GI epithelium to both the enteric and central nervous systems to modulate absorption, secretion, and mucosal blood flow.[1]

- Postoperative ileus is most commonly caused by physical manipulation of the intestines and the resultant cascade of neural and inflammatory interactions. Additional contributing factors include immobility, electrolyte abnormalities in the setting of large fluid shifts, and swelling of the wall of the intestinal wall due to excessive administration of IV fluids.[1]

- The typical course of uncomplicated ileus lasts approximately 3–4 postoperative days. This process consists of an early neurogenic phase mediated by adrenergic innervation (3–4 hours postoperatively) and a late inflammatory phase (3–24 hours postoperatively). Ileus can be complicated by opioid use for postoperative pain control. Specifically, the GI system has a significant number of mu receptors, which can lead to bowel dysfunction. These receptors can be selectively blocked by methylnaltrexone, a mu-receptor antagonist unable to cross the blood–brain barrier.[1,2]

- Depending on level of placement and dosing, epidural block utilizing local anesthetic can block sympathetic-mediated GI effects without altering parasympathetic innervation, improving GI blood flow, anastomotic perfusion, providing pain control (allowing for opioid sparing), and, overall, reducing the risk of ileus.[1]

- Blood flow in the GI system delivers hormones, removes metabolic waste, and helps to maintain the mucosal barrier, which prevents transepithelial migration of harmful chemicals and pathogens.[1]

- Twenty-five percent of cardiac output is delivered to the splanchnic system, which contains approximately one-third of total blood volume. A reservoir of blood is maintained in the venous system, which is mobilized during periods of acute blood loss. Vasopressin can also induce splanchnic vasoconstriction.[1,3]

- Laparoscopic surgery requires abdominal insufflation by CO_2, which can have multiple hemodynamic effects:[4]
  - Insufflation causes compression of IVC →initial increase in CO followed by reduced preload and a reduction in CO
  - Reduction in splanchnic blood flow → redistributed blood flow into the venous system → increased right arterial pressure (RAP)
  - CO_2 and abdominal aortic compression → sympathetic outflow → increasing systemic vascular resistance (SVR)
  - Renal artery compression → reduced renal blood flow → activation of renin–angiotensin system leading to vasopressin release → increased SVR and overall reduction in glomerular filtration rate (GFR)
  - Reduced functional reserve capacity (FRC), higher predisposal to V-Q mismatch, increased pulmonary vascular resistance (PVR) due to hypercarbia
  - Trendelenburg positioning causes further reduction in FRC and possible upper body venous engorgement, and reverse Trendelenburg positioning causes venous pooling and further reduction in preload.

- The stomach consists of three anatomical areas, from proximal to distal: fundus, corpus or body, and antrum.

- Important secretory cell types in the stomach include:
  - Parietal cell – secretes HCl[1,5]
  - Gastric (G) cell – secretes gastrin[1,5]

- Foveolar or mucous cell – secretes mucus and HCO_3^{-} [1]
- Chief cell – secretes pepsinogen, the inactive zymogen of pepsin [1]
- The stomach is protected against the caustic agents HCl and pepsin via mucus and bicarbonate. Bicarbonate production is increased via prostaglandin production, but this process is inhibited by NSAIDs. [1]
- Critically ill patients are at higher risk for stress ulcers, and stress ulcer prophylaxis is indicated for the following groups: [6]
  - High bleeding tendency (e.g., thrombocytopenia < 50 k, INR > 1.5, PTT > 2 normal)
  - Mechanical ventilation for > 48 hours (especially if not receiving enteric nutrition)
  - History of chronic liver disease, cirrhosis
  - History of prior GI bleeding or ulceration within the past year
  - TBI, spinal cord injury, or burns
  - NSAIDs or antiplatelet medications
  - 2+ of the following minor criteria: sepsis, ICU admission > 7 days, occult GI bleeding > 6 days, steroid therapy
  - See Table 34.1 for the American Society of Anesthesiologists (ASA) preoperative fasting guidelines.

Hepatic System

- The liver dual blood supply receives approximately 30% of the cardiac output. The portal vein conducts ~ 75% of hepatic blood flow and the hepatic artery receives the other ~ 25%. The liver oxygen supply is equally distributed (~ 50%) from each of these vessels. [8,9]
- Exchange of arterial and venous blood occurs in the hepatic sinusoids, the "capillaries of the liver." [8]
- The immunological Kupffer cells are present in hepatic sinusoids, acting as a filter by removing bacteria and other harmful substances from portal blood thereby preventing the entry of these into systemic circulation. [1]

Table 34.1 ASA NPO guidelines[7]

Ingested material	Minimum fasting period
Clear liquids	2 hours
Breast milk	4 hours
Infant formula, nonhuman milk, light meal*	6 hours
Everything else	8 hours

* A light meal consists of toast and clear liquids. Meals that include fried or fatty foods or meat may prolong gastric emptying time. Prolonged gastric emptying can occur in conditions that affect the GI nervous system (diabetic autonomic neuropathy) or increase sympathetic outflow (pain, trauma, labor).

- Acini are the units of liver parenchyma and composed of three progressive circulatory zones: Zone 1 (blood perfusing zone) receives blood rich in O_2 and nutrients; blood then passes through zone 2 and finally, zone 3, where the hepatocytes receive relatively O_2-poor blood. Tissue in zone 3 is most susceptible to hypoxic injury. [8]
- The hepatic arterial buffer response (HABR) refers to a compensatory increase in hepatic arterial flow when total hepatic blood flow drops, thereby preserving hepatic O_2 delivery. This response is mediated by adenosine: periods of low portal blood flow will cause buildup of adenosine, prompting hepatic arterial vasodilation to compensate for reduced portal blood flow. Disruptions in the HABR increase the possibility of hypoxic liver injury. [8]
- The liver is central to metabolism and maintenance of energy for the body. Glycogen is the main component of stored energy in the liver. When glycogen stores are depleted, hepatic gluconeogenesis occurs, enabling the liver to deliver glucose to glucose-dependent tissues, such as the brain. Oxidation of fatty acids into ketoacids increases with starvation. These compounds are released from the liver and used as energy substrates by many extrahepatic cells. [8]
- Hepatic metabolism is governed by Phase I and Phase II pathways. The Phase I pathway utilizes cytochrome P450 enzymes to oxidize, hydrolyze, or reduce medications. The Phase II pathway utilizes conjugation to make products from the Phase I pathway more water-soluble for excretion. [8]
- Ammonia is highly toxic to the many systems including the central nervous system and, without exogenous substances such as lactulose, can be eliminated only by the liver. Hepatocytes metabolize ammonia to urea, which is less toxic. [8]
- The only means of eliminating cholesterol from the body is via liver metabolism of cholesterol to bile acids. Hepatocytes produce bile acids, which eventually drain into the duodenum via the common bile duct. Bile salts are amphipathic molecules that emulsify lipophilic substances, promoting their absorption. [8]
- The terminal ileum absorbs bile acids and returns them to hepatocytes through the portal vein. This is called the enterohepatic circulation. [8]
- The liver produces many of the plasma proteins including albumin, which is the most abundant plasma protein. Albumin is the main determinant of plasma oncotic pressure and an essential vehicle of substances in the bloodstream. Hepatocytes also synthesize most of the molecular participants in coagulation pathways including vitamin K-dependent proteins (factors X, IX, VII, II, protein C, and protein S). Factor VII has the shortest half-life of these proteins (4 hours), making INR the most sensitive measurement for acute hepatic dysfunction. [8]
- Cirrhosis-induced portal hypertension causes hyperdynamic circulation. Total peripheral resistance and

systemic blood pressure decrease, with compensatory increases in cardiac output. Portosystemic shunting circumvents the hepatic filtering mechanism, and allows drugs, nitrogenous waste, and toxins to enter the central circulation.[8]

- Gradients between the inferior vena cava and the portal vein of greater the 5 mmHg qualify as portal hypertension. Gradients greater than 10 mmHg cause chronic liver injury, necrosis, fibrosis, and cirrhosis.[8,10]

- Non-selective beta blockers, such as propranolol, decrease hepatic artery blood flow, which decreases congestion in the liver. Transmitted back to the portal vein, this reduces portal pressure. These are prescribed to prevent variceal bleeding.[8]

- The only definitive treatment for end-stage hepatic disease is liver transplantation.

- Large-volume ascites can impede ventilation and reduce FRC. Large-volume paracentesis (LVP) can quickly and safely reduce abdominal mass in those patients with large-volume ascites. Hemodynamic instability can occur following LVP due to intravascular depletion secondary to rapid re-accumulation of the ascites. Albumin (5 g of albumin is given per liter of ascites removed) is commonly given to offset this response, preventing sequelae such as increased creatinine and electrolyte abnormalities.[11]

- *Hepatopulmonary syndrome* results from the formation of microscopic intrapulmonary arteriovenous dilations in patients with both chronic and acute liver failure. The mechanism is unknown but is thought to be due to increased liver production or decreased liver clearance of vasodilators, possibly involving nitric oxide. The dilation of these blood vessels causes overperfusion relative to ventilation, leading to ventilation–perfusion mismatch and hypoxemia. There is an increased gradient > 15 mmHg between the partial pressure of oxygen in the alveoli of the lung and adjacent arteries (alveolar–arterial [A–a] gradient) while breathing room air. Additionally, late in cirrhosis, it is common to develop high output failure, which leads to less time in capillaries per red blood cell, exacerbating hypoxemia. This condition improves following liver transplantation.[8]

- *Portopulmonary hypertension* is pulmonary arterial hypertension that occurs in patients with concomitant portal hypertension. Diagnosis requires a right heart catheterization demonstrating mPAP > 25 mmHg and a PVR > 240 dynes/s/cm with a pulmonary capillary wedge pressure (PCWP) < 15 mmHg. The pathophysiology is unclear, but treatment typically consists of PVR reduction by PDE-5 inhibitors, prostacyclin analogs, and endothelin receptor antagonists. This condition does not necessarily resolve with transplantation, and an mPAP > 45 mmHg is considered an absolute contraindication to liver transplantation.[8]

- *Hepatorenal syndrome (HRS)* is a "pre-renal" condition due to decreased intravascular tone leading to inadequate volume status perceived by the juxtaglomerular apparatus, causing the secretion of renin and the activation of the renin–angiotensin system, and resulting in the vasoconstriction of vessels systemically and in the kidney. However, the effect of this is insufficient to counteract the mediators of vasodilation in the splanchnic circulation, leading to persistent "underfilling" of the renal circulation and worsening kidney vasoconstriction, leading to renal failure. Diagnosis is one of exclusion after other causes of renal failure have been ruled out. HRS can be rapidly fatal (< 1 month). Liver transplantation is considered definitive treatment for HRS.[8]

ERPs/ERAS®[12]

- Enhanced recovery programs (ERPs) and Enhanced Recovery After Surgery (ERAS®) programs are multidisciplinary perioperative care programs initially developed for patients undergoing colorectal and cardiac surgery and aim to decrease postop mortality and morbidity by ensuring continuity of care, reducing care variability, and minimizing organ dysfunction. ERPs include preoperative teaching in plain language and counseling on modifiable habits including smoking, drug use, and alcohol consumption.

- Preoperatively, avoidance of fasting and ensuring adequate hydration and energy supply are encouraged to prevent insulin resistance associated with in surgical stress. Often this is performed with a preoperative carbohydrate drink.

- Intraoperatively, administration of antithrombotic prophylaxis and use of pneumatic compression devices decrease risk of DVT. Appropriate antibiosis is completed within 1 hour of surgical incision to prevent surgical site infections.

- Epidural/spinal analgesia and reduction of surgical invasiveness have reduced neuroendocrine, metabolic, inflammatory, and immunological changes associated with surgery.

- Preemptive strategies to minimize the risk of postoperative nausea and vomiting (PONV) help to avoid early feeding delays and encourage postoperative ambulation (decreasing rates of ileus and length of hospital stay).

- Postoperatively, early nutrition and opioid-sparing multimodal analgesia are encouraged. A multidisciplinary approach to optimize each patient's care should avoid routine bedrest and emphasize early, safe ambulation.

- Strategies to minimize ileus should include early enteral feeding, cautious and short-term use of gastric tubes, opioid-sparing analgesia, use of laxatives and prokinetics, and goal-directed fluid therapy to avoid/prevent bowel edema.

**

The authors would like to acknowledge Bryan Hill, Brian Chang, and Jeron Zerillo for their contributions to the previous version of this chapter.

References

1. Mar LO, Sassan Sabouri A. Gastrointestinal physiology and pathophysiology. In Gropper MA, Miller RD, Cohen NH, et al., editors. *Miller's Anesthesia*, 9th ed. Elsevier, 2020; chapter 15, pp 403–419.

2. Boeckxstaens GE, de Jonge WJ. Neuroimmune mechanisms in postoperative ileus. *Gut* 2009;**58**(9):1300–1311.

3. Bown LS, Ricksten S-E, Houltz E, Sondergaard S, Rizell M, Lundin S. Vasopressin-induced changes in splanchnic blood flow and hepatic and portal venous pressures in liver resection. *Acta Anaesthesiol Scand* 2016;**60**(5):607–615.

4. Atkinson TM, Giraud GD, Togoika BM, Jones DB, Cigarroa JE. Cardiovascular and ventilatory consequences of laparoscopic surgery. *Circulation* 2017;**135**(7):700–710.

5. Schubert ML. Regulation of gastric acid secretion. In Johnson LR, Ghishan FK, Kaunitz JD, et al., editors. *Physiology of the Gastrointestinal Tract*, vol. 2, 5th ed. Academic Press, 2012; chapter 47, pp 1281–1309.

6. Weinhouse GL. Stress ulcers in the intensive care unit: diagnosis, management, and prevention. In Finlay G, editor.*UpToDate*. UpToDate Inc., 2022 Available at: www.uptodate.com/contents/stress-ulcers-in-the-intensive-care-unit-diagnosis-management-and-prevention#H929814

7. Practice guidelines for preoperative fasting and the use of pharmacologic ggents to reduce the risk of pulmonary aspiration: application to healthy patients undergoing elective procedures: an updated report by the American Society of Anesthesiologists Task Force on Preoperative Fasting and the Use of Pharmacologic Agents to Reduce the Risk of Pulmonary Aspiration. *Anesthesiology* 2017;**126**(3):376–393.

8. Njoku DB, Chibilian HV, Kronish K. Hepatic physiology, pathophysiology, and anesthetic consideration. In Gropper MA, Miller RD, Cohen NH, et al., editors. *Miller's Anesthesia*, 9th ed. Elsevier, 2020; chapter 16, pp 420–443.

9. Rutkauskas S, Gedrimas V, Pundzius J, Barauskas G, Basevicius, A. Clinical and anatomical basis for the classification of the structural parts of the liver. *Medicina* 2006;**42**(2):98–106.

10. Blibel, W, Chopra, S, Curry, MP. Portal hypertension in adults. In Robson KM, editor. *UpToDate*. UpToDate Inc., 2022. Available at: www.uptodate.com/contents/portal-hypertension-in-adults

11. Bernardi M, Caraceni P, Navickis RJ, Wilkes MM. Albumin infusion in patients undergoing large-volume paracentesis: a meta-analysis of randomized trials. *Hepatology* 2012;**55**(4):1172–1181.

12. Baldini T, Miller G. Enhanced recovery protocols & optimization of perioperative outcomes. In Butterworth JF, Wasnick JD, Mackey DC, editors. *Morgan and Mikhail's Clinical Anesthesiology*, 6th ed. McGraw-Hill, 2018; chapter 48, pp 1111–1132.

Renal Anatomy and Physiology

35

Michael D. Lazar and Ryan Barnette

Water: Distribution, Balance, Compartments

Body Fluid

- Body compartments: **60–40–20 rule**
  - Total Body Water (TBW): 60% of body weight
  - Intracellular Fluid (ICF): 40% of body weight
  - Extracellular Fluid (ECF): 20% of body weight
- TBW%: ↑ in babies and ↓ in elderly and obesity
- **Plasma osmolality**: 285–295 mOsm/kg = 2 (Plasma Na^+) + Glucose/18 + BUN/2.8

Note: Glucose and BUN contributions are minimal and thus osmolality can be approximated by serum Na^+.

- **Osmoreceptors**: In the hypothalamus respond to changes in the *tonicity* of body fluid.
- **Baroreceptors**: In the right atria and great veins respond to changes in intravascular volume. These receptors prompt the inhibition or stimulation of antidiuretic hormone (ADH or vasopressin) release from the posterior pituitary. ADH acts at *V1 receptors* on *vascular smooth muscle* resulting in *vasoconstriction* and *V2 receptors* on the *renal collecting tubule cells* to increase aquaporin channels and the *reabsorption of H_2O*.
- **Strong Ion Difference (SID)**: Used to assist in categorizing disorders of acid–base balance. Cations predominate in plasma resulting in net positive +40 charge.[1]

$$SID = [strong\ cations] - [strong\ anions]$$

$$= [Na^+ + K^+ + Ca^{2+} + Mg^{2+}] - [Cl^- + lactate^-]$$

- Decrease SID → acidosis
  - Free water excess secondary to hyponatremia
  - Diarrhea
  - Increase in anions such as lactic acid or ketoacids
- Increase SID → alkalosis
  - Dehydration resulting in contraction alkalosis
  - Anion loss (i.e., chloride ions via emesis)
- SID of Normal Saline (NS) = 0 → resuscitation with NS can cause hyperchloremic metabolic acidosis

Electrolytes

Sodium

- Hyponatremia (Na < 135 meq/L)
  - Symptoms: Neurological symptoms due to cerebral swelling such as headache, vomiting, gait disturbance, seizures
  - Causes: Evaluation begins with assessment of TBW
    - Hypovolemic hyponatremia→ renal vs. extrarenal losses
    - Euvolemic hyponatremia → adrenal/thyroid insufficiency, SIADH, medications
    - Hypervolemic hyponatremia → congestive heart failure, liver cirrhosis, renal failure, nephrotic syndrome
  - Treatment: Typically asymptomatic when Na^+ > 125 meq/L. Conservative correction indicated with normal saline, salt tabs, fluid restriction. If associated with seizures or severe neurological symptoms correction can be made with hypertonic saline.
  - Goal correction: 4–6 meq/L increase over 24 hours, not to exceed 8–9 meq/L in a 24-hour period; more rapid correction results in risk of osmotic demyelination

- Hypernatremia (Na >145 mEq/L)
  - Symptoms: Lethargy, seizures, coma
  - Causes: Pure water loss, hypotonic fluid loss (water loss exceeds Na+ loss)
  - Treatment: With D5W after calculating water deficit.
    - Acute hypernatremia can be corrected at 1 mEq/L/hr for the first 6–8 hr to prevent the potential cerebral dehydration and demyelination.
    - Chronic hypernatremia can be corrected by 8 mEq/L/day.2

$$Water\ deficit = Total\ body\ water\ [I] \times \left(\frac{Serum\ Na^+}{140} - 1\right)$$

Potassium

- Hypokalemia (< 3.5 mEq/L)
  - Signs/symptoms: Severe muscle weakness, flattened T waves/U waves on ECG

- Causes: Medications (aminoglycosides, thiazide/loop diuretics, laxative abuse), GI losses (diarrhea, suctioning), renal tubular acidosis, magnesium deficiency
- Treatment: Potassium chloride – maximum of 60 mEq/L infused through peripheral vein. Up to 200 mEq/L through central veins in critical care setting.[3]
- Hyperkalemia (> 5.1 mEq/L)
  - Signs/symptoms: May manifest as muscle weakness and paralysis
    - 6–7 meq/L → peaked T waves
    - 10–12 meq/L → prolonged PR, widening QRS, Vfib, and asystole.[4]
  - Causes: Most K^+ exists intracellularly, therefore increases are likely due to transcellular shifts such that occur in acidotic states. Other causes include aldosterone antagonism, reperfusion of ischemic vascular beds, and renal failure.
  - Treatment: (1) *Stabilize cardiac membranes* with calcium, (2) promote intracellular shift of potassium with alkalosis (i.e., hyperventilation, bicarbonate), insulin with glucose, and beta-agonism, (3) promote K^+ excretion with loop diuretics, resin exchange, (4) hemodialysis.

Calcium

- Hypocalcemia (total serum calcium < 8.5 mg/dL, ionized calcium < 4.6 mg/dL)
  - 40% serum calcium is ionized → metabolically active
  - 60% serum calcium is complexed with albumin
  - Signs/symptoms: Paresthesias, muscle spasms, cardiac dysrhythmias, seizures, QT prolongation on ECG
  - Chvostek's sign – tapping facial nerve elicits facial muscle contraction
  - Trousseau's sign – carpal spasm
  - Causes: Vitamin D deficiency, hypoparathyroidism, chronic renal failure
  - Treatment: calcium gluconate/chloride[5]
- Hypercalcemia (total serum calcium > 14 mg/dL, ionized Ca > 5.8 mg/dL)
  - Signs/symptoms: lethargy, weakness, nausea, vomiting, abdominal pain, urinary stones, QT shortening, hypertension, psychiatric symptoms, polyuria
  - Causes: Most common are malignancy or hyperparathyroidism. Others include medications such as diuretics and lithium.
  - Treatment: Intravenous fluids, loop diuretics, and bisphosphonates.

Magnesium

- Hypomagnesemia (serum magnesium < 1.7mg/dL) – May cause concomitant hypokalemia, hypocalcemia

- Causes: Poor intake (i.e., chronic alcoholics, malnutrition), medication induced (i.e., diuretics, laxatives), hypercalcemia
- Signs/symptoms: Fatigue, cardiac arrhythmia, nystagmus, athetosis, muscle weakness/cramps, confusion, nervous system irritability
- Treatment: Raise serum levels > 2 mg/dL, also replace potassium and calcium
- Hypermagnesemia (serum magnesium > 2.3 mg/dL)
  - Causes: Intake (i.e., diuretics, laxatives), renal insufficiency, magnesium administration, rhabdomyolysis, lithium toxicity, adrenal insufficiency
  - Signs/symptoms: Hyporeflexia, weakness, vomiting, flushing, urinary retention, respiratory and myocardial depression (> 10 meq/L), heart block, potentiation of neuromuscular blocker by impaired release of acetylcholine at neuromuscular junction
  - Treatment: Stop intake, calcium to antagonize action, loop diuretic

Phosphorus

- Hypophosphatemia (serum phosphate < 2.5 mg/dL)
  - Causes: Chronic alcoholism, intravenous hyperalimentation (TPN), urinary phosphate wasting (i.e., Fanconi syndrome), chronic antacid use
  - Signs/symptoms: Metabolic encephalopathy, delirium, seizures, cardiac arrhythmias, respiratory weakness due to diaphragm weakness, dysphagia, ileus, decreased red- and white-blood cell function
  - Energy source for ATP therefore hypophosphatemia results in muscle weakness, leftward shift of the oxyhemoglobin curve (due to decrease in 2,3-DPG (diphosphoglycerate) levels.
- Hyperphosphatemia (serum phosphate > 4.5mg/dL)
  - Causes: Excessive intake, tumor lysis syndrome, rhabdomyolysis, acute/chronic kidney disease, hypoparathyroidism, acromegaly, bisphosphonates, vitamin D toxicity
  - Signs/symptoms: Also causes hypocalcemia therefore similar signs and symptoms as hypocalcemia such as cardiac arrhythmias, muscle spasms, acute renal failure
  - Acute severe hyperphosphatemia associated with symptomatic hypocalcemia can be life threatening
  - Treatment: Acute: Normal saline (although may worsen hypocalcemia), hemodialysis. Chronic: Low-phosphate diet, phosphate binders

Anatomy of the Kidney

- The kidneys are located in the retroperitoneum and are made up of three regions. The outer cortex, the inner medulla, and the innermost papilla, which empties into calyces that form the ureter (Table 35.1).

- The functional unit of the kidney is the nephron, which is made up of the glomerulus and the renal tubule. The glomerulus contains a group of capillaries intimately involved with the Bowman's capsule and is the site of plasma filtration. The renal tubule is made up of Bowman's capsule, proximal convoluted tubule, descending and ascending loop of Henle, distal convoluted tubule and the collecting ducts.

Renal Physiology

See Figure 35.1 for details of renal physiology.

Renal blood flow (RBF) = ~20% of C.O. *O₂ consumption is dependent on perfusion.*

Table 35.1 Renal cortex and medulla functions

Renal cortex	Renal medulla
1. Receives the majority of blood flow,	1. Low flow
2. Shorter loops of Henle	2. Longer loops of Henle associated with powerful concentration gradient for optimal reabsorption and secretion
3. Most specialized for filtration.	3. Most susceptible to ischemia

Right and left renal arteries → interlobar a. → arcuate a. → interlobular a. → afferent arteriole enters the glomerulus where ultrafiltrate is formed → exit the glomerulus as the efferent arteriole, which contributes a network of capillaries that surrounds the tubule throughout its length allowing for the continued secretion and reabsorption of substances based on a variety of direct and indirect influences.

Renal Plasma Flow (RPF) = RBF × (1 – Hct)

Filtration fraction = the percentage of filtrate in the Bowman's space relative to the renal plasma flow = GFR/RPF × 100 = ~20%

- Afferent arteriole: Dilated by *prostaglandins* so increases RPF and GFR
- Efferent arteriole: *Constricted* by *angiotensin* so decreases RPF but increases GFR
- Catecholamines increase FF by constricting afferent and efferent arterioles

GFR is directly proportional to RPF and dependent on the glomerular filtration pressure. As RPF decreases below a critical point GFR decreases substantially, thus the relationship is *not linear.*

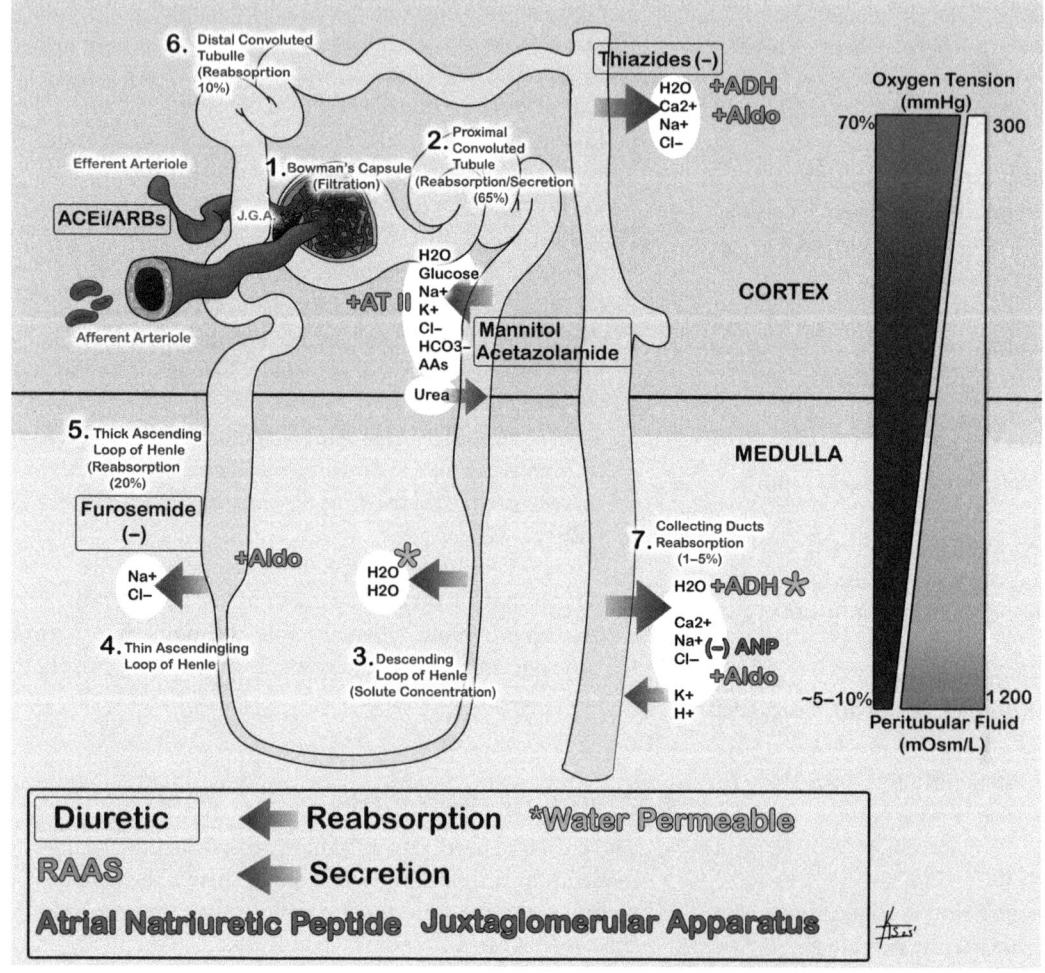

Figure 35.1 Nephron system. A black and white version of this figure will appear in some formats. For the color version, please refer to the plate section.

Control of RBF

1. Autoregulation occurs between MAPs 80–180 mmHg. MAPs < 50 mmHg result in sharp decline in GFR.
2. Tubuloglomerular feedback: macula densa cells sense decreased $[Cl^-]$ at distal tubule, low BP, or sympathetic stimulation of B_1 receptors → secrete renin
3. Cardiac atria cells sense increased volume → secrete atrial natriuretic peptide (ANP) → relaxes smooth muscle in the afferent arteriole → ↑ GFR
4. Angiotensin II, prostaglandins and catecholamines affect GFR
5. Neuronal and paracrine regulation via sympathetics from levels T4–L1 and dopamine

GFR is a reflection of overall renal function. Through the passive ultrafiltration of plasma across the glomerular membrane, the kidney is able to regulate total body salt and water content, electrolyte composition, and eliminate waste products of protein metabolism. Alterations in GFR can occur either with changes to any aspect of the Starling forces, or through a change in RPF. The forces responsible for glomerular filtration are similar to the forces that operate in systemic capillaries – the Starling forces. GFR can be calculated by *inulin clearance* (completely filtered and not secreted or reabsorbed). However, in clinical practice *creatinine clearance* is measured as an estimate of GFR.

Starling Equation

$$GFR = K_f[(P_{GC} - P_{BS}) - \pi_{GC}]$$
$$Net\ filtration = K_f([P_c - P_i] - \sigma[\pi_c - \pi_i])$$

K_f = filtration coefficient

P_{GC} = hydrostatic pressure in glomerular capillary

P_{BS} = hydrostatic pressure in Bowman's space

π_{GC} = oncotic pressure in glomerular capillary

P_c = capillary hydrostatic pressure

P_i = interstitial hydrostatic pressure

σ = reflection coefficient

π_c = capillary oncotic pressure

π_i = interstitial oncotic pressure

Tubular Resorption

See Figure 35.1 for details.

- Proximal tubule
  - 65–75% Na^+, water and Cl^- are reabsorbed.
  - Secretion of hydrogen and reabsorption of bicarbonate ions.
  - Secretes organic cations like creatinine
  - As glucose clearance exceeds > 160–200 mg/dL exceeds proximal tubules ability/threshold for reabsorption resulting in glucosuria.
  - Drugs: Carbonic anhydrase inhibitors (i.e., acetazolamide)
- Loop of Henle (LOH)
  - 25–35% ultrafiltrate makes its way to the LOH
  - 15–20% Na+, Ca^{2+} and Mg^{2+} reabsorbed
  - Drugs: Loop diuretics
- Distal Tubule
  - PTH-regulated Ca^{2+} reabsorption
  - Aldosterone mediated Na+ reabsorption
  - Drugs: Thiazides and thiazide-like diuretics (i.e., hydrochlorothiazide, metolazone)
- Collecting Duct
  - Site of sodium and H_2O reabsorption mediated by aldosterone
  - Drugs: Potassium sparing diuretics (i.e., spironolactone, amiloride)

Note: Vasopressin receptor inhibitors (i.e., conivaptan) work at both distal tubule and collecting duct

The kidneys secrete the following hormones:
- Erythropoietin (EPO)
- Renin
- Prostaglandins
- 1, 25-OH_2 Vitamin D

Renin–Angiotensin–Aldosterone System (RAAS)

Release of renin depends on beta-adrenergic stimulation, changes in afferent arteriolar wall pressure, and changes in Cl^- flow past the macula densa. Renin acts on angiotensinogen (made in the liver) to form angiotensin I (ATI) (in the lungs). Angiotensin converting enzyme (ACE) acts on AT I form angiotensin II (ATII) that is responsible for blood pressure regulation and aldosterone secretion.

ADH – produced in hypothalamus → transported to posterior pituitary for release in response to increased serum osmolarity → increases water resorption via aquaporin channel insertion in cells of the collecting tubule.[6]

- Diabetes insipidus:
  - Central – decreased secretion of ADH
  - Nephrogenic – kidneys unresponsive to ADH.
    - Associated with chronic renal disease, lithium toxicity, hypercalcemia, hypokalemia.[7]
- **SIADH (Syndrome of Inappropriate ADH)**: Excessive ADH secretion by the posterior pituitary
  - Euvolemic hyponatremia – increased diuresis secondary to atrial natriuretic peptide, inhibition of RAAS
  - Urine Na > 20 mEq/L, low serum uric acid

Drug Clearance

Three mechanisms
- Glomerular filtration
- Active secretion by the renal tubules
- Passive reabsorption by the tubules

Drugs may be metabolized by the liver into water-soluble molecules for excretion by the kidney. Alkalinization or acidification of urine can ionize and trap molecules within the tubule for excretion.
- Weak bases → trapped in acidic environments
  - Treatment: Ammonium chloride
- Weak acids (ex. aspirin) → trapped in basic environments
  - Treatment: Bicarbonate

Renal Function Tests

Blood–Urea–Nitrogen (BUN)

Protein digestion in the liver produces urea, which aids in the excretion of nitrogenous waste products such as ammonia in the kidneys. It is a surrogate of renal health and is partially reabsorbed at the proximal tubule. When flow to the kidneys is reduced in conditions, such as hypovolemia, the reabsorption is increased and BUN levels rise. Besides intravascular volume status, the BUN levels are *altered with nutritional status, pregnancy, hepatic disease, GI hemorrhage, among others.*

Azotemia = increased BUN and creatinine

Creatinine Clearance

Cockcroft–Gault Equation

$$= \frac{(140 - \text{age}) \times \text{wt (kg)}}{\text{Serum creatinine (mg/dL)} \times 72} (\times 0.85 \text{ for women})$$

Creatinine is secreted by the renal tubules. Therefore, *creatinine clearance* is an overestimation of GFR.

Urinalysis

1. RBC – indicates of glomerular filtration dysregulation. (e.g., trauma, infections, tumors)
2. WBC– infection
3. Proteinuria – parenchymal disease
4. Fatty casts – nephrotic syndrome
5. Ketones – DKA, starvation
6. Urine-specific gravity: (range: 1.003–1.03) indirect measure of hydration
7. Urine osmolality: (350–500 mOsm) indirect measure of hydration
8. Urine sodium: (20–40 mEq) indirect measure of sodium excretion

   Oliguria = urine output < 0.5 cc/kg/hr
   Anuria = UOP < 100 mL/day (Table 35.2)

Fractional Excretion of Sodium (FENa⁺): Utilized to assist in differentiating prerenal, intrarenal, and postrenal etiologies of acute renal failure.

$$\text{FENa}^+ = \frac{\text{Na}_{\text{urine}} \times \text{creatinine}_{\text{plasma}} \times 100}{\text{Na}_{\text{plasma}} \times \text{creatinine}_{\text{uninary}}}$$

>1% = intrarenal or postrenal
<1% = prerenal

Renal Pathology

Acute kidney injury (AKI) = abrupt loss of kidney function resulting in retention of urea and other nitrogenous waste products and in the dysregulation of extracellular volume and electrolytes.

AKI defined according to KDIGO (Kidney Disease Improving Global Outcomes):
- Increase in serum creatinine by > 0.3 mg/dL within 48 hr; or
- Increase in serum creatinine to > 1.5× baseline, which is known to have occurred within the prior 7 days; or
- Urine volume < 0.5 mL/kg/hr for 6 hr (Table 35.3)

Prerenal kidney injury occurs with decreased perfusion to the kidneys, which may occur due to hypotension, blood loss, heart failure, and liver disease.

Contrast-Induced Nephropathy (CIN)

- Injury to the kidneys is multifactorial
- Risk factors: Diabetes mellitus, chronic kidney failure, concomitant exposure to other nephrotoxic agents, dehydration, advanced age.
- Prevention: Normal saline infusion 100 mL/hr × 12 hr prior to exposure is the only intervention supported by most literature. The literature is inconclusive on the effectiveness of N-acetylcysteine, and bicarbonate.

Table 35.2 Renal Function Tests

Test of glomerular function	Normal values	Causes of pathology
BUN	8–20 mg/dL	Dehydration, protein intake, GI bleeding, catabolism
Serum creatinine	0.5–1.2 mg/dL	Age, muscle mass, catabolism
Creatinine clearance	120 mL/min	Age, medications

Table 35.3 AKI according to KDIGO

Test	Postrenal	Renal	Prerenal
BUN:creatinine	< 15	< 15	> 20
FENa	> 4%	> 1%	< 1%
Urine Na	> 40	> 20	< 20
Urine osmolality	< 350	< 350	> 500

Chronic Kidney Disease (CKD)

CKD is divided into different stages of disease according to the GFR and presence of albuminuria:

1. Stage 1 disease is defined by a normal GFR (> 90 mL/minute/1.73 m^2) and persistent albuminuria
2. Stage 2 disease is a GFR between 60 and 89 mL/minute/1.73 m^2 and persistent albuminuria
3. Stage 3 disease is a GFR between 30 and 59 mL/minute/1.73 m^2
4. Stage 4 disease is a GFR between 15 and 29 mL/minute/1.73 m^2
5. Stage 5 disease is a GFR of <15 mL/minute/1.73 m^2 or ESRD
   - Causes: Diabetes mellitus, chronic hypertension, glomerulonephritis, obstructive, toxicity, hepatitis B/C, and HIV
   - Signs and symptoms of chronic kidney insufficiency typically manifest when GFR <15 mL/min and when present may indicate end stage renal disease (ESRD).

End-Stage Renal Disease

Hyperkalemia, hypocalcemia, metabolic acidosis, uremia (a cause of platelet dysfunction), hyperphosphatemia, anemia (decreased erythropoietin and iron deficiency)

- Treatment → dialysis vs. *continuous veno-venous hemofiltration (CVVH)*
- Indications (AEIOU)

  Acidosis (pH < 7.1)

  Electrolyte abnormalities (hyperkalemia > 6.5)

  Ingestion of toxic substance that can be dialyzed

  Overload (volume)

  Symptomatic **U**remia (> 30 mg/dL)

- CVVH: Convection and ultrafiltration, reserved for critically ill patients that would not tolerate cardiovascular stress associated with conventional dialysis. Greater overall clearance and volume removal compared to hemodialysis (24-hour removal compared with 3–4 hours)
- Hemodialysis – diffusion of substances across a semipermeable membrane.
  - Adverse effects: Hypotension (too much fluid removed), "dialysis disequilibrium" (rapid fluid and

urea shifts resulting in cerebral edema, headache, coma), hypocalcemia, fever, hypokalemia-induced arrhythmias, bleeding (due to heparinization)[8]
  - Electrolyte disturbances: Hypokalemia/magnesemia/calcemia, increased pH due to bicarbonate infusion, hyper or hyponatremia.[8]

Acid–Base Balance and the Kidney

The kidneys are essential in the management of acid–base balance in the body through the reabsorption of HCO_3^- and the excretion of H^+ (or NH_4^+).

HCO_3^- reabsorption (primarily at the proximal tubule)

- Na^+/H^+ exchanger at the luminal membrane of cells pumps H^+ ions into the lumen → combines with filtered HCO_3^- → forms $H_2CO_3^-$ → breaks down into CO_2 and H_2O, which are reabsorbed into the cell where they are converted via carbonic anhydrase back to HCO_3^- and H^+. The bicarbonate is reclaimed and the H^+ is used to repeat the cycle.
- Contraction alkalosis – activation of renin–angiotensin system results in angiotensin II mediated stimulation of the Na^+/H^+ exchanger → increase reabsorption of HCO_3^-.
  - Seen with diuretic use and as a complication of vomiting

H^+ Excretion (primarily at the distal tubule and collecting duct) hydrogen combines with HPO_4^{2-}, NH_3, and Cl^-.

- H^+ ATPase – stimulated by aldosterone
- H^+/K^+ ATPase

Respiratory Alkalosis

- Initial change: ↓PCO_2 due to increased alveolar ventilation
- Compensatory response: ↓HCO_3
  - Acute → Intracellular buffering, for every 10 mmHg change in PCO_2 bicarbonate will fall **2 mEq/L.**
  - Chronic → decreased renal reabsorption of bicarb, for every 10 mmHg change in PCO_2 bicarb will fall **5 mEq/L**
- Causes: Hyperventilation secondary to pneumonia, pulmonary edema, PE, salicylates, pregnancy, sepsis, anxiety

Respiratory Alkalosis

- Initial change: ↑PCO_2
- Compensatory response: ↑HCO_3^-
  - Acute → intracellular buffering, **1 mEq/L** ↑HCO_3^- for every 10 mmHg change in PCO_2.
  - Chronic → generation of new bicarb due to excretion of ammonium, **4 mEq/L** ↑HCO_3^- for every 10 mmHg change in PCO_2.
- Causes: hypoventilation secondary to sedatives, neuromuscular pathology, airway obstruction, COPD/asthma

Table 35.4 Useful equations

✓Henderson–Hasselbach equation	$pH = pKa + \log [A^-]/[HA]$
✓Winters formula	$P_{CO_2} = 1.5\,(HCO_3^-) + 8 \pm 2$
Estimates expected change in CO_2 in metabolic acidosis.	
✓Anion Gap	$(AG) = Na^+ - (Cl^- + HCO_3^-) = 10\text{--}15$ (normal value)
Acidemia = pH < 7.36	
Alkalemia = pH > 7.44	

Note: "1–2–4–5" rule: change of 1, 2, 4, 5 mEq/L for acute acidosis, acute alkalosis, chronic acidosis, chronic alkalosis, respectively

Metabolic Alkalosis

- Initial change: ↓HCO_3^-
- Compensatory response: ↓ PCO_2 via decreased ventilation
  - Causes: GI suctioning, vomiting, loop/thiazide diuretics, primary aldosteronism

Metabolic Acidosis

- Initial change: ↓HCO_3^-
- Compensatory response: ↓PCO_2 via increased ventilation, $PCO2 = (1.5\,[HCO_3^-]) + 8\ 2$ = expected compensation
- Causes: "MUDPILES" and "HARDUPS"
  - Causes of anion gap metabolic acidosis (**MUDPILES**):
    - Methanol, uremia, diabetic ketoacidosis, propylene glycol, infection/isoniazid, lactic acid, ethylene glycol, salicylates[9]
  - Causes of non-anion gap metabolic acidosis (**HARDUPS**):

- Hyperalimentation (TPN), acetazolamide/topiramate, renal tubular acidosis/CKD, diarrhea, ureterosigmoid conduit, pancreatico-enteric fistula, saline
- Treatment: Alkalinize urine to trap ionic species for excretion, correct acidemia, hemodialysis in critical cases.
  - Salicylate poisoning: Tinnitus, tachypnea (CNS stimulation → respiratory alkalosis), tachycardia, sweating, nausea/vomiting, hyperthermia, altered mentation.
  - Ethylene glycol poisoning: Ingredient in antifreeze, ingestion symptoms include altered mentation, seizures, pulmonary edema, kidney failure associated with calcium oxalate crystals. Metabolism by alcohol dehydrogenase generates toxic formic acid.
  - Methanol: Metabolized by alcohol dehydrogenase into toxic formaldehyde resulting in symptoms that include nausea/vomiting.
    - Treatment: EtOH and fomepizole compete for alcohol dehydrogenase-limiting metabolism of methanol and ethylene glycol.

Acid–Base Tips

See Table 35.4 and accompanying text for equations and useful tips.

- Acid–base disorder workup? Obtain pH, PCO_2, HCO_3.
- First, determine primary disorder.
- Second, calculate anion gap.
- Third, determine whether compensation is expected.

The respiratory system compensates for acid–base disturbances rather quickly, whereas the renal system's response is delayed.

References

1. Neligan PJ. Monitoring and managing perioperative electrolyte abnormalities, acid–base disorders, and fluid replacement. In Longnecker DE, Brown DL, Newman MF, Zapol WM, editors. *Anesthesiology*, 2nd ed. McGraw-Hill, 2012; chapter 35.

2. Liamis G, Filippatos TD, Elisaf MS. Evaluation and treatment of hypernatremia: a practical guide for physicians. *Postgrad Med* 2016;**128**(3): 299–306.

3. Wee T, Goldberg M, Gulati A, Schleyer A. Hypokalemia. 2010, September 15. Available at: https://eresources.library.mssm.edu:2073/#!/content/medical_topic/21-s2.0-1014738

4. Hyperkalemia. OpenAnesthesia. Last updated April 3, 2023. Available at: www.openanesthesia.org/keywords/hyperkalemia/

5. Regmi S, Silva P, Pollak E, Lash R. Hypocalcemia. 2012. Available at: https://eresources.library.mssm.edu:2073/#!/content/medical_topic/21-s2.0-1014736

6. SIADH electrolytes. OpenAnesthesia. (n.d.). Retrieved March 7, 2017, from https://selfstudyplus.openanesthesia.org/kw/entry/14051

7. Diabetes insipidus intracranial surgery. OpenAnesthesia. (n.d.). Retrieved March 7, 2017, from https://selfstudyplus.openanesthesia.org/kw/entry/13547

8. Hemodialysis effects. OpenAnesthesia. (n.d.). Retrieved March 7, 2017, from https://selfstudyplus.openanesthesia.org/kw/entry/14051

9. Metabolic acidosis: etiology. OpenAnesthesia. (n.d.). Retrieved March 5, 2017, from https://selfstudyplus.openanesthesia.org/kw/entry/-KJIGu7f9QcFZFfOJ-A7

Renal Pharmacology

Sanford Littwin

Diuretics

Carbonic Anhydrase Inhibitors: Acetazolamide, Methazolamide
- Site of Action: Proximal tubule
- Mechanism: Inhibits the activity of carbonic anhydrase (enzyme that converts $CO_2 + H_2O \rightleftarrows HCO_3 + H^+$)
  - Reduces hydrogen ion secretion at renal tubule, with increased excretion of sodium, potassium, bicarbonate, and water
- Adverse Drug Reactions: Inhibits sodium resorption, interferes with hydrogen excretion
  - Chronic administration may lead to *hyperchloremic, hypokalemic acidosis*
  - Alkalinized urine may lead to nephrolithiasis
  - Peripheral neuropathy, sulfa allergy
- Rarely used in clinical practice
- Can be used to treat glaucoma to prevent production of aqueous humor

Loop Diuretics: Furosemide, Torsemide, Ethacrynic Acid, Bumetanide
- Site of Action: Thick ascending limb of the loop of Henle
- Mechanism: inhibits Na^+, K^+, $2\ Cl^-$ transport system
  - blocks more ions, therefore produces more diuresis in comparison to other diuretics
- Adverse Drug Reactions: Inhibits sodium and chloride resorption, augments secretion of potassium
  - Chronic administration may lead to *hypochloremic, hypokalemic metabolic alkalosis*
  - Ototoxicity, hypokalemia, sulfa allergy, gout
  - Hyperuricemia (gout), hypocalcemia, hypomagnesemia, hyperglycemia, pancreatitis, hypokalemia, ototoxicity
- Used for moderate to severe fluid retention and hypertension
- Brief duration of action (lasts approximately 4–6 hours)
- Has a more immediate effect than any other diuretic medication
- Used in acute clinical situations of volume overload, especially when water retention affects pulmonary physiology

Thiazides: Hydrochlorothiazide, Chlorthalidone, Metolazone
- Site of Action: Distal tubule and connecting segment

- Mechanism: Blocks Na^+/Cl^- co-transporter
  - Leads to increase in urinary sodium and eventual diuresis
- Adverse Drug Reaction: Inhibits sodium resorption, augments secretion of potassium
  - Leads to hypokalemia (through acceleration of sodium-potassium exchange)
  - May lead to hyperglycemia, hyperlipidemia, hyperuricemia (gout), hypomagnesemia, hypercalcemia
  - Chronic administration may lead to hypochloremic, hypokalemic metabolic alkalosis
- Used for mild to moderate hypertension

Potassium-Sparing Diuretics: Spironolactone, Triamterene, Amiloride, Eplerenone
- Site of Action: Cortical collecting tubule
- Mechanism: Aldosterone-sensitive sodium channels. Works via two different mechanisms:
  - Spironolactone: Competitively inhibits the mineralocorticoid receptor aldosterone, which increases the synthesis and activity of the Na^+/K^+ pump
  - Amiloride and triamterene: Directly decrease sodium channel activity
- Adverse Drug Reactions: Inhibits sodium resorption and sodium-potassium exchange (preventing loss of potassium)
  - Chronic administration may lead to *hyperkalemia, gynecomastia, hirsutism*
- Spironolactone
  - Onset of action may take several days for full effect
- Amiloride; triamterene
  - Quick onset

Osmotic Diuretics: Mannitol, Glycerin
- Site of Action: Proximal tubule
- Mechanism: Freely filtered, nonreabsorbable, nonmetabolized sugar alcohol
  - Remains in the tubular lumen, creating osmotic gradient of water into lumen
- Adverse Drug Reactions: Hyperosmolality which reduces cellular water, increased excretion of water, volume depletion and hypernatremia

- ○ High doses lead to hyperosmolar plasma, extracellular volume expansion, dilutional *hyponatremia, hyperkalemia,* and metabolic acidosis
- Used to prevent renal failure
- Used to reduce intracranial pressure
  - ○ Does not cross blood–brain barrier
    - ▪ Water is pulled from intracranial interstitial space into the blood

Dopaminergic Agents

Dopamine

- Mechanism: Mixed agonist effects with dopaminergic, α and β receptors.
  - ○ *Dopaminergic*: Effects mediated by increased cAMP.
    - ▪ Low infusion rate (1 to 5 mcg/kg/min): Increased renal blood flow and urine output
    - ▪ Intermediate dosage (5 to 15 mcg/kg/min): Increased renal blood flow, heart rate, cardiac output, and blood pressure

- ▪ High dosage (greater than 15 mcg/kg/min): Alpha-adrenergic effects predominate, vasoconstriction, increased blood pressure
- ○ *α-alpha:* (> 5 microgram/kg/min)
  - ▪ α1 stimulation leading to vasoconstriction
  - ▪ Theoretically decreased renal blood flow
- ○ *β-beta*: (3–5 microgram/kg/min dosing)
  - ▪ Direct and indirect β 1 and β 2 stimulation
  - ▪ Increased cardiac contractility and cardiac output

Fenoldopam

- Mechanism: Selective D_1 receptor agonist
  - ○ Decreases blood pressure
  - ○ Increases renal blood flow, creatinine clearance, urinary flow and sodium excretion
  - ○ Does not directly cause increased cardiac contractility but may lead to reflex tachycardia

Further Reading

Hropot M, Fowler N, Karlmark B, Giebisch G. Tubular action of diuretics: distal effects on electrolyte transport and acidification. *Kidney Int* 1985;**28**:477.

Jain A, Chen H. ROSE-AHF and lessons learned. *Curr Heart Fail Rep* 2014;**11** (3):260–265.

Rose BD. Diuretics. *Kidney Int* 1991;**39**:336.

Sica DA, Carter B, Cushman W, Hamm L. Thiazide and loop diuretics. *J Clin Hypertens (Greenwich)* 2011;**13** (9):639–643. doi:10.1111/j.1751-7176.201 1.00512.x.

Weber RR, McCoy CE, Ziemniak JA, et al. Pharmacokinetic and pharmacodynamic properties of intravenous fenoldopam, a dopamine1-receptor agonist, in hypertensive patients. *Br J Clin Pharmac* 1988;**25**(1):17–21.

Hematologic System: Coagulation, Anticoagulation, Antiplatelet, and Thrombolytics

Raj Parekh and Travis Burnett

Hemostasis

- **Primary Hemostasis:** Formation of the platelet plug (Figure 37.1)
  - Injured endothelium exposes procoagulant subendothelial matrix which *binds to platelets.*
  - Platelet Adhesion: Occurs via *von Willebrand Factor (vWF)* and transmembrane glycoproteins (GP)
  - Platelet Activation: Platelets become activated by exposed subendothelium and *thrombin*, leading to conformational changes causing multiple events.
    - ADP-rich granules released, allowing ADP to bind platelet receptors (i.e., P2Y$_{12}$) to recruit more platelets
    - Arachidonic acid produced and converted to thromboxane A$_2$ by COX-1
  - Platelet Plug: Fibrinogen cross-links with GPIIb/IIIa receptors on platelets to form the *platelet plug.*
- **Secondary Hemostasis:** Coagulation factors *produce fibrin,* which cross-links to stabilize the platelet plug (Figure 37.2).

  - Extrinsic Pathway: Exposed tissue factor in the endothelium will *activate thrombin* (factor IIa) and factor IXa.
  - Intrinsic Pathway: Thrombin activates *factors X, XI, and VIIIa.*
  - Common Pathway: Thrombin also activates *factor V.*

Three common groups of drugs (anticoagulants, antiplatelet agents, and thrombolytic agents) are used to treat and prevent particular vascular diseases. Older anticoagulants include unfractionated heparin, low molecular weight heparin, and warfarin, whereas newer oral anticoagulants include direct thrombin inhibitors and factor Xa inhibitors. Indications for newer drugs are continually changing as new data are published and reviewed by the FDA. The same is true for antiplatelet agents where more effective drugs are being discovered and used in everyday practice.

Anticoagulants

Unfractionated Heparin (UFH)[1–4]

- Mechanism:
  - *Binds antithrombin III* and induces conformational change that facilitates its ability to primarily inactivate

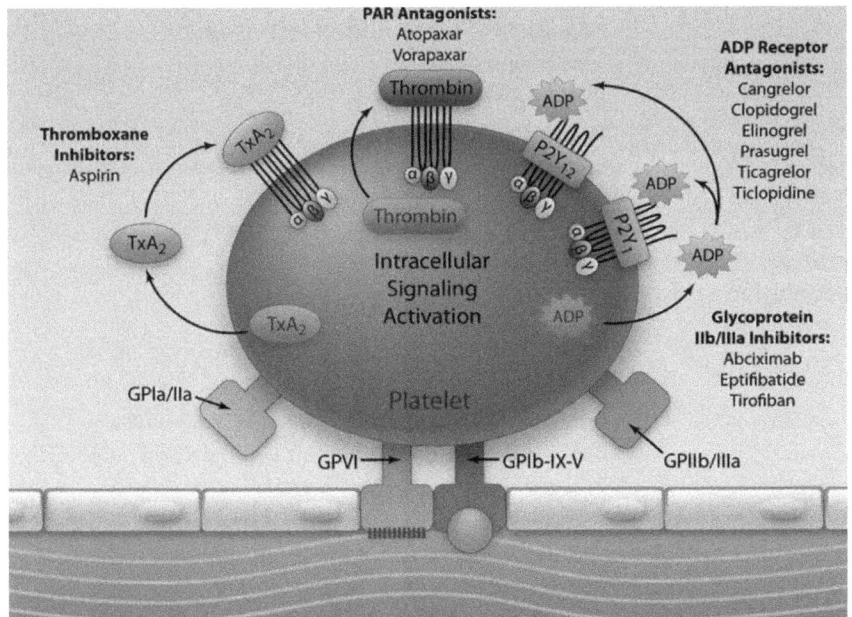

Figure 37.1 Formation of a platelet plug. A black and white version of this figure will appear in some formats. For the color version, please refer to the plate section.

The three pathways that makeup the classical blood coagulation pathway

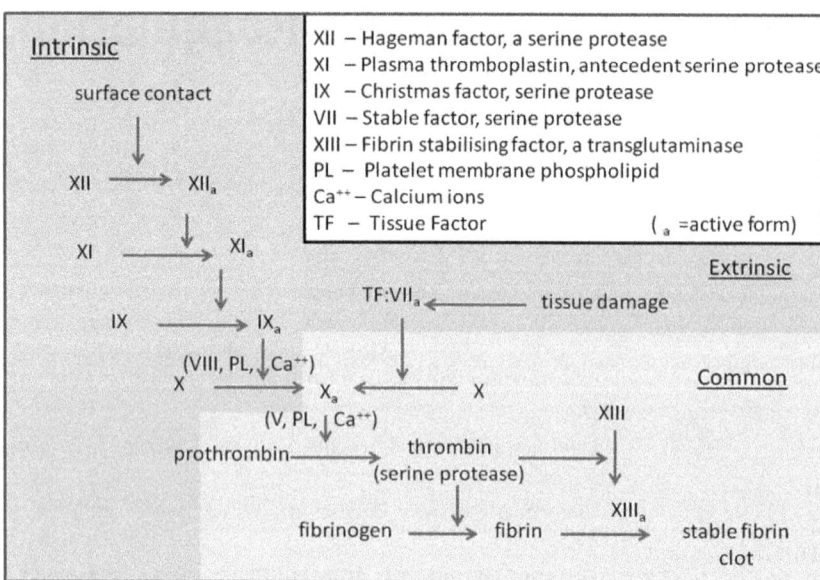

Figure 37.2 Coagulation cascade. Data from Pallister CJ, Watson MS. Haematology, 2nd ed. Pallister and Watson Scion Publishing Ltd., 2010.

thrombin (factor IIa) and factor Xa but also *inactivates factors VII, IX, XI, and XII.*

- ○ Inactivating thrombin prevents the conversion of fibrinogen to fibrin.
- Advantages: Preferred in renal failure
- Disadvantages: Hereditary or acquired antithrombin III deficiency can result in heparin resistance, such that normal doses of heparin fail to provide adequate anticoagulation.
  - ○ Risk of heparin-induced thrombocytopenia (HIT) – two types, see Table 37.1
    - Bleeding
    - Rapid bolus → moderate ↓SVR and BP (unclear reason)
- Reversal: With protamine – common reversal dose is 1 mg of protamine per 100 units of heparin

Low Molecular Weight Heparin (LMWH)[1,2,5,6]

- Mechanism:
  - ○ Binds and *enhances* effects of *antithrombin III*
  - ○ LMWH-antithrombin III complex binds to and preferentially *inactivates factor Xa.*
  - ○ Has shorter saccharide units than unfractionated heparin and so make LMWH ineffective in inhibiting thrombin directly
- Advantages: Does not require regular PTT screening and so can be used for outpatient treatment.
- Disadvantages:
  - ○ Increased risk of bleeding with long-term use
  - ○ Risk of HIT, monitor platelet count periodically (lower risk compared with UFH)
  - ○ Decreased kidney function could significantly increase plasma level.

Warfarin[1,2,7,8]

- Mechanism:
  - ○ Inhibits *vitamin K epoxide reductase* in the liver, which reduces the *gamma carboxylation of vitamin K-dependent coagulation factors*
  - ○ Decreases the amount of vitamin K-dependent clotting proteins: *Factors II, VII, IX, and X and anticoagulant proteins C+S* (hence a transient pro-coagulant effect)
- Drug Interactions:
  - ○ CYP450 inducers: St. John's wort, barbiturates, carbamazepine, phenytoin, rifampin → *decreased warfarin effects*
  - ○ CYP450 inhibitors: Levofloxacin, omeprazole, amiodarone → *increased warfarin effects*
- Disadvantages:
  - ○ Bleeding
  - ○ Warfarin-induced skin necrosis: Protein C with a half-life of 6 hours has quick decline in plasma, resulting in initial shift toward clotting
  - ○ Crosses the placenta (Table 37.2)

Direct Thrombin Inhibitors[1,2]

- Mechanism: Bind directly to thrombin (factor IIa) which:
  - ○ Prevent the conversion of fibrinogen to fibrin
  - ○ Prevent the activation of factors V, VIII, IX, and XIII
  - ○ Prevent the activation of platelets
- Indications: Include treatment and prevention of venous thromboembolism (VTE), atrial fibrillation, acute coronary syndrome, and HIT (Table 37.3)

Table 37.1 Types of HIT

Type
HIT type I: • *Non-immune mediated* • Rapid onset (2–5 days) • *< 50% decrease platelets* • Resolves on its own	**Protamine reversal:** *acid–base neutralization*–protamine (+) antagonizes heparin (−) **Protamine reactions:** • Type 1: *systemic hypotension* secondary to rapid administration causing *mast cell and histamine release* • Type 2: *anaphylaxis from IgE mediated* dose-independent reaction in a patient with *previous exposure* • Type 3: *pulmonary hypertensive crisis* via protamine-heparin complex stimulation of *thromboxane A2 release*
HIT type II: • *IgG reaction* to platelet factor 4-heparin (PF4) complexes • Onset 5–14 days • *Systemic thrombosis* (venous and arterial) • Discontinue heparin and start alternative IV anticoagulant (i.e., direct thrombin inhibitor)	

Table 37.2 Heparin, LMWH, and warfarin[1–4,6,8]

Type	Onset	Half-Life	Metabolism	Monitoring	Reversal
Heparin IV, SQ	IV: immediate SQ: 20–30 min	30–60 min	Inactivated in liver and kidney	PTT ACT (high dose)	Protamine
LMWH SQ	20–60 min	3–6 hr	Renal clearance	Factor Xa assay[a]	Protamine[b]
Warfarin PO, IV	90 min	35–40 hr	Hepatic (CYP450)	PT/INR	Non-urgent: vitamin K Urgent: FFP, prothrombin complex concentrate (PCC)

[a] Routine monitoring typically unnecessary.

[b] Less reliable reversal agent than for heparin.

Factor Xa Inhibitors

- Mechanism: Bind to factor Xa, which prevents it from converting prothrombin to thrombin
- Same potential indications as direct thrombin inhibitors (Table 37.4)

Antiplatelet Agents[2,14]

Aspirin

- Mechanism:
  - Irreversible *inhibitor of COX-1 and COX-2*
  - Prevents formation of thromboxane (potent platelet aggregator)
- Indication: Secondary prevention of cardiovascular events in patients with coronary artery disease, peripheral vascular disease, cerebrovascular disease
- Disadvantages (dose related): Dyspepsia → peptic ulcers with bleeding/perforation

Dipyridamole

- Weak antiplatelet agent on its own, but extended-release formulation combined with low-dose aspirin is used for prevention of stroke in patients with transient ischemic attacks (TIA)

- Mechanism:
  - *Inhibits phosphodiesterase* → blocks the breakdown of cAMP
  - Increased cAMP → reduce intracellular calcium → inhibits platelet activation

GP IIB/IIIA Inhibitors

- Mechanism: Prevents binding of fibrinogen and vWF to GP IIb/IIIa receptors, causing inhibition of platelet aggregation
- Reversal: None (control by discontinuation of drug)

ADP Receptor Antagonists

- Mechanism: Interferes with fibrinogen binding to platelets and thus *inhibits ADP-induced primary and secondary platelet aggregation* (Table 37.5)

Antithrombotic Agents

Tissue Plasmin Activators (tPa)[14]

- Also serves as *anticoagulant*: Fibrinolysis generates increased amounts of circulating fibrin degradation products → *inhibit platelet aggregation* by binding to platelet surfaces

Table 37.3 Direct thrombin inhibitors[1,2,9–11]

Type type	Mechanism	Half-life	Metabolism	Monitoring	Notes
Argatroban IV	*Reversible* binding to catalytic site of thrombin	45 min	Hepatic	PTT, ACT	– Preferred in renal insufficiency
Dabigatran PO	*Prodrug* converted in liver; binds *reversibly* to thrombin	12–14 hr	Renal clearance	Dilute thrombin time, PTT	– Peak effect in 2 hr – Dose adjustment in renal insufficiency – Reversal with idarucizumab (Praxbind) – Activated charcoal and hemodialysis can also aid in non-emergent reversal
Hirudin IV, topical	Binds *irreversibly* to thrombin	40–80 min	Renal clearance	ECT (ecarin clotting time)	– Naturally occurring peptide found in leeches
Bivalirudin IV	Binds *reversibly* to thrombin	25 min	Peptidase degradation, renal excretion	Low-dose: PTT High-dose: ACT	– Studied for use as heparin substitute in cardiac surgery with HIT type II
Lepirudin IV (infusion)	Binds *irreversibly* to thrombin	60 min	Renal	PTT	– Recombinant form of hirudin – Accumulates in renal failure – *Fatal anaphylaxis* (if treated again within 3 months of exposure)

Table 37.4 Factor Xa inhibitors[1,2,5,11–13]

Type	Mechanism	Half-life	Metabolism	Monitoring	Notes
Fondaparinux IV	Pentasaccharide unit binds and activates antithrombin III	21 hr	Cleared unchanged by kidneys	*Not required	– Does NOT cause HIT – Increased risk of bleeding with long term use
Rivaroxaban PO	*Reversibly* binds and inhibits factor Xa, preventing conversion of prothrombin to thrombin	5–9 hr	33% renal clearance 66% fecal/bilary	– Anti-Xa assay – Dilute PT assay	– Peak effect 2.5–4 hr – Emergent reversal with PCC4 or PCC3 plus FFP – Avoid with CrCl < 15 mL/min
Apixaban PO	*Reversibly* binds and inhibits factor Xa, preventing conversion of prothrombin to thrombin	15 hr	25% renal clearance 75% fecal/biliary	– Anti-Xa assay – Dilute PT assay	– Peak effect 1–2 hr

- Avoid surgery or puncture of noncompressible vessel within 10-day period after use
- Native:
  - Streptokinase, urokinase
  - Potent activators of plasmin
  - Mechanism: Cleave bond from plasminogen to form plasmin
- Exogenous:
  - Alteplase, tenecteplase
  - Mechanism: More fibrin selective; less selectivity for circulating plasminogen

Alternatives to Transfusion

- Normovolemic Hemodilution[15]
  - Principle: If RBC concentration decreased, total RBC loss is reduced when a large amount of blood is lost and cardiac output maintained because intravascular volume maintained
  - Mechanism:
    - 1–2 units removed just prior to surgery via large-bore IV
    - Replace with crystalloid/colloids: Patient remains normovolemic, but now with Hct 21–25%
    - Blood stored in CPDA (citrate–phosphate–dextrose–adenine) bag at room temperature (up to 6 hr) to preserve platelet function
    - Blood should be infused in reverse order of removal: First unit has highest Hct, platelets, and clotting factors and is preferably transfused last.
  - Effects:
    - Decrease in blood viscosity → increase tissue perfusion and reduce intraoperative RBC loss
    - Decreased arterial O_2 content → compensatory tachycardia and increased cardiac output → increased myocardial O_2 consumption → potential risk of myocardial ischemia

- Sequestration:[15]
  - Principle: Pooling of blood in vascular space until it is needed
  - Mechanism:
    - Tourniquets placed on the upper and lower extremities allow blood to be isolated from the general circulation.
    - Sequestered volume replaced with crystalloid/colloid
    - When tourniquets released, blood bolus returns to circulation
  - Effects:
    - Volume overload may occur with tourniquet release.
    - Greater tourniquet time → greater amount of acidic blood returned to circulation
    - Risk of stasis and thrombosis in sequestered extremities
- Autotransfusion:[15]
  - Preoperative:
    - Collection 4–5 weeks prior to procedure
    - Minimum requirements to donate 1 unit: Hct ≥ 34% or Hgb ≥11 g/dL
    - Requires concurrent iron supplementation and erythropoietin therapy
    - Advantages:
      - Reduced risk of infection and transfusion reaction
      - Conservation of blood resources
      - Blood can be frozen indefinitely for later use
    - Disadvantages:
      - Expensive
      - Does not necessarily reduce need for allogenic transfusion
      - Does not reduce certain risks: Immunological reactions due to clerical errors, bacterial contamination, improper storage

Table 37.5 Antiplatelet drugs[2,14]

Type	Mechanism	Half-life	Metabolism	Monitoring	Notes
Abciximab IV	GP IIB/IIIA inhibitor	30 min	Proteolytic cleavage (unbound)	Not recommended	– 24–48 hr for platelets to normalize
Eptifibatide IV	GP IIB/IIIA inhibitor	2.5 hr	Renal clearance/ urinary excretion	Not recommended	– 8 hr for platelets to normalize
Tirofiban IV	GP IIB/IIIA inhibitor	2 hr	Negligible metabolism (excreted in urine unchanged)	Not recommended	– 8 hr for platelets to normalize
Clopidogrel PO	Prodrug metabolized by P450 to irreversibly inhibit platelet $P2Y_{12}$ receptors	6 hr	Hepatic (active and inactive metabolites)	Not recommended	– Steady state in 7 days – 60% platelet inhibition – Preferred to ticlopidine (better safety profile) – Higher incidence of heightened platelet reactivity (HPR) and hence treatment failure then prasugrel
Ticlodipine PO	Inhibits ADP receptor mediated platelet activation	13 hr	Hepatic (active metabolite)	Not recommended	– Steady state in 14–21 days – Black Box Warning: agranulocytosis, TTP, aplastic anemia – Not available in United States
Prasugrel PO	P2Y-12 receptor irreversible inhibitor	4 hr	Rapid intestinal and serum metabolism via ester hydrolysis, then CYP450 to active metabolite	$P2Y_{12}$ assay, TEG	– Peak effect 1 hr – 90% platelet inhibition – Contraindicated if prior TIA/stroke
Ticagrelor PO	Reversible ADP analogue on P2Y-12 receptor	7–9 hr	Hepatic via CYP34A	$P2Y_{12}$ assay, TEG	– Peak effect 2–4 hr

○ Intraoperative (Cell Saver)
○ Requires estimated blood volume needs to be > 1,000–1,500 mL to be effective
○ Mechanism:
  ▪ Blood loss aspirated into reservoir and mixed with heparin
  ▪ RBCs are concentrated and washed to remove debris and anticoagulant
  ▪ Salvaged blood concentrate reinfused to patient contains RBC and normal saline with Hct 50–60%
○ Advantages:
  ▪ Often accepted by Jehovah's Witnesses
  ▪ Valuable in patients with alloantibodies
  ▪ Limits exposure to pathogens
○ Disadvantages:
  ▪ Contraindications: Septic contamination, malignancy
  ▪ Complications: Dilutional coagulopathy (coagulation factors, platelets, and calcium are not salvaged), hemolysis, air embolism, DIC, reinfusion of excess anticoagulant

Blood Substitutes:[15]

Can carry and release oxygen and offer benefit for short periods, there is still a lack of evidence of their safety and efficacy for longer periods (30 days)

• Polymerized Hemoglobin-Based Oxygen Carriers (HBOCs):
  ○ Hemoglobin molecules polymerized for longevity
  ○ Advantage: Ability to load hemoglobin at physiological PaO_2 (just like normal Hgb)
  ○ Disadvantages:
    ▪ Hypertension: Complication of clinical trials due to inhibition of endogenous NO
    ▪ Toxicity to myocardium, liver, and kidneys documented (currently offered on a compassionate use basis)
• Perfluorocarbon Emulsions (PFCEs):
  ○ Hydrophilic liquids with fluoride and carbon atoms
  ○ Advantage: Can dissolve significant amounts of gases, including O_2 and CO_2
  ○ Disadvantage: Linear O_2 dissociation curve, thus supplemental O_2 and supraphysiological PaO_2 required to maximize oxygen delivery
• Neither type has been released for clinical use

Erythropoietin:[15]

• Glycoprotein hormone produced by peritubular cells of the kidney
• Mechanism: Acts as a cytokine for RBC production in the bone marrow by *promoting blast cell maturation*
• Use:
  ○ Preoperative anemia for elective, non-cardiac surgery → decreases need for intraoperative blood transfusions, and overall morbidity and mortality rates
  ○ Jehovah's Witnesses (off-label)
  ○ Stimulate erythropoiesis in CKD patients
• Typically takes 2 weeks or more to gain as much as 2 g/dL of Hgb concentration
• Recombinant erythropoietin is very expensive
• Black Box Warning: Death, MI, stroke, venous thromboembolism
• Must dose with supplemental iron (Table 37.6)

American Society of Regional Anesthesia and Pain Medicine (ASRA) Guidelines for Anticoagulation/Antiplatelets and Neuraxial Anesthesia
See Tables 37.7 and 37.8.

Table 37.6 Immunosuppressive and antirejection drugs[16,17]

Type	Mechanism	Side effects	Notes
Prednisone	Inhibit T cell interaction	*Cushing's disease*, poor wound healing, bone disease, glucose intolerance, hypertension, cataracts	– Useful in treatment and prevention of acute rejection
Muromonab-CD3	Inhibit T cell interaction	Fever, anaphylactic reactions, and pulmonary edema, cytokine release syndrome	– Primarily used for induction therapy for solid organ transplant
Antithymocyte globulin	Inhibit adhesion molecules	*Anaphylaxis*, leukopenia, fever, nausea, chills	– Used for induction therapy and treatment of acute kidney rejection
Cyclosporine	Inhibit cytokine synthesis	*Nephrotoxicity*, hepatotoxicity, *hypertension* and neurotoxicity	– Induction and maintenance – *P450 interactions*: CYP3A – Alters barbiturate, benzodiazepine, fentanyl and isoflurane requirements

Table 37.6 (cont.)

Type	Mechanism	Side effects	Notes
			– Enhance neuromuscular blockade (NMB) – *Require monitoring of drug level* (renal and hepatic function can be affected)
Tacrolimus	Inhibit cytokine synthesis	*Nephrotoxicity,* neurotoxicity, hypertension, glucose intolerance, *lowers seizure threshold*	– Maintenance and rescue therapy for refractory acute rejection of liver transplant – *P450 interactions*: CYP3A – *Require monitoring of drug level* (renal and hepatic function can be affected)
Sirolimus	Inhibit cytokine synthesis	Myelosuppression, hyperlipidemia	– Used for maintenance, combined with other drugs to avoid permanent renal damage – Long half life – *P450 interactions*: CYP3A4
Azathioprine	Inhibit DNA synthesis	Myelosuppression, hepatic dysfunction, pancreatitis	– Used for maintenance – Antagonizes NMB in renal failure
Mycophenolate mofetil	Inhibit DNA synthesis	Myelosuppression, diarrhea, vomiting,	– Used for maintenance and chronic rejection – Never combine with azathioprine (risk of myelosuppression)

Table 37.7 ASRA antiplatelet guideline summary[18]

Antiplatelet agent	When neuraxial block can be performed after agent stopped	Restarting agent with neuraxial catheter in situ	Restarting agent after neuraxial block/catheter removal
Aspirin	No additional precautions	No additional precautions	No additional precautions
NSAIDs	No additional precautions	No additional precautions	No additional precautions
Clopidogrel	5–7 days	Can maintain for 1–2 days providing no loading dose (start 24 hr postoperative)	Immediately (loading dose: 6 hr)
Prasugrel	7–10 days	Not recommended	Immediately (loading dose: 6 hr)
Ticlodipine	10 days	Can maintain for 1–2 days providing no loading dose (start 24 hr postoperative)	Immediately (loading dose: 6 hr)
Ticagrelor	5–7 days	Not recommended	Immediately (loading dose: 6 hr)
Cangrelor	3 hr	Not recommended	8 hr
Abciximab	24–48 hr	Contraindicated within 4 weeks of surgery	No specific guidance
Tirofiban	4–8 hr	Contraindicated within 4 weeks of surgery	No specific guidance
Eptifibatide	4–8 hr	Contraindicated within 4 weeks of surgery	No specific guidance
Dipyridamole	24 hr for extended-release formulation	Not recommended	6 hr
Cilostazol	2 days	Not recommended	6 hr

Table 37.8 ASRA anticoagulation guideline summary[18]

Anticoagulant	When neuraxial block can be performed after drug is stopped	Restarting therapy with neuraxial catheter in situ	Restarting therapy after neuraxial block/catheter removal
Heparin and LMWH			
UFH subcutaneous	If > 4 days of UFH: obtain platelet count. – Low-dose prophylaxis (5,000 units BID/TID): 4–6 hr and after coagulation status assessed – High-dose prophylaxis (7,500–10,000 units BID or < 20,000 units daily total): 12 hr and after coagulation status assessed – Therapeutic dose (> 10,000 units per dose; > 20,000 units daily total): 24 hr and after coagulation status assessed	If > 4 days of UFH: obtain platelet count in addition to following guidance before catheter removal. – Low dose: Acceptable to give while catheter in situ; Catheter removal 4–6 hr after administration – High dose (doses > 5,000 units or daily total >15,000): Analyze risk/benefit in that patient and consider neurological observation regimen	1 hr (low dose; no specific guidance on high dose)
UFH intravenous	If > 4 days of UFH: perform platelet count. 4–6 hr and normal coagulation status	If > 4 days of UFH: perform platelet count before catheter removal. 4–6 hr after administration	1 hr
LMWH	If > 4 days of UFH: perform platelet count. – Prophylactic dose: 12 hr – Treatment dose: 24 hr and consider anti-factor Xa level	If > 4 days of UFH: perform platelet count. – Prophylactic dose: Catheters do not represent additional risk; first dose acceptable 24 hr after catheter placement; remove catheter 12 hr after last dose – Treatment dose: Not recommended	– Prophylactic dose: 4 hr – Treatment dose: 24 hr after low bleeding risk surgery/neuraxial block placement and 48–72 hr after high bleeding risk surgery; catheters should be removed at least 24 hr after needle/catheter placement, and first dose should be given at least 4 hr after catheter removal
Parenteral heparin alternatives			
Fondaparinux	Only where: single-needle pass, atraumatic needle placement, avoidance of indwelling neuraxial catheters	Avoid	6 hr
Argatroban	Avoid	N/A	N/A
Bivalirudin	Avoid	N/A	N/A
Oral anticoagulant agents			
Rivaroxaban	72 hr; if earlier, consider rivaroxaban or anti-factor Xa level (safe residual level for central nerve block unknown)	Not recommended. With unanticipated administration, hold rivaroxaban dosing for 22–26 hr or assess an anti-factor Xa assay calibrated to rivaroxaban before catheter removal	6 hr
Edoxaban	72 hr; if earlier, consider edoxaban or anti-factor Xa level (safe residual level for central nerve block unknown)	Not recommended. With unanticipated administration, hold edoxaban dosing for 20–28 hr or assess an anti-factor Xa assay calibrated to edoxaban before catheter removal	6 hr
Apixaban	72 hr; if earlier, consider apixaban or anti-factor Xa level (safe residual level for central nerve block unknown)	Not recommended. With unanticipated administration, hold apixaban dosing for 26–30 hr or assess an anti-factor Xa assay calibrated to rivaroxaban before catheter removal	6 hr
Dabigatran	120 hr; if no additional risk factors for bleeding: – CrCl > 80 mL/min: 72 hr – CrCl 50–79 mL/min: 96 hr – CrCl 30–49 mL/min: 120 hr – CrCl < 30 mL/min: Avoid	Not recommended. With unanticipated administration, hold dabigatran dosing for 34–36 hr or assess the dTT or ECT before catheter removal	6 hr

Table 37.8 (cont.)

Anticoagulant	When neuraxial block can be performed after drug is stopped	Restarting therapy with neuraxial catheter in situ	Restarting therapy after neuraxial block/catheter removal
Warfarin	Ideally stop INR 5 days before and INR "normalized"	– Low-dose therapy: Check INR daily with routine sensory and motor neurological testing – INR 1.5–2.9: Catheter acceptable with caution – INR ≥ 3.0: Hold warfarin	After catheter removal, suggest continuing neurological observations for 24 hr
Thrombolytic agents			
Alteplase and streptokinase	48 hr and documented normal clotting (including fibrinogen)	Not recommended. If unexpectedly given, measure fibrinogen to guide timing of catheter removal	No recommendation, but note that original contraindications to these drugs state should not be given for 10 days after puncture of non-compressible vessels

References

1. Badr R. *Hematologic System: Anticoagulatns: Mechanism of Action, Comparison of Drugs, Drug Interactions, Monitoring of Effect, Side Effects and Toxicity.* In Learnly: Online Anesthesia Basic Science Curriculum. Stanford AIM Lab, Stanford, CA, 2017.

2. Oprea AD. *Hematologic System: Pharmacology: Antithrombotic and Anti-Platelet Drugs: Mechanism of Action, Comparison of Drugs, Drug Interactions, Monitoring of Effects, Side Effects and Toxicity.* In Learnly: Online Anesthesia Basic Science Curriculum. Stanford AIM Lab, Stanford, CA, 2017.

3. Miller RD, editor. *Miller's Anesthesia*, 6th ed. Churchill Livingstone/Elsevier, 2010; pp 357–358.

4. Heparin (unfractionated). In Lexi-Comp Online™, Lexi-Drugs Online™. Hudson (OH): Lexi-Comp, Inc. Accessed via UpToDate 2017 Feb 27.

5. Miller RD, editor. *Miller's Anesthesia*, 6th ed. Churchill Livingstone/Elsevier, 2010; p 358.

6. Enoxaparin. In Lexi-Comp Online™, Lexi-Drugs Online™. Hudson (OH): Lexi-Comp, Inc. Accessed via UpToDate 2017 Feb 27.

7. Miller RD, editor. *Miller's Anesthesia*, 6th ed. Churchill Livingstone/Elsevier, 2010; p 357.

8. Warfarin. In Lexi-Comp Online™, Lexi-Drugs Online™. Hudson (OH): Lexi-Comp, Inc. Accessed via UpToDate 2017 Feb 27.

9. Miller RD, editor. *Miller's Anesthesia*, 6th ed. Churchill Livingstone/Elsevier, 2010; pp 358–359.

10. Dabigatran. In Lexi-Comp Online™, Lexi-Drugs Online™. Hudson (OH): Lexi-Comp, Inc. Accessed via UpToDate 2017 Feb 27.

11. Leung LLK. Direct oral anticoagulants (DOACs) and parenteral direct-acting anticoagulants: dosing and adverse effects. In Tirnauer JS, editor. *UpToDate.* UpToDate, Inc., last updated March 2024.

12. Apixiban. In Lexi-Comp Online™, Lexi-Drugs Online™. Hudson (OH): Lexi-Comp, Inc. Accessed via UpToDate 2017 Feb 27.

13. Rivaroxaban. In Lexi-Comp Online™, Lexi-Drugs Online™. Hudson (OH): Lexi-Comp, Inc. Accessed via UpToDate 2017 Feb 27.

14. Miller RD, editor. *Miller's Anesthesia*, 6th ed. Churchill Livingstone/Elsevier, 2010; p 359.

15. Peiris P. *Hematologic System: Alternatives to Transfusion.* In Learnly: Online Anesthesia Basic Science Curriculum. Stanford AIM Lab, Stanford, CA, 2017.

16. Cox Williams E, McFayden G. *Hematologic System: Pharmacology: Immunosuppressive and Anti-Rejection Drugs.* In Learnly: Online Anesthesia Basic Science Curriculum. Stanford AIM Lab, Stanford, CA, 2017.

17. Freeman B, Berger, J. *Anesthesiology Core Review.* McGraw-Hill Education, 2014; pp 503–505.

18. NYSORA. Regional anesthesia in anticoagulated patients. 2022. Available at: www.nysora.com/topics/sub-specialties/regional-anesthesia-in-anticoagulated-patients/

Transfusions

Russell J. Krom

Indications for Blood Transfusion

- Excessive Blood Loss (> 30% blood volume):
  - Healthy patients may lose up to 20% of blood volume before signs of hypovolemia occur due to compensatory vasoconstriction.[1]
    - When anemia develops, there is:
      - ↑ Cardiac output (CO) secondary to ↓ systemic vascular resistance (SVR)
      - Redistribution of blood flow to organs with greater oxygen requirements (e.g., brain, heart)
        - Oxygen delivery remains constant until the hematocrit (Hct) drops below 30%.[1]
      - An increase in oxygen extraction that allows O_2 delivery despite the lower O_2 tension
        - This usually begins to occur when the Hct < 25%.[1]
  - In patients with ongoing hemorrhage, a massive transfusion protocol is recommended, regardless of laboratory values, with either whole blood or a 1:1:1 ratio of red blood cells, fresh frozen plasma, and platelets until the hemorrhage is controlled.[2]
- Maximum Allowable Blood Loss (MABL):
  - MABL= Estimated Blood Volume (EBV) × (initial Hct – minimum acceptable Hct) / initial Hct (Table 38.1)[1]
- Signs of Inadequate Perfusion:[2]
  - Unstable vital signs (e.g., hypotension, tachycardia)
  - Signs of end-organ dysfunction (e.g., rise in lactate, increasing base deficit, decreasing urine output)
- Laboratory Indicators:
  - Morbidity and mortality increase when hemoglobin (Hgb) falls below 7 g/dL.[1,2,3]
    - In healthy adults, transfuse when Hgb < 7 g/dL.

Table 38.1 Estimated blood volume by age[1,2]

Age group	Blood volume (mL/kg)
Premature infant	90–105
Full-term newborn	80–90
Infant (3 months–1 year)	70–80
Child (1 year–12 years)	70–75
Adult female	60–65
Adult male	65–70

- In patients with cardiac disease, transfuse when Hgb < 9 g/dL.
  - Increased mortality is seen in this patient population using a restrictive-threshold transfusion strategy compared to a liberal strategy.

Blood Collection and Processing

- Whole Blood Collection:[1]
  - Centrifugation is used to separate whole blood into components.
  - Blood may also be separated via *apheresis*, where one component is collected and the remaining returned to the donor (Figure 38.1).
- Leukoreduction:[1,2]
  - Removes white blood cells (WBC) from the red blood cells (RBC) and platelets
  - Reduces risk of human leukocyte antigen (HLA) alloimmunization preventing *febrile reactions*
  - Reduces risk of cytomegalovirus (CMV) transmission to less than 0.1%
- Washing:[1]
  - Washing cellular components with saline is done to remove plasma in patients with *allergic transfusion reactions,* particularly patients with *IgA deficiency.*
- Irradiation:[1]
  - Units are exposed to gamma irradiation to damage donor WBC DNA and prevent cellular immune response to recipient tissue.
  - Used to prevent transfusion-related *graft versus host disease* (GVHD)

Blood Product Components, Preservation, and Storage

- Packed Red Blood Cells (PRBCs):[1,2]
  - 1 unit PRBCs = 250–300 mL and Hct 70–80%
  - Transfusion of 1 unit PRBCs = roughly 1 g/dL increase in adult hemoglobin concentrations
  - Can be stored at 1–6°C for 21–35 days or up to 42 days with additive solution
  - RBC preservation solution:
    - Citrate: Anticoagulation effect by binding calcium and inhibiting initiation of coagulation cascade

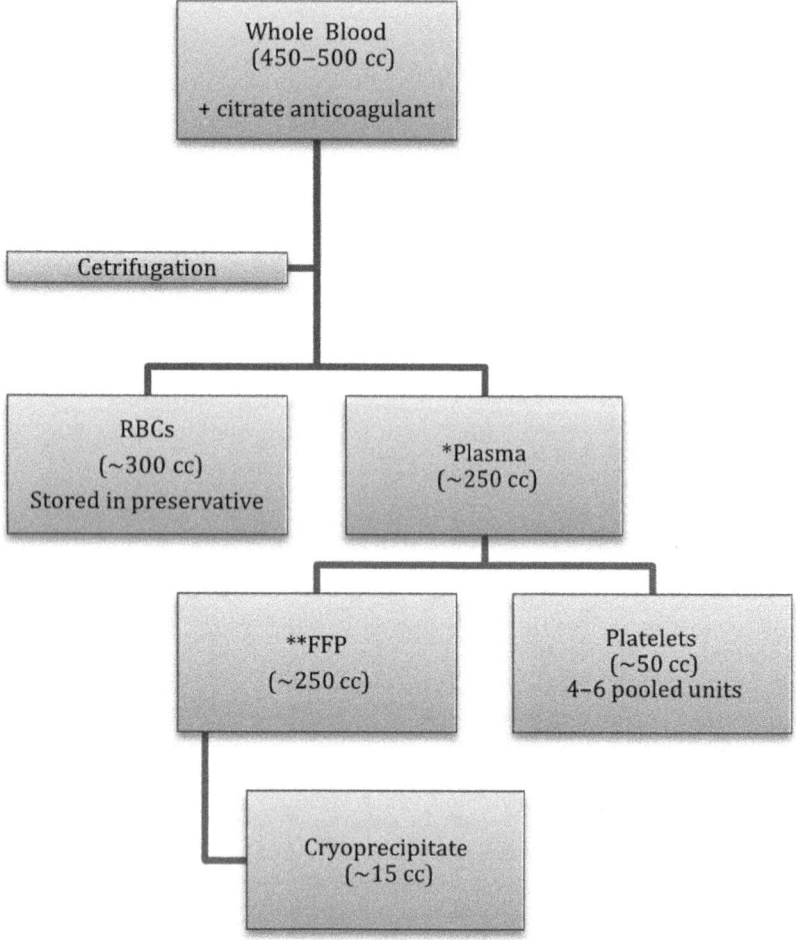

* Plasma is centrifuged again to separate platelet rich plasma from supernatant. The supernatant must be frozen within 6 hours in order to make FFP
** FFP is thawed and added to fibrinogen-rich precipitate to make cryoprecipitate

Figure 38.1 Processing and separation process of whole blood.[1]

- Phosphate: Buffer
  - Dextrose
  - Adenine
- Storage of blood products can result in the following derangements:
  - Depletion of 2,3-DPG within 2 weeks→ leftward shift of oxygen dissociation curve
  - Increased K^+ secondary to hemolysis
  - Citrate toxicity:
    - Can cause a reduction in ionized calcium levels
      - Signs include hypotension, narrow pulse pressure, prolonged QT interval, widened QRS complexes, and flattened T waves
    - Likely to occur in the setting of hypothermia, liver disease, and pediatric patients
    - Citrate is metabolized into bicarbonate → can cause metabolic alkalosis
    - Fresh frozen plasma (FFP) and platelets contain the highest citrate content
    - Treatment: Calcium

- Platelets:
  - Blood Preservation and Storage:[2]
    - Stored at room temperature for up to 5 days to preserve function
    - Increased risk of bacterial growth
    - Platelet-related sepsis occurs as frequently as 1 in 5000 transfusions and can be fatal
  - Preparation for Transfusion:[1]
    - Typically, multiple units of platelets are derived from a single donor via plasmapheresis.
      - The expected increase in platelet count after receiving a "pack" is 30,000 to 60,000.
  - Indications for platelet transfusion: Transfuse if platelet count is:[1,2]
    - < 100,000/µL
      - If patient is to undergo surgery at a critical site (e.g., spine, ophthalmological procedures)
    - < 75,000/µL
      - If patient is undergoing massive transfusion
      - For insertion or removal of epidural catheter

- < 50,000/μL
  - If patient is in disseminated intravascular coagulation (DIC)
  - Prophylactically, if patient is undergoing an invasive procedure
  - In a stable patient with coagulopathy or other signs of active bleeding
- < 10,0000/μL
  - Generally, in any patient, even if stable and without any signs of active bleeding or coagulopathy
- Fresh Frozen Plasma (FFP):
  - Blood Preservation and Storage:[2]
    - FFP is the fluid portion obtained from a single unit of whole blood that is frozen within 6 hours of collection.
    - All coagulation factors are present in FFP.
      - Factors V and VIII are the most labile, and thus freezing within 6 hours in required.
  - Preparation for Transfusion:[2]
    - Dosing should depend on PT, aPTT, or thromboelastography (TEG)/thromboelastometry (ROTEM) values
      - INR of FFP is approximately 1.5 and therefore it is impossible to correct an elevated INR to below 1.5 with FFP alone.
    - ABO compatibility testing is necessary with FFP.
  - Indications[2]
    - Liver dysfunction with clinical signs of bleeding
    - DIC with clinical signs of bleeding
    - Bleeding associated with massive transfusion
    - Emergent reversal of vitamin K antagonists, such as warfarin
    - Heparin resistance secondary to antithrombin (AT) deficiency when AT concentrate is not available
    - Correction of inherited factor deficiencies when there is no specific factor concentrate (e.g., factor V)
    - Correction of acquired multi-factor deficiencies with evidence of bleeding or in anticipation of major surgery or an invasive procedure
- Cryoprecipitate:
  - Blood Preservation and Storage:[1]
    - The fraction of plasma that precipitates when FFP is thawed that is then centrifuged is called cryoprecipitate (cryo).
    - This product contains fibrinogen, vWF, factor VIII, and factor XIII.
  - Preparation for Transfusion:[1]
    - Contains more fibrinogen per volume than FFP
    - Does not require ABO compatibility testing.
  - Indications:[1]
    - Hemophilia A (cryo contains high concentrations of factor VIII in a small volume)
    - Hypofibrinogenemia (cryo contains more fibrinogen than FFP)

Blood Filters and Pumps

- Blood filters are utilized during all transfusions to remove clots and cell aggregates that form during collection and storage.[1,4]
  - Standard blood infusion sets contain 170–260 micron filters to siphon debris.
  - Leukocyte filters are available for transfusion when leukocyte-reduced red cells or platelets are not available.
  - Platelets should be administered through large-pore filters (> 150 microns); they should not be transfused though sets which have already been used for blood due to aggregation.[4]
  - FFP and cryoprecipitate can be transfused via a standard blood filter
- Mechanical pumps are available to help with appropriate transfusion rates for special populations, particularly neonates and pediatric patients.[1,2]
  - Pressure bags should be used with rapid transfusion (5 min/unit) if needed.
    - Inflating the bag to about 200 mmHg is usually sufficient.
    - Pressure of > 300 mmHg can cause lysis of the RBCs.

Effects of Cooling and Heating: Blood Warmers

- Blood Warmers:
  - Administration of cooled blood products can result in hypothermia.[1,2]
    - Hypothermic patients have increased risk of platelet and coagulation factor dysfunction, arrhythmias, myocardial depression, as well as increased blood loss and risk of postoperative infections.
  - Specially designed warmers are used to rewarm the blood prior to administration.
  - Unrecognized malfunction of warmers may result in hemolysis of the erythrocytes, especially when overheating occurs.

Volume Expanders

- Crystalloids: Solutions that contain water and electrolytes that distribute freely within intravascular (33%) and interstitial compartments (67%)[2]
  - Balanced Salt Solutions:[1,2]
    - Salt solution with electrolyte composition similar to extracellular fluid (ECF) (e.g., lactated Ringer's [LR], Plasma-Lyte, Normosol)
    - HYPOtonic with regard to sodium
    - Buffer is usually included – generated bicarbonate in vivo
    - Includes small quantities of other electrolytes

- Plasma-Lyte is acceptable for dilution of PRBCs; however, LR should be avoided due to its calcium content, as well as its hypotonicity, which can cause cell lysis.
  - Normal Saline (0.9% NaCl):[1,2]
    - Slightly HYPERtonic
    - Contains more chloride than the ECF→ in large quantities, can result in mild hyperchloremic metabolic acidosis
    - No buffers or other electrolytes
    - Ideal solution for dilution of pRBCS given it is almost isotonic
    - Preferred solution in patients with brain injury, hypochloremic metabolic alkalosis, or hyponatremia
  - Hypertonic Salt Solutions:[2]
    - Na+ concentration ranges from 250 to 1,200 mEq/L
    - Create an osmotic gradient that helps move water from extravascular to intravascular space
    - Useful in minimizing tissue edema in patients with prolonged bowel surgery, burns, brain injuries
    - Not used for resuscitation measures given the short intravascular half-life and the potential for hemolysis at the point of injection from high osmolality
  - 5% Dextrose:[2]
    - Functions as free water, since dextrose is metabolized
    - Iso-osmotic
    - Used to correct hypernatremia
    - May be used to prevent hypoglycemia in diabetic patients who have been given insulin (Table 38.2)
- Colloids: Solutions composed of large-molecular weight (MW) substances that remain intravascular longer than crystalloids
  - 5% Albumin:[2]
    - Oncotic pressure of ~20 mmHg, half-life about 16 hours, but can be as short as 2–3 hours in pathological conditions
    - Minimal risk of infection with appropriate preparation methods
    - Contraindicated in patients with a damaged blood–brain barrier (head trauma, TBI, etc.)
  - Hydroxyethyl Starch (HES):[1,2]
    - Synthetic colloid solution that is a modification of natural polysaccharide

- HES preparations are described by their concentration, average molecular weight, molar substitution, and C_2 to C_6 ratio.
- Generally, the higher the molecular weight and molar substitution, the more prolonged the volume effect, but with more potential side effects
- Side effects vary with different HES preparations. They can include:
  - Coagulation disturbances: HES interferes with vWF, factor VIII, and platelet function
  - Renal toxicity: Usually with the older, high MW preparations
  - Tissue storage: Manifests as pruritus in up to 22% of patients
- Associated with increased mortality and AKI rates in critically ill patients
  - Carries a Black Box Warning against using HES in critically ill and septic patients

Preparation for Transfusion

- Compatibility Testing:[1,2]
  - Type and Screen (T&S):
    - ABO compatibility determines which antigens and antibodies are present on the patients red blood cell and serum.
    - RBCs are checked for "Rh factor" to avoid anti-D alloimmunization.
      - Type and screened blood is typed for A, B, and Rh antigens and screened for common antibodies.
        - Universal PRBC Donor: O–
        - Universal PRBC Recipient: AB+
        - Universal FFP Donor: AB+
        - 85% of the population is Rh+
        - Female patients of the parturient age should receive only Rh– blood to minimize the risk of developing antibodies to the Rh+ antigen (Rh sensitivity), as this can result in erythroblastosis fetalis.
    - The chance of a significant hemolytic reaction with the use of typed and screened blood is approximately 1 in ~40,000 units.
  - Type and Cross (T&C):[1,2]
    - Major: Donor's erythrocytes are incubated with the recipient's plasma.
      - This checks for IgG antibodies (Kell, Kidd, Duffy).
    - Minor: Incubation of the donor's plasma with the recipient's erythrocytes
    - Agglutination occurs if either the major or minor cross-match is incompatible.
    - Delayed hemolytic transfusion reactions commonly involve these antibodies.

Table 38.2 Fluid compositions[1,2]

Fluid	pH	Osmolarity (mOsm/L)	Na+ (mEq/L)	K+ (mEq/L)
NaCl (0.9%)	6.0	308	154	0
Lactated Ringer's	6.5	273	130	4
Plasma-Lyte	7.4	294	140	5
5% Albumin	7.4	330	145	< 2

Blood Donation and Salvage

- Autologous Blood:[1]
  - Two primary reasons for the use of autologous blood:
    - To decrease or eliminate complications from allogeneic blood transfusions
    - To conserve blood resources
  - Autologous Blood Donation:
    - Indications: Patients in whom it would be difficult to find compatible blood types, patients who refuse allogenic blood transfusion, and adolescent scoliosis surgery
    - Contraindications: Children < 10 years of age, active infection, aortic stenosis, recent myocardial infarction or stroke, uncontrolled hypertension
    - Criteria: Patient-donors must have a hemoglobin of at least 11 g/dL.
    - Most patients can donate 10.5 mL/kg of blood approximately every 5 to 7 days (maximum, 2 to 4 units), with the last unit collected at least 72 hours before surgery to permit restoration of plasma volume.
- Uncross-Matched Blood:[1]
  - In emergency situations where blood compatibility testing cannot be completed, the option is to administer O-negative (universal donor) PRBCs.
  - The incidence of a serious reaction without a cross-match is < 1%.
- Perioperative Blood Cell Salvage:[1]
  - Acute Normovolemic Hemodilution (ANH):
    - This is the process of extracting multiple units of blood in the early intraoperative period and replacing the volume with crystalloid solution.
    - The formula for MABL is used to calculate the volume that can be safely removed down to a target Hct of 27% (depending on the cardiovascular status of the patient).
    - Through hemodilution, fewer red blood cells will be lost per milliliter of blood loss during surgery.
    - At the end of surgery, the patient's concentrated, undiluted blood, which is high in hematocrit and oxygen-carrying capacity, clotting factors, and functional platelets, is reinfused.
    - Blood must still be anticoagulated with citrate
  - Cell Saver:
    - An external semi-automated device that collects blood from the surgical field into a reservoir that contains anticoagulant (heparin or citrate)
      - The blood is then filtered and centrifuged.
      - The remaining RBCs are washed from other blood components, surgical debris, and remaining anticoagulant, and delivered to a saline reservoir for future administration.
    - The blood can be stored for up to 6 hours at 4°C.
    - Most cell-savers provide RBC concentrates with Hct of 60%–70%.
    - Has reduced need for allogenic blood transfusion in major surgeries (e.g., orthopedic, spine fusion, and off-pump high-risk cardiac surgery) in patients with blood loss greater than 20% blood volume (or 1 L)
    - Complications: Dilutional coagulopathy, reinfusion of excessive anticoagulant (heparin), hemolysis, air embolism, and DIC
    - Contraindications: Microbial contamination of surgical field or malignant disease at operative site
- Designated Donor:[1]
  - Directed donations can be made by family or friends for a specific patient.
  - This method can potentially decrease the number of donor exposures by using the same donor.
  - Risk of infection is still considered the same, and so blood is still processed and tested as with any other blood donation.
  - Cellular components from blood relatives must be irradiated to prevent the risk of GVHD from closely matched donor lymphocytes that are not rejected by the recipient.
- Special Considerations:[1,2]
  - Jehovah's Witness patients do not accept blood transfusion, nor do they store their own blood for either autologous or allogeneic donation.
    - Albumin is accepted among certain patients, but a discussion is usually had with regard to this product.
    - Intraoperative blood salvage is sometimes a possible form of blood conservation, so long as the machine utilized maintains continuity of blood with the patient.

Synthetic and Recombinant Hemoglobin

- Blood Substitutes:
  - Hemoglobin-based oxygen-carrying solutions (e.g., Hemopure)[1,5]
    - Several hemoglobin solutions have been made from pools of human or bovine hemoglobin, or from recombinant hemoglobin, all of which are chemically modified to facilitate O_2 off-loading.
    - This, however, is still under investigation and no FDA-approved Hb substitute has been approved for clinical use.

References

1. Barash P, Cullen B, Stoelting R, et al. *Clinical Anesthesia*, 8th ed. Lippincott Williams & Wilkins, 2017.

2. Pardo MC Jr, Miller RD. *Basics of Anesthesia*, 7th ed. Elsevier Saunders, 2018.

3. Murphy GJ, Pike K, Rogers CA, et al. Liberal or restrictive transfusion after cardiac surgery. *N Engl J Med* 2015;**372**:997–1008.

4. Blood Safety and Conservation Team. Blood transfusion policy and procedures. Oxford University Hospitals, NHS Trust, 2012. Available from: www.transfusionguidelines.org.

5. Varnado CL, Mollan TL, Birukou I, et al. Development of recombinant hemoglobin-based oxygen carriers. *Antioxid Redox Signal* 2013 **18**:2314–2328.

Reactions to Transfusions

Patrick Maffucci, Lyle Nolasco, Marc Sherwin, and Natalie Smith

See Table 39.1 for a summation of reactions to transfusions.

Complications of Transfusions

Infections See Table 39.2.

- Hepatitis:
  - Most cases are anicteric
  - Hepatitis B most common
  - *Hepatitis C is the more serious*: progresses to chronic hepatitis, cirrhosis in 20% of carriers, hepatocellular carcinoma in 5% of carriers.[6]
  - Treatment: Ledipasvir-Sofosbuvir > 96% cure rate for some genotypes[7]
- Cytomegalovirus (CMV):
  - Typically asymptomatic or causes mild systemic illness except in high-risk patients
  - Patients at risk: Pregnant, premature neonates, immunodeficient/immunosuppressed, allograft recipients, splenectomy[8]
  - CMV safe products: Plasma components, seronegative donors, leukoreduced components
- Bacterial:
  - Incidence: One of the leading causes of transfusion-related mortality, more common with platelets (stored at room temperature) than packed red blood cells (PRBCs)
    - Positive bacterial cultures in *PRBC* – 1:7000[6]
    - Sepsis from PRBC transfusion 1:250,000[6]
    - Positive bacterial cultures in *platelets* – 1:2000[6]
    - Sepsis from platelet transfusion – 1:25,000[6]
  - Prevention: Transfuse blood products within 4 hours of removal from blood bank[6]
- Other Infectious Diseases (theoretical transmission but no available tests):
    - Malaria, Chagas, severe acute respiratory syndrome (SARS), Creutzfeldt–Jakob disease[7]

Citrate Intoxication

- Citrate is added to PRBCs as citrate phosphate dextrose adenine-1 (CPDA) to prevent clot formation by chelating calcium.[9]
- Intoxication occurs most commonly in massive transfusion, especially when giving fresh frozen plasma (FFP).
  - Transfusion rate > 1 mL/kg/min, which is equivalent to 1 PRBC every 10 min[9]

- Signs and Symptoms:
  - Liver metabolizes citrate into *bicarbonate.*
    - In patients with liver dysfunction, citrate will chelate recipient calcium causing hypocalcemia.[9]
  - Hypocalcemia, metabolic alkalosis, hypotension, narrow pulse pressure, increased left ventricular end diastolic pressure (LVEDP) and central venous pressure (CVP), and EKG changes (prolonged QT, widened QRS, flattened T wave)
- Risk Factors: Massive transfusion, hypothermia (metabolism halved when temperature decreases from 37°C to 31°C), hyperventilation, impaired hepatic blood flow, and pediatric patients[9]
- Treatment: Intravenous *calcium gluconate or calcium chloride*

Electrolyte and Acid–Base Abnormalities

- Blood storage leads to: ↓ pH, ↓ 2,3 DPG, and ↑ K$^+$.
- Hyperkalemia:
  - As high as 19–50 mEq/L in blood stored for 21 days[9]
  - Risks for hyperkalemia: Trauma, impaired renal function, and neonates[9]
- Hypocalcemia:
  - Associated with citrate intoxication – see above
- Acidosis:
  - Storage media very acidotic (ex. CPDA = pH 5.5)[9]
  - Lactate and pyruvate accumulate with storage.
  - High partial pressure of CO_2 (150–200 mmHg) – not typically clinically relevant with adequate ventilation
  - pH of 21-day blood storage ~6.9[9]
- Alkalosis:
  - Citrate metabolized to bicarbonate leading to metabolic alkalosis

Massive Transfusion

- Definition: When greater than 20 units of PRBCs are given within 24 hours (approximately 1 blood volume in a 70 kg patient)
  - Alternative definitions: > 50% blood volume transfused in 4 hours, 150 mL/min blood loss, 4 units in 1 hour[10]
- Massive Transfusion in Trauma:
  - Trauma patients present with platelet dysfunction and dysregulation of pro-/anti-coagulant and fibrinogen pathways (acute traumatic coagulopathy)

Table 39.1 Types of reactions

	Febrile non-hemolytic transfusion reaction	Allergic transfusion reaction (ATR)	Acute hemolytic transfusion reaction (AHTR)	Delayed hemolytic transfusion reaction (DHTR)
Presentation	– Fever (≥ 38°C and change of ≥1°C from pre-transfusion) and/or chills, headache, nausea, and vomiting – Occurs *during or within 4 hours after* transfusion completion – No evidence of hemolysis[1]	– **Mild (~90% of reactions):** Isolated, pruritic, urticarial lesions occurring *during or within 2 hours* of transfusion – **Severe (anaphylaxis):** acute, life threatening, systemic reactions with respiratory compromise, hypotension, and GI symptoms occurring within *seconds to 45 minutes of transfusion initiation*[2]	– Variable clinical manifestations, from minimal hemolysis without clinical sequelae to brisk hemolysis with DIC, fever, hypotension, renal failure with oliguria/anuria, shock, and death – Occurs *within 24 hours* – In anesthetized patients, hemoglobinuria may be the only sign[4]	– Fever, chills, jaundice, malaise, back pain and, infrequently, renal failure[5] – Occurs *3–10 days* after transfusion[5]

Mechanism of Action	– Fever caused by *release of cytokines* (IL-1β, IL-6, and TNF-α) from *activated monocytes and macrophages*
	– Cytokines lead to prostaglandin E2 production, which acts on the hypothalamus to increase body temperature
	– Mediated by immune and non-immune pathways:
	  Immune: donor leukocytes activated by recipient antibodies OR recipient leukocytes stimulated by recipient antibody:donor antigen immune complexes
	  Non-immune: passive transfusion of cytokines that accumulate in plasma portions during storage[1]
		– Type-1 hypersensitivity reaction (*IgE-mediated*): donor allergens activate recipient mast cells/basophils by binding IgE complexed with Fc receptors on granulocyte cell membranes
		– Atopic disease in donor does not contribute to reaction except rarely when IgE for specific allergens (*e.g.,* peanut) are passively transfused
		– Anaphylactic reactions reported in patients with deficiencies of haptoglobin, C3, and C4[2]
			– Transfusion of *ABO-incompatible RBCs* into patients with *anti A and/or B antibodies*
			– anti A/B IgM and IgG → activation of complement cascade → anaphylatoxins (C3a & C5a) and membrane attack complex formation leading to RBC lysis
			– RBC lysis leads to cell free hemoglobin, which scavenges nitric oxide, causing vasoconstriction & altered capillary responses to hypoxia
			– Free RBC stroma can cause DIC and acute renal failure[4]
				– Exposure to a *minor RBC antigen* after history of transfusion or pregnancy
				– Primary immune response: not clinically significant
				– Anamnestic response: the offending antigen is re-exposed → rapid production of IgG antibody responsible for hemolysis[5]

Diagnosis/Test	– No specific tests: diagnosis of exclusion – Exclude hemolytic reactions, ABO incompatibility, septic transfusion reactions (obtain culture), TRALI, medication reactions[1]	– Significant overlap with features of other transfusion reactions – Absence of fever and presence of cutaneous features (urticaria, angioedema) are strong indicators for allergic-type reaction – Test for IgA deficiency, presence of *anti-IgA*, or other markers of type I hypersensitivities (*e.g.,* tryptase) if severe allergic reaction[2]	– Combination of clinical signs/symptoms (as listed above) and laboratory findings – Positive direct antiglobulin test (DAT) – Signs of hemolysis: hemoglobinuria & hemoglobinemia, spherocytes, ↑ LDH, ↑ bilirubin, ↓ haptoglobin – Signs of DIC: ↓ fibrinogen and ↓ platelets[4]	– Positive DAT and/or positive identification of alloantibody via antibody screen – DAT done with anti-IgG and anti-C3 reagents – Subsequent serologic testing of recipient pre-transfusion sample and/or transfused product may be necessary – Laboratory findings: reticulocytosis, unconjugated hyperbilirubinemia, and urine urobilinogen[5]
Incidence	– Historically was most common transfusion reaction (43–75%) – Pre-storage leukoreduction decreased the incidence to <0.2% for both RBCs and platelets – Risk factors: hematologic malignancies, frequent transfusions, non-leukoreduced products, older platelets (4–5 days) higher incidence than ≤3-day old (4.6% vs. 1.1%)[1]	– Overall occur in 0.03–0.61% of RBC transfusions, 0.3–6% of platelet transfusions, and 1–3% of plasma transfusions – Anaphylaxis occurs in 1:20,000–47,000 transfusions and accounts for 5% of transfusion related deaths – Factor VIII, IX, vWF, and other recombinant concentrates occurs in 1:5000 doses[2]	– Cause of 0.41% of all reported adverse transfusion reactions – Among transfusion related deaths, 5% were from ABO-incompatible transfusion – Of ABO-incompatible transfusions, 50% of recipients are asymptomatic, death in 2–7%[4]	– Occurs in 1:1,500 transfusions – Delayed serologic transfusion reactions (anamnestic response identified serologically without clinical evidence of hemolysis) up to 4x more common[5]

Treatment	– Immediately *stop the transfusion* – Administer acetaminophen for anti-pyretic effect – Avoid aspirin and NSAIDs (contraindicated with platelet transfusions) – Meperidine (20-50mg IV) for severe rigor if not on monoamine oxidase inhibitor (MAOI) or have End Stage Renal Disease (ESRD) due to risk of seizures from normeperidine metabolite[1]	– **Mild:** Stop transfusion temporarily and administer *antihistamine*; may resume if symptoms cease – **Severe:** Stop transfusion, prepare to intubate, administer epinephrine 100ug IV bolus every 3–5 minutes, anti-histamines, H2 receptor antagonists, and glucocorticoids[2]	– *Stop transfusion*, check clerical work to ensure correct blood type, product, and patient – Send the transfused product back to blood bank along with sample from recipient – Check for: Hemolysis, DAT, ABO type – Supportive care: Intravenous fluid, diuretic to maintain urine output, consider dopamine infusion for hypotension – Plasma, platelets, cryoprecipitate as needed for active bleeding & DIC[4]	– Unnecessary unless symptomatic anemia is present – If minor antigen is not identified and transfusion is required, the benefit/risk should be weighed[5]
Prevention	– Leukoreduction (pre- or post-storage) – Pre-storage leukoreduction is the best method of prevention – Removal of plasma supernatant in platelets is effective for prevention but is not superior to pre-storage leukoreduction and may compromise platelet function – Premedication (*e.g.*, acetaminophen or diphenhydramine) is ineffective when using leukoreduced blood products[1]	**- Patients without history of ATR:** No benefit to premedication **- Patients with history of ATR:** Premedication may be beneficial to ameliorate symptoms; for patients with history of moderate-severe reactions, washing or plasma-reducing RBCs/plasma may be indicated **- Patients with history of ATR to platelets:** concentrating platelets via plasma reduction reduces incidence by 75%, washing platelets reduces incidence by 95% -IgA deficient patients should receive washed products or those from IgA deficient donors[2,3]	– Give ABO-compatible products and follow guidelines for checking products prior to transfusing – Perform Root Cause Analysis and corrective action plans[4]	– Permanent record-keeping of all clinically significant antibodies – "Active" RBC type and screen in those possibly requiring transfusion or who are pregnant – Administration of rituximab before transfusion in patients with history of severe DHTR can be considered5

Table 39.2 Infection risk with blood transfusions

Risk	
Hepatitis B virus (HBV)	1:200,000
Human immunodeficiency virus-1 and -2 (HIV)	1:1,900,000
Hepatitis C virus (HCV)	1:1,900,000
Human T-lymphotropic virus (HTLV-II)	1:2,600,000

Data from Fluid management & blood component therapy. In Butterworth JF IV, Mackey DC, Wasnick JD, editors. *Morgan & Mikhail's Clinical Anesthesiology*, 7th ed. McGraw-Hill / Medical, 2022; chapter 51; Zou S, Stramer SL, Dodd RY. Donor testing and risk: current prevalence, incidence, and residual risk of transfusion-transmissible agents in US allogeneic donations. *Transfus Med Rev* 2012;26(2):119–128.

- ○ Resuscitation focused on damage control (surgically), permissive hypotension, rapid rewarming, judicious crystalloid administration, early blood component replacement, and antifibrinolytics
- ○ Literature is mixed, but fixed ratio component therapy (FRCT) is generally recommended.
  - ▪ FRCT: typically 1:1:1 or 1:1:2 of plasma:platelets: RBCs
  - ▪ Laboratory and viscoelastic testing can also be used to guide transfusion ratios.
- • **Massive Transfusion in Non-traumatic Hemorrhage:**
  - ○ Resuscitation guided by specific pathology of hemorrhage (e.g., hemorrhage during liver transplantation worsened by dilution of coagulation factors in setting of cirrhosis vs impaired coagulation during and after cardiopulmonary bypass in the setting of anticoagulation and platelet dysfunction)
- • **Complications of Massive Transfusion:**
  - ○ Coagulopathy:
    - ▪ Coagulation factors can be significantly diluted after massive transfusion with PRBCs alone
    - ▪ Platelets and fibrinogen have been shown to decrease significantly during massive transfusion
    - ▪ Citrate intoxication & hypocalcemia (see above)
    - ▪ Acid–base disturbances (see above)
  - ○ Hypothermia:
    - ▪ Unwarmed blood products will decrease patient's temperature.
    - ▪ Prevent by warming blood through plastic coils or cassettes in warm water
    - ▪ Hypothermia can worsen coagulopathy.

Pulmonary Complications
- • Transfusion-Related Acute Lung Injury (TRALI)
  - ○ Definition:
    - ▪ TRALI Type I: New acute lung injury within 6 hours of transfusion, without any other risk factors for acute respiratory distress syndrome (ARDS)[11]
    - ▪ TRALI Type II: New acute lung injury within 6 hours of transfusion, but in the setting of other ARDS risk factors or preexisting mild ARDS[11]

- ○ Diagnosis of TRALI Type I:[11,14]
  - ▪ Evidence of hypoxemia:
    - • $PaO_2/FiO_2 < 300$ or $SaO_2 < 90\%$ on room air
  - ▪ New diffuse bilateral infiltrates on imaging (CXR, CT, lung US)
  - ▪ No evidence of left atrial hypertension
    - • Based on echocardiogram or pulmonary arterial catheter measurement, when possible
    - • However, if left atrial hypertension is present, it must not be a significant cause of hypoxemia
  - ▪ Occurs within 6 hours of transfusion
  - ▪ Rapid development of tachypnea, cyanosis, dyspnea, fever, and frequently hypotension[15]
  - ▪ Physical exam findings include diffuse crackles, decreased breath sounds on auscultation, hypoxemia, acute decrease in pulmonary compliance (increase peak and plateau airway pressures in mechanically ventilated patients)[15]
  - ▪ No risk factor for ARDS
- ○ Diagnosis of TRALI Type II:[11]
  - ▪ Meets criteria for TRALI Type I
  - ▪ But has risk factors for ARDS (e.g., sepsis, aspiration pneumonitis, pulmonary contusion, trauma, burns, smoke inhalation)[11]
  - ▪ Or alternatively, if mild ARDS (P/F ratio between 200 and 300) is present, patient must be stable for 12 hours prior to transfusion until experiencing respiratory decompensation within 6 hours of transfusion
- ○ Mechanism of Action:
  - ▪ Direct Antigen–Antibody Mediated Reaction:[13,16]
    - • Donor alloantibodies cause activation of recipient's immune system leading to inflammatory cascade
    - • Alloantibodies lead to recipient neutrophil and monocyte activation leading to increased lung vasculature permeability[15,19]
    - • HLA and HNA antibodies have NOT been identified in at least 15–20% of TRALI cases[12,16]
  - ▪ "Two-Hit" and "Multi-Causal" Models:[11,12,15,20]
  - ▪ Two-Hit Model:
    - • First hit: Patient-specific risk factors lead to neutrophil "priming" → enhanced neutrophil response
    - • >Examples of first hit include: chronic heart and lung disease, end stage liver disease, mechanical ventilation with high airway pressures, smoking, chronic alcohol use, extremes of age, positive fluid balance, major surgery[11,12]
    - • Second hit: Neutrophil activation through non-antibody mediated pathways (interleukins, lypophospitidylcholines, extracellular vesicles, etc.)[12]

- Multi-Causal Model: Similar to two-hit model; however, multi-causal models take into account the cumulative effect of multiple priming "hits"[20]
  - Final Common Pathway:
  - Neutrophil activation → release of inflammatory mediators → endothelial activation and breakdown of the endothelial-cell lung barrier → pulmonary edema and lung injury[18]
  - *Neutropenia* is a common, early finding in TRALI secondary to neutrophil sequestration within the lungs.[15]
  - Blood Products Implicated in TRALI:
    - Historically, plasma-containing products carried the highest risk of TRALI (i.e., FFP and platelets).[16]
      - Now all plasma is tested for HLA/HNA antibodies and risk of TRALI is lower (see below).
      - ALL blood products, including RBCs, have been implicated.[17]
    - Previously parous female donors are more likely to have HLA and HNA antibodies.
      - Exposed to paternal antigens from the fetus during pregnancy[18,21,22]
      - Plasma and whole blood transfusions in the United States now primarily come from male donors, nulliparous females, and females who have tested negative for HLA and HNA antibodies.[23]
  - Incidence:
    - Second most common cause of transfusion-related death, accounting for 21%[24]
    - Estimated incidence of 1 in 5,000 blood products[15,19]
  - Treatment:
    - Stop transfusion, supportive care, resolves within 72–96 hours[16,26,27]
    - Treatment strategies virtually identical to ARDS protocol[11,12]
      - Low tidal volumes, low plateau pressures, high FiO_2, and positive end-expiratory pressure (PEEP)
      - Prone positioning and inhaled nitric oxide may be used to improve V/Q matching.
      - Extracorporeal membrane oxygenation (ECMO) may be utilized in cases where oxygenation is severely impaired.
  - Prevention:
    - Avoid unnecessary transfusions.
    - Utilizing point of care testing (e.g., thromboelastography [TEG]) to guide transfusion management may decrease transfusions.[27,29]
- Transfusion-Associated Circulatory Overload (TACO)
  - 2021 Definition from CDC's National Healthcare Safety Network:[30]

- Three or more of the following within 12 hours of transfusion:
  - At least one of:
    - New or worsening respiratory distress
    - New or worsening pulmonary edema based on imaging (CXR, US, CT) or clinical exam
  - Plus:
    - Increased brain natriuretic peptide (BNP) or NT-pro BNP
    - Cardiovascular changes not otherwise explained (e.g., high CVP, hypertension, tachycardia, wide pulse pressure)
    - Fluid overload
- The 2021 CDC definition also further delineated definite, probable, and possible transfusion associated circulatory overload (TACO) as follows:[30]
  - Definite TACO – no alternative explanation for circulatory overload
  - Probable TACO – transfusion of blood products is believed to be a contributor to overload; however, the patient received other fluids or has a cardiac history that may also be contributing.
  - Possible TACO – the patient has a cardiac history that is the likely reason for overload
  - Presentation:
    - Increased CVP, evidence of left heart failure on echocardiogram, increased BNP / NT-pro BNP, imaging (e.g., CXR, CT, lung US) evidence of pulmonary edema[28,31,32]
    - Physical Exam Findings: Tachycardia, hypertension, hypoxemia, diaphoresis, anxiety, dyspnea, jugular venous distension, rales, rhonchi and/or wheezing, use of accessory muscles
  - Mechanism of Action:
    - Volume overload
  - Incidence:
    - Most common cause of transfusion-related death, accounting for 34% of all transfusion related mortality[24]
    - Incidence: approximately 1% of patients transfused12,[24]
    - More common in elderly (70–85 years old), pregnant patients, infants, patients with cardiac disease, renal disease, or chronic obstructive pulmonary disease (COPD)[25,28,33]
  - Treatment:
    - Most cases resolve within 24–72 hours.[33]
    - Stop the transfusion, administer supplemental oxygen, sit patient upright, consider diuretic therapy.[28,33]
  - Prevention:
    - Decreased risk with slower transfusion rate[25]
    - Consider splitting future transfusions into smaller aliquots.[28]

Immunosuppression

- Transfusion can reduce immunoresponsiveness and propagate inflammation.
  - ◦ Increased risk of postoperative bacterial infection, cancer recurrence, and mortality with transfusions[6]

- ◦ Renal transplant patients with preoperative blood transfusion have post-transfusion immunosuppression, which improves graft survival.[6]

References

1. Maramica I. Febrile nonhemolytic transfusion reactions. In Shah B, Hillyer C, Gil M, editors. *Transfusion Medicine and Hemostasis*, 3rd ed. Elsevier, 2019; chapter 61, pp 385–388.

2. Savage W. Allergic transfusion reactions. In Shah B, Hillyer C, Gil M, editors. *Transfusion Medicine and Hemostasis*, 3rd ed. Elsevier, 2019; chapter 62, pp 389–392.

3. Goss C. Washed blood products. In Shah B, Hillyer C, Gil M, editors. *Transfusion Medicine and Hemostasis*, 3rd ed. Elsevier, 2019; chapter 46, pp 281–284.

4. Kleinman S, Caulfield T, Chan P, et al. Toward an understanding of transfusion-related acute lung injury: statement of a consensus panel. *Transfusion* 2004;**44**(12):1774–1789.

5. Zerra P, Josephson C. Delayed hemolytic transfusion reactions. In Shah B, Hillyer C, Gil M, editors. *Transfusion Medicine and Hemostasis*, 3rd ed. Elsevier, 2019; chapter 64, pp 397–400.

6. Fluid management & blood component therapy. In Butterworth J IV, Mackey D, Wasnick J, editors. *Morgan and Mikhail's Clinical Anesthesiology*, 7th ed. McGraw-Hill / Medical, 2022; chapter 51.

7. Tong MJ, El-Farra NS, Reikes AR, Co RL. Clinical outcomes after transfusion-associated hepatitis C. *N Engl J Med* 1995;**332**(22):1463–1466.

8. Preiksaitis JK, Brown L, McKenzie M. The risk of cytomegalovirus infection in seronegative transfusion recipients not receiving exogenous immunosuppression. *J Infect Dis* 1988;**157**(3):523–529.

9. Dudley M, Miller R, Turnbull J. Patient blood management: transfusion therapy. In Gropper MA, Miller RD, Cohen NH, Absalom AR, editors. *Miller's Anesthesia*, 9th ed. Elsevier, 2020; chapter 49, pp 1546–1578.

10. Dunbar N, Seheult J, Yazer M. Massive transfusion. In Shah B, Hillyer C, Gil M, editors. *Transfusion Medicine and Hemostasis*, 3rd ed. Elsevier, 2019; chapter 58, pp 365–369.

11. Vlaar APJ, Toy P, Fung M, et al. A consensus redefinition of transfusion-related acute lung injury. *Transfusion* 2019;**59**(7):2465–2476.

12. McVey MJ, Kapur R, Cserti-Gazdewich C, et al. Transfusion-related acute lung injury in the perioperative patient. *Anesthesiology* 2019;**131**(3):693–715.

13. Toy P, Gajic O, Bacchetti P, et al. Transfusion-related acute lung injury: incidence and risk factors. *Blood* 2012;**119**(7):1757–1767.

14. Kleinman S, Caulfield T, Chan P, et al. Toward an understanding of transfusion-related acute lung injury: statement of a consensus panel. *Transfusion* 2004;**44**(12):1774–1789.

15. Silliman CC, McLaughlin NJD. Transfusion-related acute lung injury. *Blood Rev* 2006;**20**(3):139–159.

16. Triulzi DJ. Transfusion-related acute lung injury: current concepts for the clinician. *Anesth Analg* 2009;**108**(3):770–776.

17. Looney MR, Gropper MA, Matthay MA. Transfusion-related acute lung injury: a review. *Chest* 2004;**126**(1):249–258.

18. Bux J, Sachs UJ. The pathogenesis of transfusion-related acute lung injury (TRALI). *Br J Haematol* 2007;**136**(6):788–799.

19. Sachs UJ, Wasel W, Bayat B, et al. Mechanism of transfusion-related acute lung injury induced by HLA class II antibodies. *Blood* 2011;117(2):669–677.

20. Middelburg RA, van der Bom JG. Transfusion-related acute lung injury not a two-hit, but a multicausal model. *Transfusion* 2015;**55**(5):953–960.

21. Eder AF, Herron R, Strupp A, et al. Transfusion-related acute lung injury surveillance (2003-2005) and the potential impact of the selective use of plasma from male donors in the American Red Cross. *Transfusion* 2007;**47**(4):599–607.

22. Gajic O, Rana R, Winters JL, et al. Transfusion-related acute lung injury in the critically ill: prospective nested case-control study. *Am J of Respir Crit Care Med* 2007;**176**(9):886–891.

23. Sher G, Markowitz M. Association Bulletin #14–02. Association for the Advancement of Blood and Biotherapies. 2014. Available from: www.aabb.org/docs/default-source/default-document-library/resources/association-bulletins/ab14-02.pdf. (Accessed December 13, 2022).

24. Center for Biologics Evaluation and Research. *Fatalities Reported to FDA Following Blood Collection and Transfusion Annual Summary for FY 2020*. Food and Drug Administration, 2020.

25. Bolton-Maggs PH, Cohen H. Serious hazards of transfusion (SHOT) haemovigilance and progress is improving transfusion safety. *Br J Haematol* 2013;**163**(3):303–314.

26. Yost CS, Matthay MA, Gropper MA. Etiology of acute pulmonary edema during liver transplantation: a series of cases with analysis of the edema fluid. *Chest* 2001;**119**(1):219–223.

27. Tsai HI, Chou AH, Yang MW. Perioperative transfusion-related acute lung injury: a retrospective analysis. *Acta Anaesthesiol Taiwan* 2012;**50**(3):96–100.

28. Gil MR, Hillyer CD, Shaz B, editors. *Transfusion Medicine and Hemostasis: Clinical and Laboratory Aspects*, 3rd ed. Elsevier Science, 2019.

29. Morita Y, Pretto EA. Increased incidence of transfusion-related acute lung injury during orthotopic liver transplantation: a short report. *Transplant Proc* 2014;**46**(10):3593–3597.

30. Division of Healthcare Quality Promotion, National Center for

Emerging and Zoonotic Infectious Diseases, Centers for Disease Control and Prevention, National Healthcare Safety Network Biovigilance Component Hemovigilance Module Surveillance Protocol, v.2.8. February 2023. Available from: www.cdc.gov/nhsn/pdfs/biovigilance/bv-hv-protocol-current.pdf

31. Clifford L, Jia Q, Subramanian A, et al. Characterizing the epidemiology of postoperative transfusion-related acute lung injury. *Anesthesiology* 2015;**122**(1):12–20.

32. Raval JS, Mazepa MA, Russell SL, et al. Passive reporting greatly underestimates the rate of transfusion-associated circulatory overload after platelet transfusion. *Vox Sang* 2015;**108**(4):387–392.

33. Roubinian NH, Hendrickson JE, Triulzi DJ, et al. Incidence and clinical characteristics of transfusion-associated circulatory overload using an active surveillance algorithm. *Vox Sang* 2017;**112**(1):56–63.

Chapter

40

Endocrine and Metabolic Systems

Joseph R. Williams, Daniel R. Mandell, and Kathirvel Subramaniam

Hormone Physiology and Common Pathology

- **Thyroid Gland**
  - Physiology:
    - Thyroid releases T4 and T3, which are iodine-containing hormones that control the metabolic rate. T4 is secreted more than T3, and most T3 formed peripherally by conversion of T4 by deiodinases. T3 is more potent.
    - T3 *increases carbohydrate and fat metabolism.* Increased metabolism will increase O_2 consumption, CO_2 production, and minute ventilation.
  - Hyperthyroidism:
    - Most common etiology – Grave's disease and adenoma
    - Signs and symptoms: weight loss, diarrhea, weakness, stiffness, heat intolerance, nervousness, increased LV contractility, tachycardia, hypertension, atrial fibrillation in elderly patients
    - Anesthetic Management:
      - Goal is euthyroid state prior to elective anesthetic
      - Evaluate for airway compression if goiter present
      - Thyroid storm *triggered by stress of surgery.*
      - Signs/symptoms of thyroid storm are hyperthermia, tachycardia, dysrhythmia, myocardial ischemia, heart failure. Treat with *IV fluids, sodium iodide, propylthiouracil, hydrocortisone, propranolol, cooling blanket, acetaminophen*
  - Hypothyroidism:
    - Incidence ~5% population, 95% cases from primary thyroid gland failure
    - Signs and symptoms: Lethargy, slow mental function, cold intolerance, bradycardia, decreased cardiac output, decreased ventilatory response to hypoxia and hypercapnia, anemia, coagulopathy, risk of postoperative ileus
    - Anesthetic Management:
      - Patients are sensitive to most anesthetics and opioids.

- Only implement thyroid replacement in preparation for anesthesia if severe hypothyroidism or myxedema coma
- Myxedema coma characterized by stupor, hypoventilation, hypothermia, hyponatremia, hypotension. Treat with *ventilator support, levothyroxine, hydrocortisone, IV fluids and electrolyte therapy.*

- **Parathyroid Glands**
  - Physiology:
    - Regulates calcium homeostasis along with vitamin D
    - PTH increases blood calcium levels and stimulates urinary excretion of phosphate (mnemonic: PTH = phosphate trashing hormone).
  - Primary hyperparathyroidism can occur due to adenoma/hyperplasia of the parathyroid gland, secondary to hypocalcemia, or chronic renal disease.
  - Hypoparathyroidism can occur due to systemic causes or surgical removal of the parathyroid glands.
    - Postoperative hypoparathyroidism and resultant hypocalcemia present at 24–48 hours as laryngeal stridor and airway obstruction.
    - Note: Airway obstruction < 24 hours after thyroid surgery most likely related to hematoma formation
  - Primary anesthetic consideration is maintenance of serum calcium levels in the perioperative period. In hypocalcemia, follow the Rule of 10: *10 cc of 10% calcium gluconate over 10 minutes.* In hypercalcemia, *hydration with isotonic saline then furosemide*

- **Adrenal Medulla**
  - Physiology:
    - Releases primarily epinephrine, some norepinephrine
      - *Tyrosine* conversion to DOPA is the first and rate-determining step of catecholamine synthesis.
    - Stimulated by sympathetic preganglionic fibers, therefore stimulated by surgery, hypotension, hypovolemia, pain, fear, hypoglycemia, hypoxemia, hypercapnia

222

- ○ Pheochromocytoma:
  - Catecholamine secreting tumor, rare etiology of secondary hypertension (0.1%)
  - Approximately 20% may be extra-adrenal (paraganglioma)
  - Associated syndromes: Multiple endocrine neoplasia (MEN) type IIa, MEN type IIb, von Hippel–Landau syndrome, neurofibromatosis
  - Signs and symptoms: Hypertension, headaches, palpitations, tremor, diaphoresis, flushing
  - Diagnosis: Elevated 24-hour urinary *vanillylmandelic acid (VMA),* unconjugated norepinephrine/epinephrine, and plasma catecholamine levels
  - Definitive treatment is tumor resection.
  - Prior to resection, initiate alpha antagonist (ex. phenoxybenzamine, prazosin, doxazosin, etc.) and facilitate intravascular volume expansion.
    - **Note**: Avoid beta blockade until after establishing alpha blockade due to risk of unopposed alpha-mediated vasoconstriction and potential hypertensive crisis
  - Avoid histamine-releasing medications (ex. morphine, atracurium, pancuronium, etc.), as histamine is a potent catalyst for catecholamine release.
- **Adrenal Cortex**
  - ○ Three classes of corticosteroids: mineralocorticoids, glucocorticoids, and sex steroids (androgens and estrogen)
    - The precursor of all corticosteroids is *cholesterol.*
  - ○ Mineralocorticoids (secreted by zona glomerulosa)
    - Aldosterone is the primary mineralocorticoid.
      - Stimulated by angiotensin II (therefore secreted secondary to hypotension, hypovolemia), ACTH secretion, hyperkalemia
      - Mechanism is Na^+ reabsorption and K^+/H^+ secretion in renal distal tubule
      - Results in expansion of extracellular volume, decrease serum K^+, metabolic alkalosis
  - ○ Glucocorticoids (secreted by zona fasciculata)
    - Physiology:
      - Cortisol is the primary glucocorticoid.
  - ○ Release stimulated by ACTH
    - Enhance gluconeogenesis, inhibit peripheral glucose utilization → raise blood glucose
    - Fatty acid mobilization, protein catabolism, anti-inflammatory effects
    - Required for vascular and bronchial smooth muscle to respond to catecholamines
    - Most glucocorticoids promote Na+ retention and K+ excretion (mineralocorticoid effect).
  - Glucocorticoid Excess (Cushing's disease) :

- Overproduction of cortisol or exogenous glucocorticoid
- Signs and Symptoms: Truncal obesity, hypertension, hyperglycemia, increased intravascular volume, hypokalemia, fatigue, osteoporosis, weakness, hyperglycemia, emotional lability, immunosuppression, hypokalemic alkalosis
  - Adrenal Insufficiency (Addison disease):
    - Etiologies include autoimmune, sepsis, hemorrhage
    - Relative adrenal insufficiency common in critically ill surgical patients with hypotension
    - Signs and Symptoms: Fatigue, weakness, anorexia, nausea, vomit, diarrhea, hypotension, hyperkalemia
    - **Note**: When the body is under stress, the adrenal gland makes approximately 250–300 mg of cortisol in 24 hours
    - Anesthetic management includes administration of stress-dose steroids
- **Pancreas**
  - ○ Basic Physiology: Alpha cells secrete glucagon, beta cells secrete insulin
    - Rate of insulin secretion primarily determined by plasma glucose concentration
    - Insulin has multiple metabolic effects
      - Glucose and potassium entry into adipose and muscle cell → decrease plasma glucose and serum K^+
      - Increase glycogenesis and fatty acid synthesis
      - Decrease glycogenolysis, gluconeogenesis, ketogenesis, lipolysis and protein metabolism
  - ○ Perioperative Management of Diabetes:
    - Goals are to determine degree of end organ complications, glucose lowering regimen, and need for perioperative glycemic control
    - Consider anesthetic effects of early atherosclerosis in regards to coronary, cerebral, peripheral and renovascular disease
    - Autonomic neuropathy increases risk of intraoperative hypotension
    - Potential airway difficulty with poorly controlled diabetes from *decreased atlanto-occipital joint mobility (stiff joint syndrome)*
    - DKA and hyperglycemic hyperosmolar state are acute complications that should be corrected before elective surgery.
    - Management of Diabetic Ketoacidosis:
      - Insulin bolus + Insulin infusion
      - IV fluids, anticipate severe total body water deficit
      - Give potassium 10–40 mEq/hr when urine output > 0.5 mL/kg/hr

- When glucose < 250, add 5% dextrose at 100 cc/hr
- Consider bicarbonate infusion if pH < 6.9
- Major surgery in diabetic patients increases mortality/morbidity

  - In general, perioperative serum blood glucose target < 180 mg/dL

- **Anterior Pituitary**
  - Acromegaly: Excessive growth hormone production
    - Signs and Symptoms: Skin and soft tissue changes, bony/cartilage growth, compression of optic nerve and chiasma causing visual field defects, sleep apnea, difficult airway, compression of normal pituitary causing hypopituitarism, visceromegaly
- **Posterior Pituitary**
  - Syndrome of inappropriate antidiuretic hormone secretion (SIADH)
    - Signs and Symptoms: Hyponatremia, water retention, hypervolemia
    - Treatment: Treat the cause (i.e., infection, malignancy, drugs, surgery), fluid restriction, IV hypertonic saline with furosemide (Na$^+$ level should be allowed to rise slowly 0.5 meq/L/hr as aggressive Na$^+$ therapy may precipitate central pontine myelinolysis), demeclocycline, vasopressin receptor antagonists (tolvaptan and conivaptan)

  - Diabetes Insipidus:
    - Common following pituitary surgery. Usually transient but can be permanent in extensive

transfrontal resections. Additional etiologies include head trauma and tumors.
- Signs and Symptoms: Polyuria, polydipsia, hypernatremia
- Diagnosis:
  - Differential diagnosis includes excessive fluid therapy and diuresis
- Treatment includes water replacement, electrolyte monitoring/therapy, and DDAVP administration (Table 40.1)

Biochemistry of Normal Body Metabolism

- **Carbohydrates**
  - Aerobic Utilization:
    - Requires O_2
    - Glycolysis → citric acid cycle → oxidative phosphorylation
    - Results in 38 molecules of adenosine triphosphate (ATP)
  - Anaerobic Utilization:
    - No O_2 in setting of ischemic tissue
    - Glycolysis → yields 2 ATP/glucose molecule
    - End product pyruvate → lactic acid → lactic acidosis
  - Relationship to Hormones:
    - Insulin – decrease blood glucose
    - Human growth hormone – increase glucose
    - Glucocorticoids – increase glucose
    - Glucagon – increase glucose
    - Epinephrine – increase glucose
  - Stress/surgery → increase blood glucose

Table 40.1 Summary of hormones and their functions

Gland/tissue	Hormone	Function
Hypothalamus	Thyrotropin-releasing hormone (TRH)	Stimulates secretion of thyroid-stimulating hormone and prolactin
	Corticotropin-releasing hormone (CRH)	Stimulates release of adrenocorticotropic hormone
	Growth hormone-releasing hormone (GHRH)	Stimulates release of growth hormone
Anterior pituitary	Growth hormone (GH)	Stimulates protein synthesis, fatty acid mobilization, and tissue growth
	Thyroid-stimulating hormone (TSH)	Stimulates synthesis and secretion of thyroid hormones (e.g., thyroxine and triiodothyronine)
	Adrenocorticotropic hormone (ACTH)	Stimulates synthesis and secretion of adrenocortical hormones (e.g., cortisol, androgens, aldosterone)
Posterior pituitary	Antidiuretic hormone (ADH)	Increase water reabsorption by kidneys and causes vasoconstriction
	Oxytocin	Stimulates milk ejection and uterine contractions
Thyroid	Thyroxine (T4) and Triiodothyronine (T3)	Increase rates of chemical reactions in most cells, increase metabolic rate
Adrenal cortex	Glucocorticoids (cortisol)	Multiple metabolic functions, anti-inflammatory effects
	Mineralocorticoids (aldosterone)	Increase renal Na$^+$ reabsorption, K$^+$ secretion, H$^+$ secretion
Adrenal medulla	Norepinephrine, epinephrine	Sympathetic stimulation
Pancreas	Insulin	Promotes glucose entry into cells
	Glucagon	Promotes glycogenolysis and gluconeogenesis; inhibits glycogenesis
Parathyroid	Parathyroid hormone	Controls serum Ca^{2+} concentration by increasing Ca^{2+} absorption from gut, kidney and release Ca^{2+} from bone

- Protein Function:
  - Provides structure of cells and enzymes
  - Intracellular signaling molecules
    - cAMP (cyclic adenosine monophosphate)
    - cGMP (cyclic guanosine monophosphate) – relaxes smooth muscle (mechanism of nitric oxide)
- Selected Plasma Proteins:
  - Albumin:
    - Provides oncotic pressure to maintain intravascular volume
    - Transports many anesthetic drugs
  - Immunoglobulins:
    - Provide cellular immunity
  - Fibrinogen:
    - Forms fibrin clot via coagulation cascade
- Lipids:
  - Triglycerides, lipoprotein, cholesterol
    - Lipoprotein – transport form of lipids in plasma
    - Adipocytes and liver store triglycerides until needed to provide energy.
    - Cholesterol – forms cholic acid/conjugates to form bile salts and synthesize adrenal hormones

- HMG-CoA reductase is the rate-determining step of cholesterol synthesis (enzyme target of statin drugs)
  - Specific Organ Metabolism:
    - Brain – glucose primary fuel source, uses ketones during starvation. No fatty acid metabolism
    - Heart – fatty acids are main source of energy, but can also use ketone bodies and lactate. Virtually no glucose metabolism.
    - Liver – stores fatty acids and secreted primarily as very-low-density lipoproteins (VLDL) during fed state, converts fatty acids into ketone bodies during fasted state
    - Muscle – metabolize glucose, fatty acid, ketones
- Nitrogenous Compounds:
  - Urea:
    - Nitrogenous waste compound excreted by kidneys
    - Uremia may result from renal failure, GI bleeding, or diet
      - Symptoms: Altered mental status, nausea, seizures, Hypertension, pericarditis, uremic-induced platelet dysfunction

Further Reading

Barash PG, Cullen BE, Stoelting RK, et al. *Clinical Anesthesia*, 7th ed. Lippincott Williams & Wilkins, 2013.

Berg J, Tymoczko JL, Stryer LL. *Biochemistry*, 7th ed. Palgrave Macmillan, 2011.

Butterworth J, Mackey DC, Wasnick JD. *Morgan & Mikhail's Clinical Anesthesiology*, 5th ed. McGraw-Hill Education, 2013.

Hall JE. *Guyton and Hall Textbook of Medical Physiology*, 13th ed. Saunders, 2016.

Yao F-S, Hemmings HC Jr, Malhotra V, Fong J, editors. *Yao & Artusio's Anesthesiology: Problem-Oriented Patient Management*, 9th ed. Lippincott Williams & Wilkins, 2021.

Neuromuscular Physiology and Disorders

Jacqueline Donovan

Anatomy and Physiology of Neuromuscular Transmission

Prejunctional Events: The neuromuscular junction (NMJ) consists of a presynaptic motor nerve terminal and a postsynaptic skeletal muscle membrane. The space between the presynaptic junction and postsynaptic membrane is called the *synaptic cleft.* Acetylcholine (ACh) is stored in the nerve terminal in synaptic vesicles. ACh receptors (AChR) are located in the postsynaptic motor end plate opposite the nerve terminal. In the adult NMJ, there are approximately 5 million AChRs. The NMJ is the location at which electrical signals are effectively transformed into chemical signals, which in turn produce muscular contraction (Figure 41.1).

- **Acetylcholine Synthesis and Release:**
  - The choline and acetate used to form acetylcholine are located in the environment of the nerve terminal.
  - Choline is transported from the extracellular fluid and acetate is obtained from acetyl coenzyme A in the mitochondria.
  - Choline acetyltransferase is responsible for the production of acetylcholine from choline and acetate.
  - Acetylcholine is then stored in vesicles within the nerve, both at the nerve terminus and deeper within the nerve as a reserve supply.
  - Movement of and release of vesicles is dependent upon calcium flow into the nerve.
  - Calcium ions enter the nerve via P-channels where they interact with SNARE proteins to create a pore through which the acetylcholine may enter the synaptic cleft in a process known as exocytosis.
  - During continuous stimulation, calcium penetrates the nerve more deeply via L type calcium channels where it activates the VP1 vesicles (reserve supply) to be moved to the nerve terminal.
  - The rate-limiting step of this entire process is thought to be choline uptake and activity of choline acetyltransferase.
  - All the components needed to make, store, and release these chemical signals are made in the cell body of the neuron and brought to the nerve terminal by axonal transport.
  - Acetylcholine is stored in the cytoplasm until it is transported and stored in synaptic vesicles.

- There are two types of synaptic vesicles:
  - Smaller VP2 vesicles are positioned at the nerve terminal where they are ready for release of acetylcholine.
  - Larger VP1 vesicles are located further from the nerve terminal and are moved to the terminal when the VP2 vesicles have depleted their stores.

- **Modulation of Nicotinic and Muscarinic Prejunctional Receptors:**
  - ACh release into the synaptic cleft is modulated via both *positive and negative feedback loops.*
  - Presynaptic *nicotinic* receptors modulate ACh in a positive feedback loop with *increasing ACh leading to increased release.*
  - Presynaptic *muscarinic* receptors modulate ACH in a negative feedback loop with ACh *leading to decreased ACH release.*
  - When the nicotinic response is in full effect, the muscarinic response is less capable of producing a negative response.

Postjunctional Events: The AChRs are formed by a five-subunit glycoprotein in the form of a cylindrical channel consisting of two alpha (α) subunits and one each of beta (β), gamma (γ), and delta (δ) subunits. The fetal receptor has a similar composition with the epsilon (ε) subunit substituted for the γ subunit. Alterations in the conventional AChR occur in pathologies including muscle denervation, which leads to increase membrane permeability associated with hyperkalemic cardiac arrest. The receptor complexes extend through the membrane of the muscle cell, linking the cytoplasm with the extracellular fluid. Acetylcholine binds the α subunits on the extracellular side of the receptor, and channel activation requires binding of *both α subunits* in order to effect conformational change and allow passage of ions.

- **Acetylcholine Binding to Acetylcholine Receptors:**
  - The amount of acetylcholine stored in each vesicle is referred to as a quantum (10^4 molecules).
  - Each nerve impulse releases approximately 200 quanta.
  - This process is enhanced *by increasing calcium concentration.*
  - As stated above, acetylcholine binds to the *alpha subunits* of the receptors and *both alpha subunits* must be bound by acetylcholine to evoke a conformational change in the receptor.

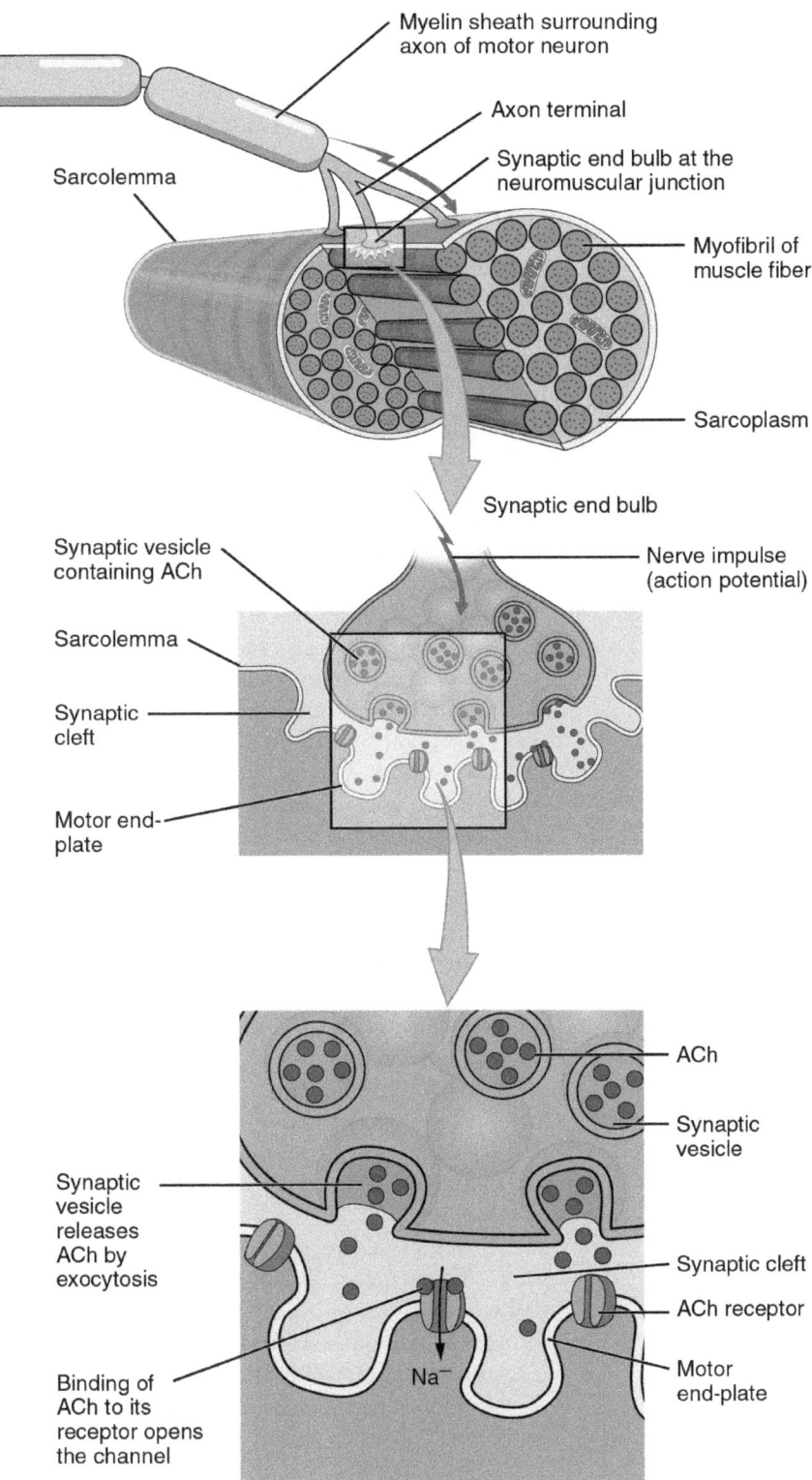

Myelin sheath surrounding
axon of motor neuron

Axon terminal

Synaptic end bulb at the
neuromuscular junction

Sarcolemma

Myofibril of
muscle fiber

Sarcoplasm

Synaptic end bulb

Synaptic vesicle
containing ACh

Nerve impulse
(action potential)

Sarcolemma

Synaptic
cleft

Motor end-
plate

ACh

Synaptic
vesicle

Synaptic
vesicle
releases
ACh by
exocytosis

Synaptic cleft

ACh receptor

Na⁻

Motor
end-plate

Binding of
ACh to its
receptor opens
the channel

Figure 41.1 Neuromuscular junction, motor end plate, and innervation. Source: OpenStax College. "Anatomy and Physiology." OpenStax CNX, OpenStax College, June 19, 2013, cnx.org/content/col11496/1.6/. A black and white version of this figure will appear in some formats. For the color version, please refer to the plate section.

- The conformational change involves a brief opening of the receptor core allowing ion flow through the receptor.
- **Ion Flow through Acetylcholine Receptor:**
  - Sodium and calcium flow into the receptor; potassium flows out of the receptor, creating an end plate potential.
- When enough receptors are bound, the end plate potential becomes strong enough to depolarize the membrane, which opens voltage gated sodium channels.
- The action potential then propagates by sodium channels opening, leading to release of calcium from the sarcoplasmic reticulum and binding of contractile proteins leading to muscle contraction.

227

Prejunctional Voltage-Gated Channels

- P type calcium channels are located at the nerve terminal.
- Voltage gated and calcium gated, potassium channels are also present, and regulate the duration of depolarization.
- High concentrations of magnesium, cadmium, and manganese can block entry of calcium through P channels.
- Nerve endings also contain slower, L-type calcium channels.
- Verapamil, diltiazem, and nifedipine block L-type calcium channels but do not affect P-type calcium channels.

Neuromuscular Pathology

Multiple sclerosis is a demyelinating disorder of the optic nerves, cerebrum, and spinal cord, particularly the spinothalamic tract and posterior columns, characterized by a variable course.

- MS has autoimmune pathophysiology that ultimately leads to the disruption of the blood–brain barrier and demyelination.
- Anesthetic management should focus on keeping patients normothermic as hyperthermia has been shown to increase the risk of a flare-up. Previous thought was that spinal anesthesia should be avoided; however, current literature has shown successful use, particularly for scheduled caesarean deliveries. It seems that dose and duration of local anesthetic may play a more important role than spinal vs. epidural. General, spinal, and epidural anesthesia have all been shown to be safe options.

Amyotrophic lateral sclerosis is a demyelinating disorder of both the anterior gray horn matter and the corticospinal tracts, and thus affects both upper and lower motor neurons.

- Clinically, patients present with progressive weakness, fasciculations, and spasticity of the extremities as well as oropharyngeal dysfunction.
- Anesthetic management must balance the risk of enhanced respiratory depression, exaggerated response to muscle relaxation, potential risk of furthering neurological damage with regional anesthesia, and risk of pulmonary aspiration. Furthermore, depolarizing anesthetics are discouraged due risk of hyperkalemic response. Despite these concerns, both general and epidural anesthesia techniques have been described with success.

Guillain–Barré syndrome is characterized by a sudden onset of lower-extremity flaccid paralysis that spreads cephalad affecting the diaphragm, upper extremities, face, and bulbar muscles, with spontaneous resolution usually within weeks.

- Autonomic dysfunction is a prominent feature, with wide swings in blood pressure, resting tachycardia, cardiac conduction abnormalities, and orthostatic hypotension being described.
- Anesthetic management should focus on maintaining hemodynamic stability, which can prove difficult due to autonomic dysfunction.

- Indirect acting vasopressors are not recommended, as they may produce exaggerated responses due to up-regulation of receptors.
- Additionally, exaggerated hyperkalemic responses can be caused by depolarizing muscle relaxants, and exaggerated hemodynamic responses can be seen with nondepolarizing muscle relaxants that have cardiac side effects.

Duchenne muscular dystrophy (DMD) results from an absence in the dystrophin protein as well as dysfunction of the dystrophin-associated protein complex, leading to instability of the sarcolemma and muscle membrane.

- Clinically, symptoms emerge between ages 2 and 5 years and include gait instability, toe-walking, difficulty climbing stairs, calf hypertrophy, and Gower's sign: using the hands to walk up the legs in order to stand.
- Loss of skeletal muscle function leads to spine instability and scoliosis, which can have profound effects on pulmonary function and diaphragm involvement further deteriorates pulmonary function.
- The loss of dystrophin, also found in smooth and cardiac muscle, eventually causes fibrosis of the basal segment of the left ventricle, ventricular hypertrophy, fibrosis of the posterior papillary muscle, and mitral regurgitation, as well as significant cardiac arrhythmia.
- Electrocardiogram changes are seen and include tall R waves in V1, deep Q waves in leads 1, V5, and V6, sinus tachycardia, and right-axis deviation.
- Patients with DMD have a frequent need for surgical procedures including scoliosis correction, muscle biopsies, contracture releases, and reduction or fixation of fractures.
- Anesthetic management should include careful preoperative planning with a multidisciplinary team to manage the risk of pulmonary and cardiac complications.
- Pulmonary function testing, resting EKG, and echocardiogram are all recommended due to the high risk for perioperative respiratory and cardiac sequelae, most notably respiratory failure and cardiac arrhythmias.
- Patients with DMD are also at risk for difficult intubations owing to macroglossia, limited cervical spine mobility, and small mouth opening.
- Additionally, diminished airway reflexes and gut motility predispose to pulmonary aspiration.
- In terms of anesthetic choice, succinylcholine and volatile anesthetics should be avoided due to risk of hyperkalemia and rhabdomyolysis.
- It was previously thought that these children were at risk for malignant hyperthermia (MH); however, this is now thought to be unlikely, as the genes are located on different chromosomes.
- It has also been noted that hyperkalemia and rhabdomyolysis present without the hypermetabolism seen in MH and thus dantrolene is not an effective treatment.

- Regional anesthesia techniques may be preferable in these patients both to avoid the use of general anesthesia and for postoperative pain management.

Becker's muscular dystrophy (BMD) is nearly identical to DMD, except that it presents later in life (adolescence) and is much less common (1 in 30,000).

Myotonic dystrophy can be classified into two types, DM1 and DM2, with DM2 presenting later in life and with milder symptoms. Both are due to CTG repeats on the 3′ untranslated region of the dystrophia myotonica-protein kinase gene on chromosome 19.

- This results in a characteristic wasting facial muscles as well as weakness of neck extensors and the external rotators of the arm.
- Additionally, proximal muscle weakness of the lower extremities, as well as hands, ankles, and pharyngeal muscles can be seen.
- Significant cardiac involvement is common with conduction delays, arrhythmias, cardiomyopathy, and valvular abnormalities.
- Anesthetic management should include assessment of cardiac function as well as pulmonary function and risk of aspiration.
- Muscular weakness, number of CTG repeats, and duration of surgery all correlated with risk of postoperative respiratory complications in a series of pediatric patients with DM1.

Mitochondrial myopathy presents a challenge due to its clinical heterogeneity, but can essentially be classified based on the five main components of mitochondrial metabolism.

- Common symptoms that are "red flags" of mitochondrial diseases include sensorineural hearing loss, short stature, diabetes mellitus, hypertrophic cardiomyopathy, axonal neuropathy, and external ophthalmoplegia.
- Anesthetic considerations for these patients involve a thorough preoperative evaluation of muscle weakness, respiratory and cardiac involvement, and degree of metabolic and endocrine abnormalities.
- All anesthetic choices have a theoretical risk in these patients.
- Extended propofol infusions may predispose to propofol infusion syndrome as both propofol and midazolam have been shown to affect mitochondria in a dose-dependent fashion.
- Volatile anesthetics and succinylcholine confer a risk of malignant hyperthermia and hyperkalemia.
- Nondepolarizing muscle relaxants predispose to extended respiratory depression as do narcotics.
- Despite this, all manner of anesthetic combinations have been described with success in the literature.

Hyperkalemic periodic paralysis (hyperKK) is a sodium channelopathy and presents with myotonia and paralysis. The hyperKK periodic paralyses are a group of autosomal-dominant disorders characterized by episodes of flaccid paralysis often triggered by an alteration in serum potassium concentration.

- During the episode of muscle weakness or paralysis, potassium ions are released from the muscle and serum potassium rises, though not always above normal levels.
- Administration of potassium, potassium-rich foods, and rest after exercise precipitate attacks.
- Patients with hyperKK should be admitted preoperatively for electrolyte management and potassium-free fluid administration.
- Potassium, succinylcholine, and anticholinesterases should be avoided, as they can all trigger episodes.

Hypokalemic periodic paralysis (hypoKK) has two subtypes. Type 1 is caused by a defect in L-type calcium channels, whereas type 2 is caused by a defect in the same gene that affects the sodium channel in HyperKK.

- The disease presents up to the third decade of life and affects proximal muscles, with bulbar and ocular muscle involvement occurring rarely.
- HypoKK is not associated with myotonia, presents with hypokalemia, and is triggered by glucose, unlike HyperKK.
- Trigger avoidance is a mainstay of treatment along with acetazolamide for type 1. Acetazolamide can precipitate attacks in type 2 hypoKK.
- Triggers often include high-carbohydrate meals, alcohol, viral infections, prolonged rest, menstruation, and pregnancy.
- Anesthetic management should exclude succinylcholine and dextrose-containing solutions, and focus on maintaining normothermia.
- Patients with hypoKK have an increased risk of postoperative pulmonary complications, and thus long-acting muscle relaxants should be avoided.
- Furthermore, there have been numerous accounts of malignant hyperthermia in patients with hypoKK and therefore an association cannot be ruled out.
- A non-triggering anesthetic and extreme vigilance are prudent.

Myasthenia gravis (MG) is an autoimmune disease affecting the alpha subunit of the muscle type nicotinic acetylcholine receptors at the neuromuscular end plate.

- Antibodies may be associated with thymoma or thymic hyperplasia in approximately 50% of patients.
- Skeletal muscle weakness ensues and can include bulbar and oropharyngeal weakness. Classically, weakness becomes worse with repetition or throughout the day and the course of the disease is punctuated by periods of relapse and remission.
- Cardiac manifestations have been described and include cardiomyopathy, arrhythmias, myocarditis, heart block, and sympathetic hyperactivity leading to wide swings in heart rate and blood pressure.
- Anesthetic management should focus on preserving neuromuscular function.

- Risk of postoperative mechanical ventilation is increased with the following: disease for more than 6 years, pyridostigmine dose greater than 750 mg total/day, previous or coexisting lung disease, and forced vital capacity less than 2.9 L.
- Risk of postoperative MG crisis has also been demonstrated with presence of bulbar symptoms, serum antibody level greater than 100 nmol/L, current MG crisis, and estimated blood loss greater than 1 liter.
- It should be noted that patients are exquisitely sensitive to nondepolarizing muscular relaxants and resistant to succinylcholine.
- Uneven distribution of muscular relaxation has also been described, making train of four monitoring difficult and less accurate, particularly if monitoring the orbicularis oculi muscle.
- Potent volatile anesthetics have been used alone successfully without the need for paralysis in many patients.
- If choosing a regional anesthetic technique, ester-type local anesthetics may show extended duration of action due the anticholinesterases patients are using preoperatively.

Lambert–Eaton myasthenic syndrome (LEMS) is caused by antibodies to voltage-gated calcium channels at the presynaptic terminal of the motor end plate, preventing release of acetylcholine and subsequent weakness.

- Unlike MG, weakness improves with repetition, as use of the muscle increases the amount of acetylcholine released.
- LEMS is commonly from a paraneoplastic syndrome with small cell lung cancer found in 50–60% of cases.
- Proximal lower limb weakness is the most common symptom, though the upper extremities, respiratory, and bulbar muscles may be affected.
- Additionally, cholinergic symptoms such as dry mouth and decreased lacrimation can be seen.
- Patients are exquisitely sensitive to both depolarizing and nondepolarizing NMBDs.
- Reversal of NMBDs may also be insufficient with anticholinesterases.
- Epidural anesthesia has been successfully described but also requires careful titration and preparedness for postoperative weakness and respiratory monitoring much like MG.

Further Reading

Dunø M, Colding-Jørgensen E. Myotonia congenita. 2005 Aug 3 [Updated 2015 Aug 6]. In Pagon RA, Adam MP, Ardinger HH, et al., editors. *GeneReviews®* [Internet]. Seattle (WA): University of Washington, Seattle; 1993–2017.

Fink J. Heredeitary spastic paraplegia. *Neurologic Clinics* 2002;**20**:711–726.

Jeevendra Martyn JA. Neuromuscular physiology and pharmacology. In Miller RD, Eriksson LI, Fleischer LA, et al., editors. *Miller's Anesthesia*, 8th ed. Elsevier, 2015; chapter 22, pp 423–443.

Makris A, Piperopoulos A, Karmaniolou I. Multiple sclerosis: basic knowledge and new insights in perioperative management. *J Anesth* 2014;**28**:267.

Marchant CL, Ellis FR, Halsall PJ, et al. Mutation analysis of two patients with hypokalemic periodic paralysis and suspected malignant hyperthermia. *Muscle Nerve* 2004;**30**:114–117.

Neuromuscular blocking agents. In Butterworth JF IV, Mackey DC, Wasnick JD, editors. *Morgan & Mikhail's Clinical Anesthesiology*, 5th ed. McGraw-Hill, 2013; chapter 11, pp 199–220.

Nozari A, Bagchi A, Saxena R, Bateman BT. Neuromuscular disorders and other genetic disorders. In Miller RD, Eriksson LI, Fleischer LA, et al., editors. *Miller's Anesthesia*, 8th ed. Elsevier, 2015; chapter 42, pp 1266–1286.

Raja Rayan DL, Hanna MG. Skeletal muscle channelopathies: nondystrophic myotonias and periodic paralysis. *Curr Opin Neurol* 2010;**23**:466–476.

Segura L, Lorenz J, Weingarten T, et al. Anesthesia and Duchenne or Becker muscular dystrophy: review of 117 anesthetic exposures. *Pediatr Anaesth* 2013;**23**:855–864.

Shaw PJ, Cudkowicz ME. Amyotrophic lateral sclerosis and other motor neuron diseases. In Goldman L, Schaffer AI, editors. *Goldman-Cecil Medicine*, 26th ed. Elsevier, 2020; pp 2522–2526.

Sinclair JL, Reed PW. Risk factors for perioperative adverse events in children with myotonic dystrophy. *Paediatr Anaesth* 2009;**19**:740–747.

Südhof TC. The molecular machinery of neurotransmitter release (Nobel lecture). *Angew Chem Int Ed Engl* 2014 Nov 17;**53** (47):12696–12717.

Thomas M, Scrutton M. Spinal anaesthesia in a patient with hereditary spastic paraplegia: case report and literature review. *Int J of Obst Anesth* 2006;**15**:254.

Xiao W, Zhao L, Wang F, et al. Total intravenous anesthesia without muscle relaxant in a parturient with amyotrophic lateral sclerosis undergoing cesarean section: a case report. *J Clin Anesth* 2017;**36**:107–109.

Special Problems or Issues in Anesthesiology

Evan Shawler, Regine Goh, Megan Meyer, Martha Schuessler, and Sanjana Vig

Physician Impairment or Disability

Substance Abuse

The *Diagnostic and Statistical Manual of Mental Disorders*, 5th edition, text revision (DSM-5-TR) diagnosis for Substance Abuse Disorder involves 11 criteria and is categorized as mild (2–3 symptoms), moderate (4–5 symptoms), or severe (6 or more symptoms).[1]

1. Taking the substance in larger amounts or for longer than you're meant to.
2. Wanting to cut down or stop using the substance but not managing to.
3. Spending a lot of time getting, using, or recovering from use of the substance.
4. Cravings and urges to use the substance.
5. Not managing to do what you should at work, home, or school because of substance use.
6. Continuing to use, even when it causes problems in relationships.
7. Giving up important social, occupational, or recreational activities because of substance use.
8. Using substances again and again, even when it puts you in danger.
9. Continuing to use, even when you know you have a physical or psychological problem that could have been caused or made worse by the substance.
10. Needing more of the substance to get the effect you want (tolerance).
11. Development of withdrawal symptoms, which can be relieved by taking more of the substance.

Facts
- Risk of addiction with physicians is the *same* as in the general population.[2,3]
  - Approximately 10–12% throughout a physician's career
- Specific risk factors in physicians:
  - Family: Genetics, positive family history of substance abuse, dysfunctional familial interactions
  - Work:
    - Residency training (including resultant alienation from friends and family)
    - Personal identity suppression by professional identity, dehumanization of physicians

- Excessive fatigue, use of stimulants, insomnia
- Self-medication for physical/psychological pain
- Access to medication
- Types of abused substances in physicians from all specialties:[2,4]
  - Alcohol 50.3%
  - Opioids 35.9%
  - Stimulants 7.9%
  - Other 5.9%
  - Multiple substance abuse 50%
- Typical patterns in addiction medicine, like progression from alcohol to marijuana to cocaine, is not seen in anesthesiology. Anesthesiologists display increased association with anesthesia drugs such as fentanyl, nitrous oxide, benzodiazepines, ketamine, lidocaine, ephedrine, cocaine, propofol.

Anesthesia and Addiction[4]
- Anesthesiologists represent approximately 2.5 times the rate of the average physician in rehabilitation facilities.
- Incidence of overdose death and suicide was comparable to other physician specialties.
- Methods of obtaining illicit substances:
  - False recording on anesthesia record
  - Substituting syringes
  - Keeping waste
  - Breaking ampules
  - Poor accountability
- Figure 42.1 shows commonly abused medications among anesthesiologists and the time it takes to detect abuse.[4]
- Highest incidence of addiction during first 5 years of delivering anesthesia:
  - Data collected from the ABA suggests 0.86% of residents are diagnosed with SUD.
- Risks of Substance Abuse:[4]
  - Physical:
    - Declining health or loss of life. High mortality rate for anesthesiologists (2.21 × more likely to commit suicide by drug overdose, and 2.79 × more likely to experience drug-related death)[3]

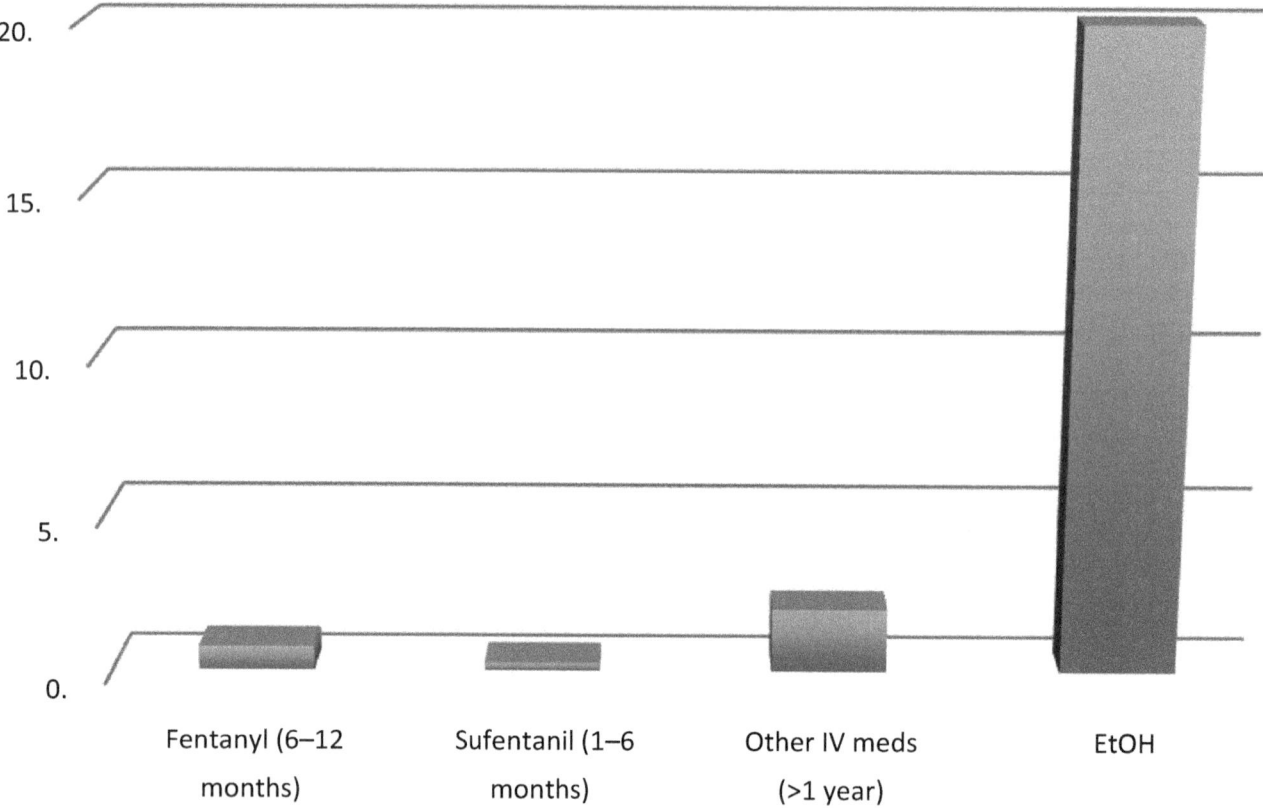

Figure 42.1 Commonly abused medications among anesthesiologists and time to detection (years).

- ■ Mortality rates of relapse upwards of 9%[4]
  - ○ Patients:
    - ■ Increased malpractice claims, decline in quality of patient care
  - ○ Work:
    - ■ Loss of licensure, professional standing, career
  - ○ Life:
    - ■ Loss of family, self esteem
    - ■ Loss of ability to gain health or disability insurance
- Detection: Self-reporting is exceedingly rare. More commonly direct observation of abuse or audits, but unfortunately suicide and accidental death are increasingly observed.[4]
- Re-entry: Physicians have better outcomes recovering from addiction than non-physician counterparts, including prescription opioid abuse. However, some evidence suggests re-entry to the workforce is risky and ineffective.[4,5]
  - ■ 15 × less likely to finish residency, 10 × decrease in achieving board certification, 7 × increase in adverse licensure actions
  - ■ There is an overall relapse rate of 43% over a 30-year period.
  - ■ First symptom of relapse can be death (16% of cases).[4]

Americans with Disabilities Act of 1990 (ADA)[3]

- The ADA offers some protections to anesthesiologists with addiction if enrolled in a treatment or monitoring program. If not enrolled, no protections are provided, and the ADA does not provide legal protection against drug diversion.

Fatigue

Definition(s):[6,7]

Fatigue	Chronic partial sleep deprivation	Sleep inertia
Extreme tiredness, typically resulting from *mental or physical exertion* or illness	Sleep duration of *less than five or six hours* for several consecutive nights	Awakening at certain parts of the circadian cycle creating similar effects to a period of 26 hours awake

ASA Statement on Fatigue

- Sources of fatigue: Sleep deprivation, patient severity, case volume and turnover, facility conditions, personal stressors, age, work patterns, breaks, meals, scheduling changes, wait times, and handover procedures
- Sleep deprivation causes significant, measurable cognitive impairment, as well as a decline in self-assessment ability, quality of decision making, clinical performance, vigilance, memory, motor skills, and attention.

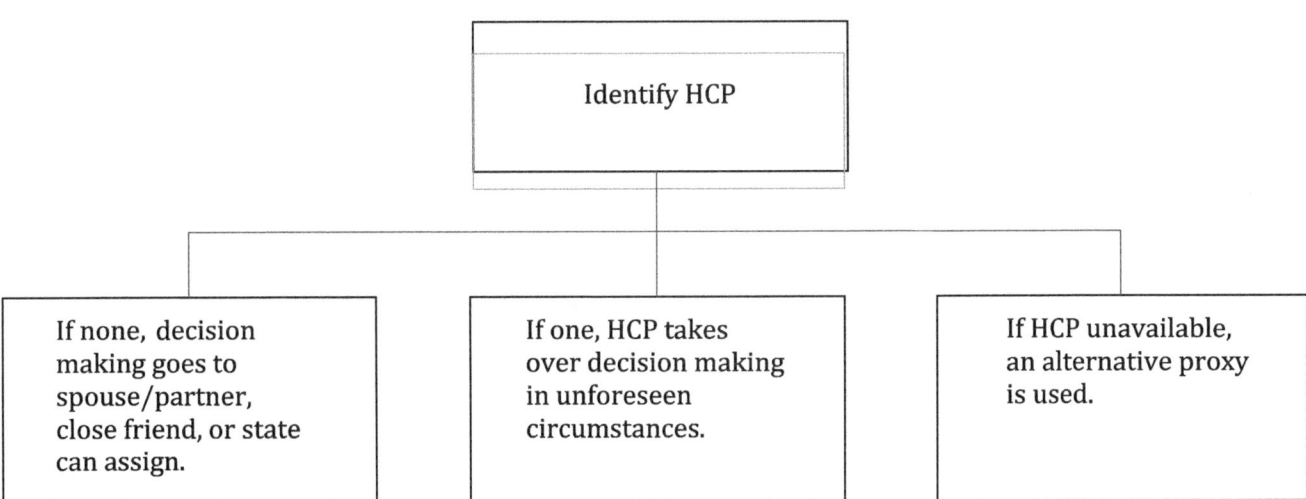

Figure 42.2 Decision tree for HCP.

- Fatigue mitigation: Sleep is the only solution, but some risk can be mitigated by system backups (alarms and reminders) and physiological actions (frequent breaks, walking, naps, and caffeine consumption). Naps less than 20–40 minutes can improve performance, but longer naps are associated with impaired alertness due to sleep inertia with the progression to deeper sleep cycles.

Aging, Visual, and Auditory Impairment

Facts[8]

- In the United States, the number of practicing physicians older than 65 years has grown 374% since 1975.[9]
  - In 2015, 23% of practicing physicians were 65 years or older.
- Aging causes normal physiological and cognitive changes that may or may not affect a clinician's ability to deliver the standard of care and is a factor that may impact clinical competence.
- In the practice of anesthesia, dexterity, visual–spatial acuity, memory, problem solving, data analysis, and lifelong learning are among the most important areas that may be compromised.
- The aging process is extremely variable. Physicians should be regularly and routinely assessed. Often this does not happen until an incident occurs.

Ethics, Practice Management, and Medico-Legal Issues

Professionalism and Licensure

Ethics[10]

- The ASA adheres to the American Medical Association's (AMA) 2001 statement on the Principles of Medical Ethics and defines one element of professionalism as the application of ethical principles to patients, colleagues, institutions, and society.

- Additionally, the ASA lists more specific guidelines for anesthesiologists to uphold while providing healthcare. These include ethical responsibilities to patients, medical colleagues, healthcare facilities, themselves, their community, and society.

Licensure[11]

- Varies state by state, required for ABA certification
- Application for license requires completion of USMLE boards, anesthesia residency, and passing of anesthesiology written and oral exams.
- Any and all conditions or restrictions filed against a practitioner must be disclosed when applying for new, or maintaining, licensure.

Advance Directives/DNR/DNI/DNAR/AND

Advance Directives[12–15]

Definition(s)
- Healthcare Proxy (HCP) – a designated person or persons to make decisions for the patient if the patient is unable (cannot be a treating physician)

Facts
- Serves as a way to prevent costly and unwanted interventions to the patient (Figure 42.2)
- Only goes into effect if the patient loses capacity for decision making
- 2009: *America's Affordable Health Choices Act* authorized reimbursement for these discussions
  - Not included in *Affordable Care Act (ACA)*, due to fear of creation of "death panels"
- *Physician Orders for Life-Sustaining Treatment (POLSTs)* can serve as a way to provide a framework especially in patients without advance directives, but do not supersede an advance directive.

233

Table 42.1 Alternatives to advance directives in the operating room

	Suspension options	
Limited attempt at resuscitation defined with regard to *Specific Procedures*	**Limited attempt at resuscitation defined with regard to *Patient's Goals and Values***	**Full attempt at resuscitation**
Patient/surrogate may elect to continue to refuse certain resuscitation procedures. Anesthesiologists must indicate which are necessary for a successful anesthetic and which are not essential (i.e., DNI must be suspended in order to provide anesthetic; however, chest compressions as part of a resuscitation effort are not necessarily essential).	Patient or surrogate allows the anesthesiologist and surgical team to use clinical judgment when determining which resuscitation procedures are appropriate based on patient goals of care (i.e., intubation is acceptable if necessary, so long as the patient can be extubated in the immediate postoperative period).	Patient or surrogate may fully suspend DNR/advance directives in the perioperative period.

DNR/DNI/DNAR/AND

Definition(s)

- DNR: Do Not Resuscitate; in the event of a cardiac arrest, do not perform CPR.
- DNI: Do Not Intubate, even outside the context of a cardiac arrest.
- DNAR: Do Not Attempt Resuscitation. Same definition as DNR. In 2005, the American Heart Association transitioned to using DNAR as a replacement for DNR to convey that natural death would occur if no interventions were attempted.[15]
- AND: Allow Natural Death. Same definition as DNR/DNAR. Recent literature encourages DNAR or AND language to convey that CPR is an attempt to save life and is not a guarantee.
- Patients who elect for a designation of DNR typically include DNI in the definition, as CPR typically includes intubation and artificial ventilation.

Facts
- DNR/DNI is a type of advance directive
- In an operating room setting, advance directives may be suspended (Table 42.1).

Patient Privacy
HIPAA Privacy Rule[16]

Facts
- *Health Insurance Portability and Accountability Act (HIPAA) of 1996:*
  ○ Set standards for protection of privacy of health information
  ○ Addresses use of protected health information (PHI)
- Requires patient permission for use, except in instances listed in Table 42.2
  ○ Applies to providers, healthcare clearinghouses, health plans
  ○ Includes all past/present/future physical or mental health problems and care received, including common identifiers

Table 42.2 Exceptions to PHI permission requirement

Instances where patient permission is NOT required when disclosing PHI
• Legal proceedings
• Prevention or control of disease/injury/disability, child/elder abuse/neglect, persons at risk for spreading or contracting a disease
• Workplace surveillance OSHA/Worker's Compensation
• Research/IRB approval
• Cadaveric organ donation
• Historical purposes > 50 years after death

Informed Consent/Decision-Making Capacity
Informed Consent[17,18]

- Definition: As highlighted in Figure 42.3. There are multiple elements required to complete consents appropriately and accurately.

- In seeking a patient's (or surrogate's) informed consent, physicians should:
  ○ Assess the patient's ability to understand relevant medical information, the implications of treatment alternatives, and to make an independent, voluntary decision.
  ○ Present relevant information accurately and sensitively
  ○ The physician should include information about:
  ○ The diagnosis (when known)
  ○ The nature and purpose of recommended interventions
  ○ The burdens, risks, and expected benefits of all options, including forgoing treatment
- Document the informed consent conversation and the patient's (or surrogate's) decision in the medical record in some manner.

Decision-Making Capacity[17-18]

Definitions(s)
- The ability to participate in care decisions is called decision-making capacity.
- This is distinct from the legal concept of competency, which only a judge has the authority to determine.

Threshold Elements	Information Elements	Consent Elements	
Competency and capacity Voluntariness	Discussion with patient Disclosure: treatment and alternatives, material risks (common vs. rare) Physician Recommendations Assessment of patient understanding	Decision by patient Autonomous authorization	

Figure 42.3 Elements of informed consent.

- Decision-making capacity can and should be assessed by anesthesiologists and other clinicians.
- Evidence for decision-making capacity includes understanding the current situation, using relevant information, and communicating a preference supported by reasons.

Patient Safety

Medical Errors/Negligence[17–20]

- Medical Errors: Assessment and Prevention:
  - Fall into three categories:
    - Slips – failure to execute
    - Lapses – memory failure
    - Mistakes – rule-based or knowledge-based
  - Include wrong patient, wrong surgery, wrong site, failure to diagnose, wrong drug/dose
- Malpractice and Negligence:
  - Malpractice is defined as professional misconduct, but specifically is referring to negligence.
  - Negligence:
    - Four components required to prove:
      - Duty:
        - The anesthesiologist owed a particular obligation to the patient.
      - Breach of Duty:
        - The anesthesiologist failed to fulfill this specific obligation to the patient.
      - Causation:
        - There is a reasonably direct correlation between the actions of the anesthesiologist and the reason for the suit.
      - Damages:

- Damages occurred as a result of the specific actions of the anesthesiologist.

- Sentinel Events:[21]
  - Defined by The Joint Commission as "a patient safety event that results in death, permanent harm, or severe temporary harm."
  - Requires immediate investigation and response.
  - Not synonymous with the term "error."
  - Hospital review of sentinel events is a component of The Joint Commission review.

- Disclosure of Errors to Patients:
  - Often a full disclosure and formal apology will decrease the likelihood of litigation.
  - Careful preparation with risk management and all involved parties should occur prior to disclosure.
  - Disclosure should occur in a private environment with all necessary parties (including family, social workers, language interpreters, clergy, etc.). Disclosure should be limited to the medical error itself, and blame should not be assigned to others. Focus should be on answering questions, the relationship with the patient and coordinating further care.

Core Competencies

The core competencies required of residents include the following:[22]

- Patient Care and Procedural Skills
- Medical Knowledge
- Practice-Based Learning and Improvement
- Interpersonal and Communication Skills
- Professionalism
- Systems-Based Practice

References

1. American Psychiatric Association. *Diagnostic and Statistical Manual of Mental Disorders*, 5th ed., text revision (DSM-5-TR). American Psychiatric Association Publishing, 2022. (Accessed 20 November 2022).

2. Berge KH, Seppala MD, Schipper AM. Chemical dependency and the physician. *Mayo Clin Proc* 2009;**84**(7)625–631.

3. Bryson EO, Silverstein JH. Addiction and substance abuse in anesthesiology. *Anesthesiology* 2008;**109**(5):905–917.

4. Tetzlaff J. SUD curriculum. *American Society of Anesthesiologists*, November 12, 2015, Available at: www.asahq.org/standards-and-guide lines/~/media/857bafdbf3f84486

b280132363342d5e.ashx. (Accessed 13 November 2022).

5. Oreskovich MR, Caldeiro RM. Anesthesiologists recovering from chemical dependency: can they safely return to the operating room? *Mayo Clin Proc* 2009;**84** (7):576–580.

6. American Society of Anesthesiologists. ASA statement on fatigue. 2021. Available at: www.asahq.org/standards-and-guidelines/statement-on-fatigue. (Accessed 20 November 2022).

7. Wong LR, Flynn-Evans E, Ruskin KJ. Fatigue risk management: the impact of anesthesiology residents' work schedules on job performance and a review of potential countermeasures. *Anesth Analg* 2018;**126**(4):1340–1348.

8. American Society of Anesthesiologists. The aging anesthesiologist. 2018. Available at: www.asahq.org/standards-and-guidelines/statement-on-the-aging-anesthesiologist. (Accessed 20 September 2022).

9. Patchen Dellinger EP, Pellegrini C, Gallagher TH. The aging physician and the medical proession: a review. *JAMA Surgery* 2017;**152**(10) 967–971.

10. American Society of Anesthesiologists. Guidelines for the Ethical Practice of Anesthesiology. 2020. Available at: www.asahq.org/standards-and-guidelines/guidelines-for-the-ethical-practice-of-anesthesiology. (Accessed 20 September 2022)

11. American Board of Anesthesiology. *Policy Book 2022.* ABA, 2022.

Available at: https://theaba.org/pdfs/Policy_Book.pdf. (Accessed 20 October 2022).

12. American Society of Anesthesiologists. ASA Statement on Suspension of DNR. 2021. Available at: www.asahq.org/standards-and-guidelines/ethical-guidelines-for-the-anesthesia-care-of-patients-with-do-not-resuscitate-orders-or-other-directives-that-limit-treatment. (Accessed 20 November 2022).

13. H.R.3200 – America's Affordable Health Choices Act of 2009: 111th Congress (2009–2010). Available at: www.congress.gov/bill/111th-congress/house-bill/3200. (Accessed 12 November 2022).

14. National POLST. POLST basics. Available at: https://polst.org/about/ (Accessed 12 November 2022)

15. Morrison LJ, Kierzek G, Diekema DS, et al. Part 3: Ethics: 2010 American Heart Association Guidelines for Cardiopulmonary Resuscitation and Emergency Cardiovascular Care. *Circulation* 2010 Nov 2;122(18 Suppl 3):S665–S675.

16. U.S. Department of Health and Human Services. Health Insurance Portability and Accountability Act of 1996. 1996. Available at: https://aspe.hhs.gov/report/health-insur

ance-portability-and-accountability-act-1996. (Accessed 13 November 2022).

17. Waisel, D, Truog RD. Informed consent. *Anesthesiology* 1997;**87**:968–978.

18. O'Leary, C. Informed consent: principles and practice. *ASA Monitor* 2010;**74**: 20–45.

19. American Society of Anesthesiologists. Revised "Manual on Professional Liability" now available online! *ASA Newsletter* 2010;**74**(8):65.

20. Ferner RE, Aronson JK. Clarification of terminology in medication errors. *Drug Safety* 2006;**29** (11):1011–1022.

21. The Joint Commission. Sentinel event. 2016. Available at: www.jointcommission.org/resources/sentinel-event/. (Accessed 18 November 2022).

22. Eno C, Correa R, Stewart NH, et al. *Milestones Guidebook for Residents and Fellows,* 2nd ed. Accreditation Council for Graduate Medical Education (ACGME). 2020. Available at: www.acgme.org/globallassets/pdfs/milestones/milestonesguidebookforresidentsfellows.pdf. (Accessed 18 November 2022).

Appendix

Jordan Abrams

ALVEOLAR GAS EQUATION

$$P_AO_2 = [(P_{ATM} - P_{H2O}) \times FiO_2] - (P_aCO_2 \div R)$$

While breathing room air at atmospheric pressure:
≈ [(760 - 47) × 0.21] - (P_aCO_2 + 0.8)
≈ 150 - (P_aCO_2 × 1.25)

↑ P_{ATM} → ↑ P_AO_2
↑ F_iO_2 → ↑ P_AO_2
↓ Temp → ↓ P_{H2O}
↓ P_{H2O} → ↑ P_AO_2
↓ P_aCO_2 → ↑ P_AO_2

P_AO_2 = alveolar partial pressure of O_2
P_{ATM} = barometric pressure (760 mmHg at sea level)
P_{H2O} = partial pressure of water (47 mmHg)
FiO_2 = fraction of inspired O_2 (21% at room air)
P_aCO_2 = partial pressure of CO_2 in arterial blood (directly measured via ABG)
R = respiratory quotient = CO_2 produced ÷ O_2 consumed

A-A GRADIENT

$$= P_AO_2 - P_aO_2$$

P_aO_2 = arterial blood partial pressure of O_2 (via ABG)
P_AO_2 = alveolar partial pressure of O_2 (via Alveolar Gas Equation)

Normal A-a Gradient
<10 (F_iO_2 ≈ 0.21)
<60 (F_iO_2 ≈ 1.00)

DRIVING PRESSURE

$$\Delta P = P_{PLATEAU} - PEEP = V_T \div C_S$$

STATIC RESPIRATORY COMPLIANCE

$$C_S = V_T \div (P_{PLATEAU} - PEEP) = V_T \div \Delta P$$

DYNAMIC RESPIRATORY COMPLIANCE

$$C_D = V_T \div (P_{PEAK} - PEEP)$$

ΔP = driving pressure; reflection of lung compliance
$P_{PLATEAU}$ = plateau pressure (via end-inspiratory hold maneuver)
PEEP = positive end-expiratory pressure (via end-expiratory hold maneuver)
V_T = tidal volume
C_S = static compliance (accounts for alveoli only)
C_D = dynamic compliance (accounts for airways & alveoli)
P_{PEAK} = peak pressure; reflection of airway resistance + lung compliance

REYNOLDS NUMBER

$$Re = (V \times \rho \times D) \div \mu$$

V = velocity
ρ = density
D = diameter
μ = viscosity

Re < 2000 = laminar flow
Re > 4000 = turbulent flow
High flow (turbulent) most affected by density
Low flow (laminar) most affected by viscosity

POISEUILLE'S LAW

$$Q = (\Delta p \times \pi \times r^4) \div (8 \times \mu \times L)$$

$$R = (8 \times \mu \times L) \div (\pi \times r^4)$$

Q = flow rate
Δp = pressure difference
r = radius
μ = viscosity
L = length
R = resistance

Poiseuille's law only relates to laminar flow.

Reynolds number predicts whether flow is laminar or turbulent.

LAW OF LAPLACE

$$T = (P \times r) \div (2 \times u)$$

T = wall tension
P = transmural pressure
r = radius
u = wall thickness (typically not considered for alveoli)

TIME CONSTANT

$$= volume \div flow$$

Machine: volume of circuit + fresh gas flow (FGF)
Lung: FRC + $V_{ALVEOLAR}$

Time Constant	1	2	3	4
% Wash-in/Wash-out	63%	84%	95%	99%

VOLATILE ANESTHETICS AT ALTITUDE

Variable bypass vaporizer (eg, Sevoflurane, Isoflurane)
• ↑ concentration (%) of agent (vapor output) than dialed
• Constant partial pressure (≈ MAC delivered)

Dual-circuit (gas/vapor blender) vaporizer (eg, Desflurane)
• Constant concentration (%) of agent (vapor output) dialed
• ↓ partial pressure

DESFLURANE REQUIRED DIAL SETTING

$$= normal\ dial\ setting \times (760\ mmHg \div Ambient\ pressure\ mmHg)$$

GAS OUTFLOW (VARIABLE-BYPASS VAPORIZER)

$$Outflow = Inflow \times SVP \div (P_{ATM} - SVP)$$

SVP = saturated vapor pressure (mmHg)
P_{ATM} = barometric pressure (760 mmHg at sea level)

Volatile Anesthetic	SVP	SVP ÷ (P_{ATM} - SVP)
Halothane	240	~½
Isoflurane	240	~½
Sevoflurane	160	~¼
Enflurane	175	~⅓

1 mL of liquid volatile agent ≈ 200 mL of vapor

Boiling Point: Desflurane = 24°C, N_2O = -88°C

Critical Temp: N_2O = 36.5°C

Anesthetic	Blood:Gas partition coefficient	Oil:Gas partition coefficient	MAC
Halothane	2.3	200	0.75%
Isoflurane	1.4	90	1%
Sevoflurane	0.69	50	2%
Enflurane	1.8	100	1.7%
Desflurane	0.42	20	6%
N_2O	0.47	1.3	104%

Blood:Gas coefficient ≈ Solubility (rate of induction/emergence)

Oil:Gas coefficient (Meyer-Overton correlation) ≈ Lipid solubility (Potency)

MAC ≈ 1/oil:gas coefficient (↓ O:G coefficient → ↓ potency → ↑ MAC)

MAC ≈ 1/P_{ATM} (↑ altitude → ↓ barometric pressure → ↑ MAC)

OXYGEN CONTENT

$$= \text{Hg-bound } O_2 + \text{Dissolved } O_2$$
$$C_vO_2 = (Hg \times 1.34 \times S_vO_2) + (P_vO_2 \times 0.003)$$
$$C_aO_2 = (Hg \times 1.34 \times S_aO_2) + (P_aO_2 \times 0.003)$$

C_vO_2 = mixed venous oxygen content
C_aO_2 = arterial oxygen content
Hg = hemoglobin
1.34 = volume of O_2 bound to 1 gram of saturated Hg
S_vO_2 = % Hg fully saturated with O_2 in venous blood
S_aO_2 = % Hg fully saturated with O_2 in arterial blood
P_vO_2 = partial pressure of O_2 dissolved in venous blood
P_aO_2 = partial pressure of O_2 dissolved in arterial blood
0.003 = solubility coefficient of O_2 dissolved in blood

OXYGEN DELIVERY

$$DO_2 = CO \times C_aO_2$$

OXYGEN CONSUMPTION

$$VO_2 = CO \times (C_aO_2 - C_vO_2)$$

OXYGEN EXTRACTION RATIO

$$ER_{O2} = (VO_2 \div DO_2) \times 100$$

DO_2 = oxygen delivered
VO_2 = oxygen consumption
ER_{O2} = oxygen extraction ratio
CO = cardiac output
C_aO_2 = arterial oxygen content
C_vO_2 = mixed venous oxygen content

FICK EQUATION

$$S_vO_2 = S_aO_2 - [VO_2 \div (CO \times Hg \times 1.34)]$$

S_vO_2 = mixed venous O_2 saturation (normal: 65-75%) $S_vO_2 \propto S_aO_2$, CO, Hg
S_aO_2 = arterial O_2 saturation $S_vO_2 \propto 1/VO_2$
VO_2 = total body O_2 consumption
CO = cardiac output
Hg = hemoglobin

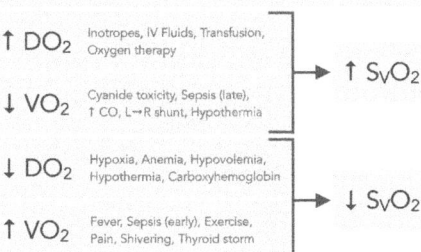

| ↑ DO₂ | Inotropes, IV Fluids, Transfusion, Oxygen therapy |
| ↓ VO₂ | Cyanide toxicity, Sepsis (late), ↑ CO, L→R shunt, Hypothermia |

→ ↑ S_vO_2

| ↓ DO₂ | Hypoxia, Anemia, Hypovolemia, Hypothermia, Carboxyhemoglobin |
| ↑ VO₂ | Fever, Sepsis (early), Exercise, Pain, Shivering, Thyroid storm |

→ ↓ S_vO_2

APNEIC TIME

$$= (FRC \times EtO_2) \div VO_2$$

FRC = functional residual capacity
EtO_2 = end-tidal oxygen percent
VO_2 = oxygen consumption

Pre-oxygenation (denitrogenation) can be achieved by Tidal volume breathing 100% O_2 over 3 mins OR by 8 vital capacity breaths over 1 minute

USEFUL 'ANCHOR' POINTS

SO₂	50%	75%	85%	90%	97%
PO₂ (mmHg)	27	40	50	60	100

MEAN ARTERIAL PRESSURE

$$MAP = CO \times SVR$$

SYSTEMIC VASCULAR RESISTANCE

$$SVR = 80 \times (MAP - CVP) \div CO$$

CARDIAC OUTPUT

$$CO = HR \times SV$$

STROKE VOLUME

$$SV = \text{Preload} \times \text{Contractility} \times \text{Afterload}$$

MAP = mean arterial pressure
CO = cardiac output
SVR = systemic vascular resistance
80 = conversion factor to change woods units 'mmHg/L/min' to metric units 'dynes/sec/cm⁵'
CVP = central venous pressure (surrogate for right atrial pressure, RAP)
SBP = systolic blood pressure
DBP = diastolic blood pressure
HR = heart rate
SV = stroke volume

Parameter	Normal Values
Cardiac Output (CO)	5-6 L/min
Cardiac Index (CI)	2.5-4 L/min/m²
Pulmonary Capillary Wedge Pressure (PCWP)	4-12 mmHg
Central Venous Pressure (CVP)	8-12 mmHg
Mixed Venous O₂ Saturation (S$_v$O₂)	75 %
Mixed Venous O₂ Partial Pressure (P$_v$O₂)	40 mmHg
Systemic Vascular Resistance (SVR)	700-1500 dynes/sec/cm⁵
Oxygen consumption (VO₂)	250 cc/min

ALLOWABLE BLOOD LOSS

$$= EBV \times (H_i - H_f) \div H_i$$

EBV = estimated blood volume
H_i = initial (starting) hematocrit
H_f = final (lowest acceptable) hematocrit

VOLUME TO TRANSFUSE

$$= EBV \times (H_{desired} - H_{current}) \div H_{transfused}$$

EBV = estimated blood volume
$H_{desired}$ = desired hematocrit
$H_{current}$ = current hematocrit
$H_{transfused}$ = hematocrit of transfused blood

Age	Estimated Blood Volume (mL/kg)
Preemie	100
Neonate	90
< 1 year	80
< 12 years	75
Men ♂	70
Women ♀	65 (~90 in pregnancy)

PLASMA OSMOLALITY

$$P_{OSM} = (2 \times Na) + (Glucose \div 18) + (BUN \div 2.8)$$

P_{OSM} = Plasma osmolality
Na = serum sodium concentration
BUN = blood urea nitrogen concentration

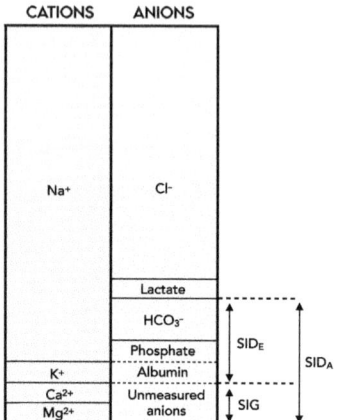

Normal SID_A = 40-45 mEq/L

Principle of electroneutrality → assumption there are unmeasured anions in serum (SID_E), primarily HCO_3^-, Phosphate, and Albumin

Cations are constituents of basic compounds (eg, NaOH, KOH)
↑ cations (or ↓ anions) → ↑ SID_A → alkalosis

Anions are constituents of acidic compounds (eg, HCl, lactic acid)
↑ anions (or ↓ cations) → ↓ SID_A → acidosis

STRONG ION DIFFERENCE APPARENT (SID$_A$)

$$SID_A = (Na^+ + K^+ + Ca^{2+} + Mg^{2+}) - (Cl^- + lactate^-)$$

STRONG ION DIFFERENCE EFFECTIVE (SID$_E$)

$$SID_E = HCO_3^+ + Phosphate + Albumin$$

STRONG ION GAP

$$SIG = SID_A - SID_E$$

SID_A = difference between abundant cations and abundant anions in serum
SID_E = measure of remaining anions

ACUTE KIDNEY INJURY

Finding	Prerenal	Intrinsic	Postrenal
BUN:Cr	>20	<15	>15
FENa (%)	<1%	>2%	>4%
UNa (mEq/L)	<10	>20	>40
UOsm (mOsm/kg)	>500	<350	<350

BUN:Cr = BUN:Creatinine ratio
FENa = Fractional excretion of sodium
UNa = Urine sodium
UOsm = Urine osmolality

APPROPRIATE ACID–BASE COMPENSATION

Metabolic Acidosis	$P_aCO_2 = 1.5 \times HCO_3^- + 8 \pm 2$
Metabolic Alkalosis	↑ $P_aCO_2 = 0.7 \times \Delta HCO_3^-$
Respiratory Acidosis (acute)	↑ $HCO_3^- = 0.1 \times \Delta P_aCO_2$
Respiratory Alkalosis (acute)	↓ $HCO_3^- = 0.2 \times \Delta P_aCO_2$
Respiratory Acidosis (chronic)	↑ $HCO_3^- = 0.3 \times \Delta P_aCO_2$
Respiratory Alkalosis (chronic)	↓ $HCO_3^- = 0.4 \times \Delta P_aCO_2$

P_aCO_2 = partial pressure of CO_2 in arterial blood   Baseline P_aCO_2 = 40 mmHg
HCO_3^- = Bicarbonate   Baseline HCO_3 = 24 mEq/L
ΔHCO_3^- = change in bicarbonate (baseline - current)
ΔP_aCO_2 = change in CO_2 (baseline - current)

ANION GAP

$$= (Na^+ + K^+) - (HCO_3^- + Cl^-)$$

Normal AG = 8-12 mEq/L

ANION GAP (CORRECTED)

$$= AG + 0.25 \times (4.5 - Albumin)$$

HCO$_3$ DEFICIT

$$= 0.2 \times Base\ Deficit \times Weight\ (kg)$$

HCO_3^- Deficit = Amount of HCO_3^- needed to correct metabolic acidosis

BODY FLUID COMPARTMENTS

Total Body Water 20-40-60 Rule:

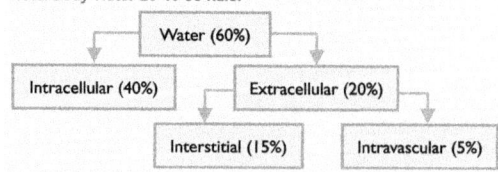

Age	Total Body Water (%)
Neonate	80
< 1 year	70
< 12 years	65
Men ♂	60
Women ♀	50
Elderly	45

BODY MASS INDEX (BMI)

$$= \text{Weight (kg)} \div \text{Height (m}^2\text{)}$$
$$= 703 \times \text{Weight (lbs)} \div \text{Height (in}^2\text{)}$$

703 = conversion factor (English → Metric)

PARKLAND FORMULA

$$= 4 \text{ mL} \times \text{TBSA (\%)} \times \text{Weight (kg)}$$

Estimated fluid requirement in a burn victim
50% volume given in first 8 hrs; remaining 50% given over next 16 hrs

TBSA = total body surface area (estimated using rule of 9's)

RADIATION INTENSITY

$$I \propto 1 \div r^2$$

I = Radiation intensity & exposure   Doubling the distance → ¼ exposure
r = Radius (distance from source)

ULTRASOUND PHYSICS

$$v = f \times \lambda$$

v = velocity   ↑ f → ↓ λ → ↑ resolution & ↓ tissue penetration
f = frequency   ↓ f → ↑ λ → ↓ resolution & ↑ tissue penetration
λ = wavelength

PRESSURE CONVERSION

$$1 \text{ atm} = 760 \text{ mmHg} = 14.7 \text{ psi} = 988 \text{ cmH}_2\text{O}$$

1 mmHg = 1.36 cmH$_2$O   **1 cmH$_2$O = 0.74 mmHg**

Keep airway pressure <20 cmH$_2$O during mask ventilation to minimize gastric insufflation

MAX RECOMMENDED INFLATION PRESSURE

LMA	60 cmH$_2$O (44 mmHg)
ETT	30 cmH$_2$O (22 mmHg)

Normal tracheal capillary pressure = 25-35 mmHg

If ETT cuff pressure > tracheal capillary pressure → tissue ischemia
Persistent ischemia → tracheomalacia & destruction of tracheal rings

BOYLE'S LAW

$$P_1V_1 = P_2V_2$$

With constant Temperature, **Volume & Pressure are inversely proportional**

CHARLE'S LAW

$$V_1 \div T_1 = V_2 \div T_2$$

With constant Pressure, **Volume & Temperature are directly proportional**

GAY-LUSSAC'S LAW

$$P_1 \div T_1 = P_2 \div T_2$$

With constant Volume, **Pressure & Temperature are directly proportional**

DALTON'S LAW

$$P_{Total} = P_1 + P_2 + P_3 \dots$$

Total gas pressure in a system = Sum of partial pressures of the component gases

HENRY'S LAW

$$\text{Solubility of gas} \propto \text{Partial pressure of gas}$$

With constant Temperature, the amount of gas dissolved in liquid is directly proportional to partial pressure of the gas

Hyperbaric oxygen increases the dissolved O$_2$ content of blood via Henry's law:
↑ atmospheric pressure → ↑ PAO$_2$ → ↑ PaO$_2$

BIS MONITORING

Wave & Range	BIS & Description
Gamma (26-80 Hz)	BIS >85 (Awake)
Beta (13-25 Hz)	
Alpha (9-12 Hz)	BIS 65-84 (Sedation, Resting with eyes closed)
Theta (5-8 Hz)	Not prominent in adults
Delta (1-4 Hz)	BIS 40-64 (Surgical anesthesia, Deep sleep)
Slow (<1 Hz)	BIS <40 (Isoelectric, possible burst suppression)

1°C ↓ in body temperature → BIS ↓ ~1 unit
Burst suppression = alternating episodes of isoelectricity & active oscillations

HERBAL SUPPLEMENTS

Supplement	Perioperative Concern
Ginger	↑ Bleeding risk
Garlic	↑ Bleeding risk
Ginkgo	↑ Bleeding risk
Ginseng	↑ Bleeding risk, Hypoglycemia
Green tea	↑ Bleeding risk
Saw Palmetto	↑ Bleeding risk
Vitamin E	↑ Bleeding risk
Black Cohosh	↑ Bleeding risk, Hepatic injury
Licorice	Aldosterone-like effect (HTN, ↓ K, ↑ Na)
Kava	↑ Sedative effects of anesthesia
Valerian	↑ Sedative effects of anesthesia
St. John's Wort	CYP P450 Induction
Echinacea	Allergic reaction/Anaphylaxis

Herbal supplements should be stopped 1-2 weeks prior to surgery
If the supplement starts with "G", then it ↑ bleeding risk

IV FLUID COMPOSITION

Fluid	Osmolality (mOsm/kg)	Na⁺ (mEq/L)	Cl⁻ (mEq/L)	K⁺ (mEq/L)	Ca²⁺ (mEq/L)	Mg²⁺ (mEq/L)	Glucose (g/L)	Lactate
Plasma	289	140	103	5	5	2	-	1
Plasmalyte	294	140	98	5	-	3	-	-
LR	273	130	109	4	3	-	-	28
0.9% NS	308	154	154	-	-	-	-	-
0.45% NS	154	77	77	-	-	-	-	-
3% NS	1026	513	513	-	-	-	-	-
D5W	253	-	-	-	-	-	50	-
D5LR	525	130	109	4	3	-	50	28
D5NS	560	154	154	-	-	-	50	-
D5½NS	406	77	77	-	-	-	50	-
Albumin	300	145	-	-	-	-	-	-

Plasmalyte also contains Gluconate (23 mEq/L) and Acetate (27 mEq/L)
Lactate in LR is converted by pyruvate in the liver to bicarb via citric acid cycle

TEG/ROTEM

Value	Measures	Normal Range	Treatment
R Time to start clot formation	Clotting factors ↑ R = ↓ Clotting Factors	<6 min	FFP
K Time until clot reaches fixed strength	Fibrinogen ↑ K = ↓ Fibrinogen	1-3 min	Cryoprecipitate
α angle Rate of fibrin accumulation	Fibrinogen	<60°	Cryoprecipitate
Maximum Amplitude (MA) Clot strength	Platelet ↓ MA = ↓ Platelets	>60 mm	Platelets and/or DDAVP
Lysis at 30 minutes (LY30) % amplitude reduction 30 mins after MA	Clot Stability ↑ LY30 = Excess Fibrinolysis	<6%	Anti-fibrinolytic (TXA or ACA)

Index